T0180542

Lecture Notes in Statistics **122**

Edited by P. Bickel, P. Diggle, S. Fienberg, K. Krickeberg,
I. Olkin, N. Wermuth, S. Zeger

Springer
New York
Berlin
Heidelberg
Barcelona
Budapest
Hong Kong
London
Milan
Paris
Santa Clara
Singapore
Tokyo

Timothy G. Gregoire
David R. Brillinger
Peter J. Diggle
Estelle Russek-Cohen
William G. Warren
Russell D. Wolfinger
(Editors)

Modelling Longitudinal and Spatially Correlated Data

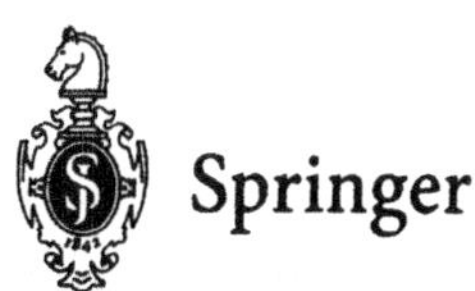

Springer

Timothy G. Gregoire
Department of Forestry
Virginia Polytechnic University
and State Institute
Blacksburg, VA 24061-0324

David R. Brillinger
Department of Statistics
University of California, Berkeley
Berkeley, CA 94720

Peter J. Diggle
Department of Mathematics and Statistics
University of Lancaster
Lancaster LA1 4YF
England

Estelle Russek-Cohen
Department of Animal Sciences
University of Maryland, College Park
College Park, MD 20742-2311

William G. Warren
Department of Fisheries and Oceans
P.O. Box 5567
St. John's, Newfoundland
Canada A1C 5X1

Russell D. Wolfinger
SAS Institute Inc.
SAS Campus Drive
Cary, NC 27513-2414

Library of Congress Cataloging-in-Publication Data
Modelling longitudinal and spatially correlated data: methods, applicatons, and future directions/Timothy G. Gregoire ... [et al.] (editors)
p. cm. — (Lecture notes in statistics; 122)
ISBN 0-387-98216-7 (softcover: alk. paper)
1. Multivariate analysis. 2. Longitudinal method. 3. Spatial analysis (Statistics) I. Gregoire, T. G. II. Series: Lecture notes in statistics (Springer-Verlag); v. 122.
QA278.M647 1997
519.5'35—dc21 97-9855

Printed on acid-free paper.

Camera ready copy provided by the editors.
Printed and bound by Braun-Brumfield, Ann Arbor, MI.
Printed in the United States of America.

9 8 7 6 5 4 3 2 1

ISBN 0-387-98216-7 Springer-Verlag New York Berlin Heidelberg SPIN 10572457

Preface

Correlated data arise in numerous contexts across a wide spectrum of subject–matter disciplines. Modeling such data present special challenges and opportunities that have received increasing scrutiny by the statistical community in recent years. In October 1996 a group of 210 statisticians and other scientists assembled on the small island of Nantucket, U.S.A., to present and discuss new developments relating to *Modelling Longitudinal and Spatially Correlated Data: Methods, Applications, and Future Directions.* Its purpose was to provide a cross–disciplinary forum to explore the commonalities and meaningful differences in the source and treatment of such data. This volume is a compilation of some of the important invited and volunteered presentations made during that conference.

The three days and evenings of oral and displayed presentations were arranged into six broad thematic areas. The session themes, the invited speakers and the topics they addressed were as follows:

- Generalized Linear Models: Peter McCullagh—"Residual Likelihood in Linear and Generalized Linear Models"
- Longitudinal Data Analysis: Nan Laird—"Using the General Linear Mixed Model to Analyze Unbalanced Repeated Measures and Longitudinal Data"
- Spatio–Temporal Processes: David R. Brillinger—"Statistical Analysis of the Tracks of Moving Particles"
- Spatial Data Analysis: Noel A. Cressie—"Statistical Models for Lattice Data"
- Modelling Messy Data: Raymond J. Carroll—"Some Results on Generalized Linear Mixed Models with Measurement Error in Covariates"
- Future Directions: Peter J. Diggle—"Spatial and Longitudinal Data Analysis: Two Histories with a Single Future?"

Each session but the last was led off by the invited speaker. Professor Diggle's presentation concluded the conference.

With the exception of Professor Laird's presentation, the text of each invited paper appears in this volume, perhaps listed under a slightly revised title. Mirroring the organization of the meeting, all written papers have been arranged by these same broad themes. However, the order of arrangement is inconsequential.

The cooperation of all authors in the timely preparation of their manuscripts is gratefully recognized. The generous assistance and advice in the processing of these manuscripts provided by Doug Bates warrants special acknowledgement.

The Organizing Committee decided early on that it was important to referee and critically evaluate the papers which were submitted for inclusion in this volume. For this substantial task, we relied on the service of numerous referees to whom we are most indebted. Among those we wish to recognize are Rick Schoenberg, Rafael Irizarry, Ed Ionides, Bin Yu, Haiganoush Preisler, and Imola Fodor.

The sponsoring organizations for the Nantucket Modelling Meeting were the Eastern North American Region of the International Biometric Society, the Section on Statistics and the Environment of the American Statistical Association, and The International Environmetrics Society. Their collective endorsement was crucial to the success of the conference.

The financial and logistical support provided by SAS Institute, Inc. and the Department of Forestry at Virginia Polytechnic Institute and State University is gratefully acknowledged, as is the many months of behind–the–scenes work capably performed by Ms. Connie Noonkester. Finally we thank Ms. Vicki Miller and Mr. Andrew Robinson for their cheerfully rendered on–site services.

Organizing Committee
Timothy G. Gregoire, Chair
David R. Brillinger
Peter J. Diggle
Abdel H. El–Shaarawi
Estelle Russek–Cohen
William G. Warren
Russell D. Wolfinger

Table of Contents

Modelling Spatio–Temporal Processes

Modelling Messy Data

Special Topics and Future Directions

Linear Models, Vector Spaces, and Residual Likelihood

Peter McCullagh*
University of Chicago
United States

ABSTRACT It is shown that, for purposes of likelihood calculation, the standard definition of residual in linear models is unsatisfactory. An alternative definition of residual as an element of a quotient space is proposed and exploited. It is shown that the standard REML, or residual, likelihood arises naturally as the normal-theory likelihood based on the 'observation' $y + \mathcal{X}$ in the quotient space. In addition, for non-normal linear models, the adjusted profile likelihood is shown to be a Laplace approximation to the distribution of the residual in the quotient space.

Keywords and phrases: Quotient space, REML, residual.

1 Vectors

1.1 Vectors and vector spaces

For most working statisticians, a vector is an ordered list of n real numbers, where n is any positive integer. Some might take a more liberal view, extending the term to include an ordered list of complex numbers, or an ordered list of character strings, The problem of determining what is and what is not a vector is very much akin to the problem of classification of animals and plants. Familiarity makes it easy to distinguish birds from non-birds, plants from animals, fruit from vegetables and so on. Yet, near the boundaries, disputes are likely to arise, for example whether a tomato is a fruit or a vegetable or both. At some point, it becomes necessary to revisit the definitions to see what is the essence of a fruit and what is the essence of a vegetable. That is what I propose to do in this section for vectors.

*Author address: Department of Statistics, University of Chicago, 5734 S. University Avenue, Chicago, IL 60637–1546 U.S.A

A few examples will serve to show that the issue is not so clear as might appear at first sight. Consider the following examples:

1. the real number π as an element of the real line.

2. the list $(3, 1, 1)$ as eigenvalues of a 3×3 symmetric matrix.

3. the probability vector $(0.2, 0.5, 0.3)$ as an element of the probability simplex in $\mathcal{R}^3$.

The standard mathematical construction of a vector begins with the definition of a vector space, which is a set of undefined elements that is closed under addition, closed under scalar multiplication, contains a zero element, and obeys certain other properties (Halmos 1974, section 2). A vector is then defined to be an element of a vector space.

According to this definition, only the first example in the preceding list constitutes a vector.

1.2 Vectors and component-vectors

Let $\mathcal{U}$ be an n-dimensional real vector space, and let $\{e_1, \ldots, e_n\}$ be a basis in $\mathcal{U}$. It may be helpful in what follows to avoid standard perceptions regarding the appearance of vectors in $\mathcal{U}$. If necessary, we will speak of elements of $\mathcal{U}$ as real-valued functions on some domain: a statistical vector, or variable, is a function from the statistical units into the real numbers. Each element of $\mathcal{U}$ is expressible as a linear combination of the basis vectors

$$v = v^1 e_1 + \cdots + v^n e_n = v^j e_j \qquad (1)$$

in which $v^1, \ldots, v^n$ are real numbers, the components of v with respect to the given basis.

With a basis in hand, equation (1) defines a 1–1 correspondence between functions $v \in \mathcal{U}$ and component-vectors $(v^1, \ldots, v^n)$ in $\mathcal{R}^n$. It is important to appreciate that $(v^1, \ldots, v^n)$, as a point in $\mathcal{R}^n$, is not the same thing as v in $\mathcal{U}$. The following example may help to clarify matters.

Let $\mathcal{U}$ be the space of harmonics on the unit circle of degree not more than two. In conventional notation,

$$\mathcal{U} = \text{span}\{e_0 = 1,\ e_1 = \cos\theta,\ e_2 = \sin\theta,\ e_3 = \cos 2\theta,\ e_4 = \sin 2\theta\}$$

is a space of dimension five. An element of $\mathcal{U}$ such as $v = \cos\theta + 4\sin^2(\theta)$ is expressible as a linear combination of basis vectors:

$$\begin{aligned} v &= 2 + \cos\theta - 2\cos 2\theta \\ &= 2e_0 + e_1 - 2e_3, \end{aligned}$$

so the associated component-vector in $\mathcal{R}^5$ is $(2, 1, 0, -2, 0)$.

2 Volume and measure

2.1 Inner products

Let $\mathcal{U}$ be a real inner product space, and let $\{e_1, \ldots, e_n\}$ be a basis. The set of inner products

$$g_{ij} = \langle e_i, e_j\rangle$$

constitutes a real positive-definite symmetric matrix G. For any vectors $u = u^j e_j$ and $v = v^j e_j$ in $\mathcal{U}$, the inner product of u and v is given by

$$\langle u, v\rangle = \langle u^i e_i, v^j e_j\rangle = u^i v^j \langle e_i, e_j\rangle = u^i v^j g_{ij},$$

which is a quadratic form in the component-vectors.

The unit cell

$$E = (0, e_1) \times \cdots \times (0, e_n),$$

a subset of $\mathcal{U}$, is in 1–1 correspondence with the unit cube in the space of component-vectors in $\mathcal{R}^n$ in the sense that for any $v \in E$ with $v = v^i e_i$, the components satisfy $0 < v^i < 1$. It does not follow, however, that the size, volume, or measure of E must be the same as the volume of the unit cube in $\mathcal{R}^n$. As we shall see, the volume of E is more appropriately set at $|G|^{1/2}$. More generally, the measure of any subset of $\mathcal{U}$ is $|G|^{1/2}$ times the volume of the image set in $\mathcal{R}^n$.

The length of the interval $(0, e_1)$ is the length, or norm, of e_1, which is $\langle e_1, e_1\rangle^{1/2}$, or $g_{11}^{1/2}$. The two-dimensional measure of the product set $(0, e_1) \times (0, e_2)$ is, in general, less than the product of the two lengths. The two-dimensional measure is in fact equal to the product $\|e_1\| \times \|\check{e}_2\|$, where $\check{e}_2$ is the orthogonal component of e_2 given by $e_2 - \langle e_2, e_1\rangle e_1/\|e_1\|^2$. Standard calculations give

$$\mu_2\big((0, e_1) \times (0, e_2)\big) = (g_{11}g_{22} - g_{12}^2)^{1/2},$$

the determinant of the 2×2 sub-matrix of inner products. Although the details are messy, this construction can be extended to give $\mu_n(E) = |G|^{1/2}$.

Both the matrix G and the definition of the unit cell are intrinsically connected with the choice of basis in $\mathcal{U}$. Suppose we were to choose a different basis, $\{x_1, \ldots, x_n\}$, so that the transformed unit cell is the product set $(0, x_1) \times \cdots \times (0, x_n)$. Each x_r is a linear combination of the original basis vectors, so we may write

$$x_r = L_r^i e_i$$

for some non-singular matrix of coefficients L_r^i. The transformed inner product matrix is

$$\langle x_r, x_s\rangle = \langle L_r^i e_i, L_s^j e_j\rangle = L_r^i L_s^j \langle e_i, e_j\rangle = L_r^i L_s^j g_{ij}.$$

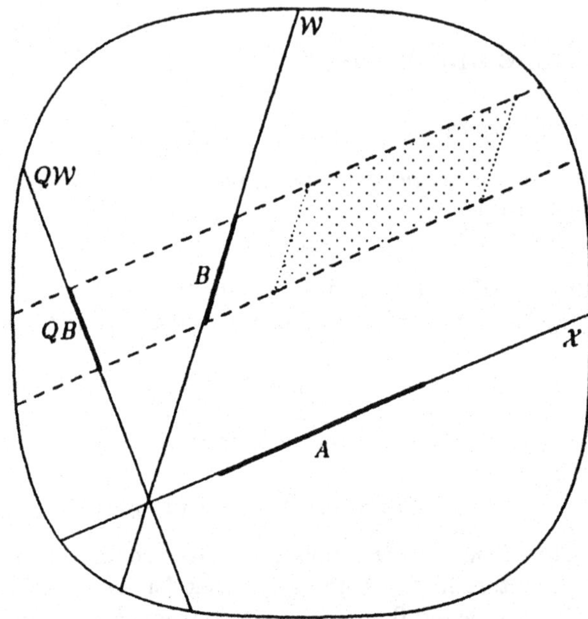

FIGURE 1. Stone diagram illustrating two complementary subspaces $\mathcal{X}$ and $\mathcal{W}$, together with the orthogonal complement $Q\mathcal{W} = \mathcal{X}^\perp$. The subsets A, B and QB are shown as heavy line segments, and the Cartesian product $A \times B$ is shown shaded. The region between the dashed lines is the set of cosets $B + \mathcal{X}$, which is the same as $QB + \mathcal{X}$. The Lebesgue measure of the product set $A \times B$ is the product of $\mu_k(A)$, the measure of A in $\mathcal{X}$ and $\mu_{n-k}(QB)$, the measure of the orthogonal projection of B in $\mathcal{X}^\perp$. The latter factor is also the Lebesgue measure of the set of cosets $B + \mathcal{X}$ in the quotient space $\mathcal{U}/\mathcal{X}$.

In matrix notation, the transformed inner product matrix is LGL^T, whose determinant is $|L|^2 \times |G|$. In other words, the Lebesgue measure of the transformed unit cell is $|G|^{1/2} \times J$, where J is the absolute value of the determinant of L.

More generally, let $\mathcal{X}$ and $\mathcal{W}$ be complementary subspaces of $\mathcal{U}$ of dimensions n and $n-k$ respectively, with $A \subset \mathcal{X}$ and $B \subset \mathcal{W}$. The measure of the product set $A \times B$ is

$$\mu_n(A \times B) = \mu_k(A) \times \mu_{n-k}(QB)$$

where Q is the orthogonal projection from $\mathcal{U}$ to $\mathcal{X}^\perp$. For present purposes, the second factor will be interpreted as Euclidean measure in the quotient space $\mathcal{U}/\mathcal{X}$. To put this in another way, the set of cosets $B + \mathcal{X}$ is a subset of the quotient space $\mathcal{U}/\mathcal{X}$. The intersection of these cosets with the complementary subspace $\mathcal{W}$ is B: the intersection with $\mathcal{X}^\perp$ is QB. The measure of the quotient set $B + \mathcal{X}$, essentially its perpendicular cross-sectional measure, is the measure of its intersection with $\mathcal{X}^\perp$. Thus we arrive at the expression

$$\mu_{\mathcal{U}}(A \times B) = \mu_{\mathcal{X}}(A) \times \mu_{\mathcal{U}/\mathcal{X}}(B + \mathcal{X}).$$

In particular, if A represents the unit cell $(0, x_1) \times \cdots \times (0, x_k)$ in $\mathcal{X}$, we have

$$J|G|^{1/2} = \mu_{\mathcal{X}}\big((0, x_1) \times \cdots \times (0, x_k)\big) \times \mu_{\mathcal{U}/\mathcal{X}}\big((0, x_{k+1}) \times \cdots \times (0, x_n) + \mathcal{X}\big).$$

The first factor is the measure of the unit cell in $\mathcal{X}$: the second factor is the measure of the unit cell in the quotient space. Consequently, since the inner product matrix in $\mathcal{X}$ is $\bar{G} = X^T G X$, the measure of the unit cell in the quotient space is

$$\mu_{\mathcal{U}/\mathcal{X}}\big((0, x_{k+1}) \times \cdots \times (0, x_n) + \mathcal{X}\big) = J|G|^{1/2}/|\bar{G}|^{1/2}.$$

In Figure 1, an abstract diagram in the style of Stone (1987), the vector space $\mathcal{U}$ is represented by an outer cartouche. Subspaces are represented by solid lines labelled $\mathcal{X}$, $\mathcal{W}$, and $Q\mathcal{W}$, which is also meant to represent $\mathcal{X}^\perp$. Cosets of $\mathcal{X}$ are represented by dashed lines parallel to $\mathcal{X}$. The region between the dashed lines is a set of cosets of $\mathcal{X}$, and hence a subset of the quotient space $\mathcal{U}/\mathcal{X}$. The Lebesgue measure of this set in $\mathcal{U}/\mathcal{X}$ is equal to the measure of its intersection with $\mathcal{X}^\perp$, that is to say $\mu_{n-k}(QB)$ rather than, say, $\mu_{n-k}(B)$. The Lebesgue measure in $\mathcal{U}$ of the product set $A \times B$ is thus computed as $\mu_{\mathcal{X}}(A) \times \mu_{\mathcal{X}^\perp}(QB)$, the latter factor being the same as $\mu_{\mathcal{U}/\mathcal{X}}(B + \mathcal{X})$, the measure of the subset $B + \mathcal{X}$ in the quotient space.

3 Linear models

3.1 Residuals

Let $\mathcal{X}$ be the space spanned by the columns of the model matrix X. We consider a linear model in which the response Y is an element of an inner product space $\mathcal{U}$, and the inner product matrix G is the inverse covariance matrix of the components of Y. The fitted value is the orthogonal projection PY of Y on to the subspace $\mathcal{X}$, and the residual, as conventionally defined, is the complementary orthogonal projection $QY = (I - P)Y$ on to $\mathcal{X}^\perp$.

For some purposes, particularly for probability calculations, these definitions are quite satisfactory. For likelihood calculations, however, there is a potentially serious obstacle, at least in those cases where the covariance matrix depends on unknown parameters or variance components in a non-trivial way. The difficulty is that, whereas the space $\mathcal{X}$ is given, the complementary space $\mathcal{X}^\perp$ depends on the values of the unknown variance components. So the residual vector in the conventional sense is not observable. It should also be borne in mind that a likelihood ratio is a ratio of densities with respect to a fixed measure on a fixed space. In the problem

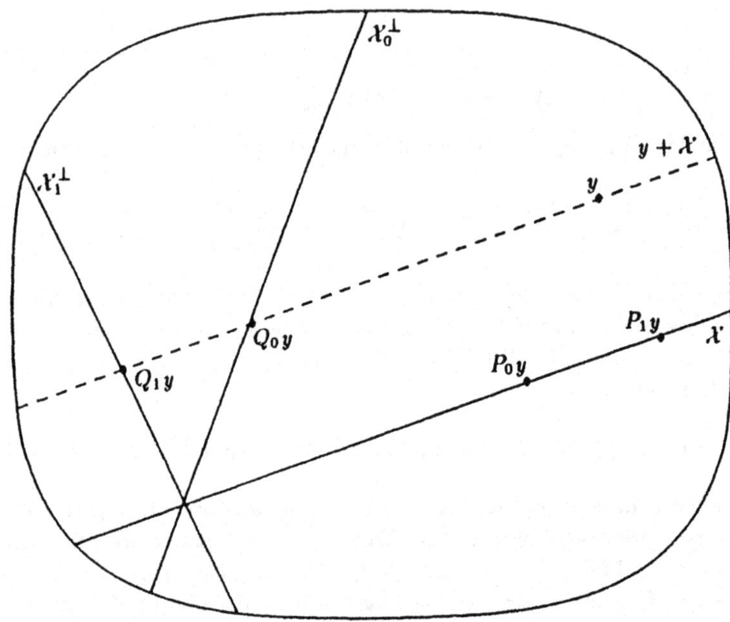

FIGURE 2. Stone diagram illustrating the least squares projections on to the space $\mathcal{X}$ for two parameter values, θ_0 and θ_1, giving rise to different inner products. The orthogonal complement of $\mathcal{X}$ under the inner product determined by θ_r is the subspace denoted by $\mathcal{X}_r^\perp$. The orthogonal projections under θ_r of y on to $\mathcal{X}$ are denoted by P_0y and P_1y. The complementary projections, denoted by Q_0y and Q_1y, are points in $\mathcal{X}_0^\perp$ and $\mathcal{X}_1^\perp$ respectively. The locus of such residuals lies in the coset $y + \mathcal{X}$ (dashed line).

under discussion, not only is the measure in $\mathcal{U}$ dependent on parameters through $|G|^{1/2}$, but the space in which the residuals sit varies from one parameter value to another. This is illustrated in Figure 2 for two parameter values θ_0 and θ_1 leading to different covariance matrices and different inner products. The easiest way to resolve this impasse is to define the residual, not as an element of $\mathcal{U}$ in the subspace $\mathcal{X}^\perp$, but as an element of the quotient space $\mathcal{U}/\mathcal{X}$. The observed residual is then equal to the coset $Y + \mathcal{X}$, the set of translates of Y by $\mathcal{X}$, in $\mathcal{U}/\mathcal{X}$. This definition is geared towards likelihood calculations: needless to say, it is not especially useful for more traditional purposes such as plotting or graphical presentation.

3.2 Normal distribution

The standard normal density in the inner product space $\mathcal{U}$ has the form

$$(2\pi)^{-n/2}\exp(-\tfrac{1}{2}\|y\|^2)\,d\mu_n.$$

Since $d\mu_n(y) = |G|^{1/2} dy$, the density of the component-vector with respect to standard Lebesgue measure in $\mathcal{R}^n$ is

$$(2\pi)^{-n/2} \exp(-\tfrac{1}{2} y^i y^j g_{ij}) \, |G|^{1/2} \, dy$$

To say the same thing in another way, the component vector is normally distributed with precision matrix, or inverse covariance matrix, G.

We now transform to a new basis in which the first k elements, $x_1, \ldots, x_k$, the columns of the matrix X, form a basis of $\mathcal{X}$ in $\mathcal{U}$. The choice of the remaining $n - k$ basis elements, $\{x_{k+1}, \ldots, x_n\}$ is immaterial provided only that the set of n elements is linearly independent. The vectors $\{Qx_{k+1}, \ldots, Qx_n\}$ form a basis in $\mathcal{X}^\perp$ and the cosets $\{x_{k+1}+\mathcal{X}, \ldots, x_n+\mathcal{X}\}$ form a basis in the quotient space. By orthogonality, $\|y\|^2 = \|Py\|^2 + \|Qy\|^2$. Further, since the null space of Q is $\mathcal{X}$, $\|Qy\|^2$ may be interpreted either as a function on $\mathcal{X}^\perp$ or as a function on the quotient space. The normal density with respect to the new basis is

$$(2\pi)^{-n/2} \exp(-\tfrac{1}{2}\|Py\|^2) \, d\mu_k(Py) \times \exp(-\tfrac{1}{2}\|Qy\|^2) \, d\mu_{\mathcal{U}/\mathcal{X}}(y + \mathcal{X})$$

In terms of the observable component vectors, this density becomes

$$(2\pi)^{-n/2} \exp(-\tfrac{1}{2}\|Py\|^2) \, |\bar{G}|^{1/2} \times \exp(-\tfrac{1}{2}\|Qy\|^2) \, J \, |G|^{1/2}/|\bar{G}|^{1/2}$$

In conventional matrix notation, $G = \Sigma^{-1}$ and $\bar{G} = X^T \Sigma^{-1} X$. The first factor gives the density of the fitted values Py in $\mathcal{X}$: the second factor gives the density of the residuals $y+\mathcal{X}$ in the quotient space. The constant factor J arises because we have not specified a basis in the quotient space.

So far as likelihoods are concerned, it must be borne in mind that the inner product in $\mathcal{U}$ is based on variances and covariances, and is therefore different for different parameter values. The Jacobian factor is arbitrary, but does not depend on unknown parameters. Consequently, the residual likelihood, also known as the restricted likelihood or the REML likelihood, (Patterson and Thompson, 1971; Harville, 1974, 1977; Corbeil and Searle, 1976) is given by the second factor in the preceding expression. Reverting to conventional matrix notation, the residual log likelihood is

$$-\tfrac{1}{2}\|Qy\|^2 + \tfrac{1}{2}\log|G| - \tfrac{1}{2}\log|\bar{G}| = -\tfrac{1}{2}R^T\Sigma^{-1}R - \tfrac{1}{2}\log|\Sigma| - \tfrac{1}{2}\log|X^T\Sigma^{-1}X|,$$

where R, the conventional residual vector, is

$$R = Y - X(X^T\Sigma^{-1}X)^{-1}X^T\Sigma^{-1}Y.$$

It is worth emphasizing that, in general, R depends on unknown parameters and is thus not observable. It is technically incorrect to say that the REML likelihood is the likelihood based on R.

3.3 *Residual likelihood for non-normal linear models*

Let Y be a random vector in an inner product space $\mathcal{U}$, whose density at $y \in \mathcal{U}$ is given by

$$f(y)\, d\mu(y).$$

It is required to find the density of the residual $Y + \mathcal{X}$ as an element of the quotient space $\mathcal{U}/\mathcal{X}$. For any product set $dy = dx \times dr$, Lebesgue measure factors into $\mu(dy) = \mu_x(dx) \times \mu_{\mathcal{U}/\mathcal{X}}(dr + \mathcal{X})$ Also, $y = x + r$ with $x \in \mathcal{X}$ and $r \in \mathcal{X}^\perp$. Consequently, the required marginal density is given by

$$\int_{\mathcal{X}} f(x + r)\, d\mu_{\mathcal{X}}(x) \times \mu_{\mathcal{U}/\mathcal{X}}(dr + \mathcal{X}).$$

The fact that $\mu_{\mathcal{X}}$ is invariant under translation means that the integrated density satisfies

$$g(r + x_0) = \int_{\mathcal{X}} f(x + r + x_0)\, d\mu_{\mathcal{X}}(x) = \int_{\mathcal{X}} f(x + x_0 + r)\, d\mu_{\mathcal{X}}(x) = g(r)$$

for each $x_0 \in \mathcal{X}$. In other words, g is constant on cosets, and hence a function on $\mathcal{U}/\mathcal{X}$.

Suppose, for example, that the density of Y in $\mathcal{U}$ takes the form

$$f(y) = K_n(c^2) p(c^2 + \|y\|^2)\, d\mu$$

for some non-negative function p, constant c, and normalization factor K_n. Then the marginal density of the residual is

$$\begin{aligned} & K_n(c^2) \int_{\mathcal{X}} p(c^2 + \|Qy\|^2 + \|x\|^2)\, d\mu_{\mathcal{X}}(x) \times \mu_{\mathcal{U}/\mathcal{X}}(dy + \mathcal{X}) \\ = & \frac{K_n(c^2)}{K_k(c^2 + \|Qy\|^2)}\, d\mu_{\mathcal{U}/\mathcal{X}}(y + \mathcal{X}) \\ = & \frac{K_n(c^2)}{K_k(c^2 + \|Qy\|^2)}\, J\, |G|^{1/2} / |\bar{G}|^{1/2}\, (dy + \mathcal{X}). \end{aligned}$$

To take a second example, suppose that Y has the multivariate t distribution on ν degrees of freedom, in which the density at y in $\mathcal{U}$ has the form

$$\frac{\Gamma((n + \nu)/2)}{\pi^{n/2}\, \Gamma(\nu/2)} (1 + \|y\|^2)^{-(n+\nu)/2}\, d\mu.$$

Then the marginal density of the residual in the quotient space is

$$\begin{aligned} & K \int_{\mathcal{X}} (1 + \|Qy\|^2 + \|x\|^2)^{-(n+\nu)/2}\, d\mu_{\mathcal{X}}(x) \times d\mu_{\mathcal{U}/\mathcal{X}}(y + \mathcal{X}) \\ = & K \Psi \int_{\mathcal{X}} (1 + \|x\|^2/\lambda^2)^{-(n+\nu)/2} \lambda^{-k}\, d\mu_{\mathcal{X}}(x) \times d\mu_{\mathcal{U}/\mathcal{X}}(y + \mathcal{X}) \end{aligned}$$

$$
\begin{aligned}
&= K\Psi \int_{\mathcal{X}} (1+\|x\|^2)^{-(n+\nu)/2}\, d\mu_{\mathcal{X}}(x) \times d\mu_{\mathcal{U}/\mathcal{X}}(y+\mathcal{X}) \\
&= K'\,\Psi\, d\mu_{\mathcal{U}/\mathcal{X}}(y+\mathcal{X}) \\
&= K'\,\Psi\, J|G|^{1/2}/|\bar{G}|^{1/2}\,(dy+\mathcal{X}).
\end{aligned}
$$

where $\Psi = (1+\|Qy\|^2)^{-(n-k+\nu)/2}$. Since $\|Qy\|^2$ is the norm of $y+\mathcal{X}$ in the quotient space, the residual may be said to have a Student t distribution, also on ν degrees of freedom, in the quotient space. The residual likelihood is thus

$$K'(1+\|Qy\|^2)^{-(n-k+\nu)/2}\,|G|^{1/2}/|\bar{G}|^{1/2},$$

in which G, $\bar{G}$ and Qy, as defined in the previous section, depend on unknown variance or dispersion parameters. Note that K' depends only on ν, so this factor can be dropped if ν is known.

More generally, suppose that the density of Y at $y \in \mathcal{U}$ is $f(y)$. Then the marginal density of the configuration, or residual, $Y+\mathcal{X}$ in the quotient space is

$$\int_{\mathcal{X}} f(y+x)\, d\mu_{\mathcal{X}}(x) \times d\mu_{\mathcal{U}/\mathcal{X}}(y+\mathcal{X}).$$

Under certain conditions, the integral over $\mathcal{X}$ can be approximated using Laplace's method. Let $l(y)$ be the log density, and suppose that, on the coset $y+\mathcal{X}$, l has a maximum at $y+\hat{x}_y$. Then, by Taylor approximation in the neighbourhood of the maximum,

$$l(y+x) \simeq l(y+\hat{x}_y) - 1/2H(x-\hat{x}_y)$$

where H represents a quadratic form on $\mathcal{X}$, generally slightly different from the inner product on $\mathcal{X}$. Let $\hat{G}$ be the matrix of this quadratic form, which may vary from one coset to another. Then the Laplace approximation is

$$\int_{\mathcal{X}} f(y+x)\, d\mu_{\mathcal{X}}(x) \simeq (2\pi)^{-k/2} f(y+\hat{x}_y)\,|\hat{G}|^{-1/2}\,|\bar{G}|^{1/2}$$

The approximate density of the residual vector is thus

$$(2\pi)^{-k/2} f(y+\hat{x}_y)\, J\,|G|^{1/2}/|\hat{G}|^{1/2}\,(dy+\mathcal{X})$$

In more familiar statistical terminology, $f(y+\hat{x}_y)\,|G|^{1/2}$ is the profile likelihood maximized over the regression parameters β in a linear model with range $\mathcal{X}$. The matrix $\hat{G}$ is the *observed* Fisher information for β for each fixed value of the dispersion parameters, and the approximate REML likelihood $f(y+\hat{x}_y)\,|G|^{1/2}/|\hat{G}|^{1/2}$ is known as the adjusted profile likelihood for the dispersion parameters (Cox and Reid, 1987). Note, however, that this derivation does not require parameter orthogonality. That is to say that the dispersion parameters need not be orthogonal to the regression parameters (Barndorff-Nielsen and McCullagh, 1993).

4 REFERENCES

[1] Barndorff-Nielsen, O.E. and McCullagh, P. (1993) A note on the relation between modified profile likelihood and the Cox-Reid adjusted profile likelihood. *Biometrika* **80**, 321-328.

[2] Corbeil, R.R. and Searle, S.R. (1976) Restricted maximum likelihood (REML) estimation of variance components in the mixed model. *Technometrics*, **18**, 31-38.

[3] Cox, D.R. and Reid, N. (1987) Parameter orthogonality and approximate conditional inference, (with discussion). *J. Royal Statistical Society, Series B* **49**, 1-39.

[4] Halmos, P. (1974) *Finite-dimensional Vector Spaces*, Springer-Verlag.

[5] Harville, D.A. (1974) Bayesian inference for variance components using only error contrasts. *Biometrika* **61**, 383-385.

Harville, D.A. (1977) Maximum likelihood approaches to variance component estimation and to related problems (with discussion). *J. American Statistical Association* **72**, 320-340.

[6] Kruskal, W.H. (1975) The geometry of generalized inverses. *J. Royal Statistical Society, Series B* **37**, 272-283.

[7] Stone, M. (1987) *Coordinate-Free Multivariable Statistics*, Clarendon Press: Oxford.

[8] Patterson, H.D. and Thompson, R. (1971) Recovery of inter-block information when block sizes are unequal. *Biometrika* **58**, 545-554.

An Assessment of Approximate Maximum Likelihood Estimators in Generalized Linear Mixed Models

John M. Neuhaus and Mark R. Segal
University of California, San Francisco
United States

ABSTRACT Generalized linear mixed models provide useful methods for estimating within-cluster associations of covariates with the expected value of the response for data gathered in clusters or groups. These models assume that, conditional on a vector of cluster-specific parameters, the responses within a given cluster follow a generalized linear model. The model further assumes that the cluster-specific parameters follow a distribution, typically multivariate normal with unknown mean vector and covariance matrix. Since the calculation of the unconditional likelihood typically involves intractable integrals, several authors have proposed approximate maximum likelihood procedures. Breslow and Clayton (1993) approximated integrals using Laplace's method while Longford (1994) proposed Taylor series approximations of the likelihood. This paper examines the performance of these approximate methods. We present several examples to show that these approximate estimates more closely resemble population-averaged (marginal) estimates than the actual mixed-effects model maximum likelihood estimates. For example, the penalized quasilikelihood estimates from the simulations and model fits in Breslow and Clayton (1993) show attentuation with respect to true values and mixture model maximum likelihood estimates that closely corresponds to the expected attenuation for population-averaged models fit to mixed-effects data. Additional simulation studies with Longford's approach and logistic models yield similarly attenuated covariate effect estimates. Since population-averaged parameters typically differ from mixed-effects parameters for non-linear models, these results suggest that the approximate methods do not consistently estimate the fixed effects parameters and that the bias can be substantial in practice. Our work suggests that the approximate methods may require modification before their asymptotic bias can be competitive with mixed-effects model methods such as the Gibbs sampler that provide consistent estimation.

1 Introduction

Clustered samples arise frequently in practice. This clustering may be due to gathering repeated measurements on experimental units as in longitudinal studies, or may be due to subsampling the primary sampling units. The latter type of design is common in fields such as ophthalmology, where two eyes form natural clusters and teratology, where one gathers data on all members of a litter. The data consist of an outcome variable Y_{ij} together with a p-dimensional vector of covariates X_{ij}. The data are gathered in clusters or groups, and i=1, ..., m indexes clusters while j=1, ..., n_i indexes units within clusters. Clustered data tend to exhibit intracluster correlation which the analysis must address in order to obtain valid inferences.

The goal of studies with clustered data is often to assess the association of within-cluster changes in the covariate with within-cluster changes in the expected value of the response, $E(Y_{ij})$. For example, one might want to estimate how much an individual's probability of experiencing respiratory symptoms changes in response to changes in environmental conditions. Generalized linear mixed models (Breslow and Clayton 1993) provide a useful approach to assess within-cluster covariate effects. Under this model class, within the ith cluster, the Y_{ij} are independent and follow a generalized linear model with parameters that vary between clusters. That is, given a vector of parameters specific to the ith cluster, b_i, the conditional density of Y_{ij} is of the form $f(y_{ij}|b_i) = \exp[\{y_{ij}\theta_{ij} - c(\theta_{ij})\}\phi + d(y_{ij}, \phi)]$ where c and d are functions of known form. In addition, we assume that $E(Y_{ij}|b_i) = g^{-1}(Z_{ij}b_i + \beta X_{ij})$, where Z_{ij} is a specified covariate vector. The function g links the linear predictor to the expected response and is assumed to be strictly monotone and differentiable. Interest focuses on the parameter β which measures the change in the conditional expectation within the ith cluster corresponding to a unit increase in the covariate, that is

$$\beta = g[E(Y|X+1, b)] - g[E(Y|X, b)].$$

The model further assumes that the random effects b follow a distribution G, typically multivariate normal with mean vector 0 and covariance matrix $\Sigma(\theta)$.

The likelihood for generalized linear mixed models is

$$\text{L}(\beta, \text{G}) = \prod_{i=1}^{m} \int \prod_{j=1}^{n_i} f(Y_{ij} = y_{ij} \mid b,\ X_{ij})\ dG(b) \tag{1}$$

and one would like to estimate model parameters by maximizing (1). However, the integral is typically intractable and numerical integration methods are infeasible except when b is low dimensional, for example, one or two dimensions. Thus, several authors have suggested using approximations to (1) that one can maximize to obtain approximate maximum likelihood estimators of the covariate effects β and the parameters θ of the random effects distribution.

This paper examines the performance of two such approximate approaches: an approach involving a Taylor series expansion of (1) about $b = 0$ (Goldstein 1991; Longford 1994) and an approach involving a Laplace integral approximation (Breslow and Clayton 1993). Section 2 describes the two approximate approaches and presents expressions for the bias of the approximate MLEs with respect to the true MLEs for the case of a single random effect. Section 3 presents a comparison of the approximate and t rue MLEs obtained from two example data sets, while Section 4 contains a discussion of our findings.

2 Likelihood Approximations

2.1 Taylor Expansion about $b = 0$

Goldstein (1991) and Longford (1994) proposed to approximate the log-likelihood

$$\log \mathrm{L}(\beta, \mathrm{G}) = \sum_i \log \int \prod_j f(Y_{ij} = y_{ij} \mid b, X_{ij}) dG(b) \tag{2}$$

by

$$\sum_i \int \log f_2(Y_{ij} = y_{ij} \mid b,\ X_{ij}) dG(b), \tag{3}$$

where $\log f_2(Y_{ij} = y_{ij} \mid b,\ X_{ij})$ is a second order Taylor expansion of $\log \prod_j f(Y_{ij} = y_{ij} \mid b,\ X_{ij})$ about $b = 0$. Note the exchange of the logarithm and integration operations between (2) and (3). Since $\log \mathrm{E}(Z) \neq \mathrm{E} \log(Z)$ for a random variable Z, this exchange may be the source of substantial error in the approximation.

The approximation (3) is a quadratic form in b. Since it is standard to assume b follows a multivariate normal distribution, one can analytically evaluate the integral in (3) to obtain the approximation

$$\begin{aligned} \log \mathrm{L}(\beta, \mathrm{G}) \ \approx\ & \sum_i \sum_j \log f(Y_{ij} = y_{ij} \mid b = 0,\ X_{ij}) \\ & -0.5 \log|G| + 0.5\, e' \left(W_0 - {V_0}^{-1}\right) e \end{aligned} \tag{4}$$

where W_0 is a diagonal matrix with entries $var(Y_{ij} \mid b = 0)$, $G = I + Z'W_0Z\Sigma$, $e = {W_0}^{-1}[y - E(Y \mid b = 0)]$ and $V_0 = Z'\Sigma Z + {W_0}^{-1}$.

Goldstein (1991) and Longford (1994) obtained estimating equations for β and θ by differentiating (4) with respect to these parameters ignoring the dependence of the weights W_0 on β. This introduces another source of error into the Taylor approximate approach. The differentiation yields

$$\frac{\partial \text{log L}}{\partial \beta} = X^T V_0{}^{-1} e = 0, \tag{5}$$

and another estimating equation for θ. Note that (5) is of the same form as the generalized estimating equations proposed by Liang and Zeger (1986). The results of Liang and Zeger show that the Taylor approximation estimators (5) consistently estimate the parameters of the marginal or population-averaged model, $E(Y|X)$, fit to clustered data. Note that Breslow and Clayton (1993) describe these Taylor approximation approaches as marginal quasi-likelihood methods (MQL) to emphasize their connection to the marginal expectation of the response. Zeger, Liang and Albert (1988), Neuhaus, Kalbfleisch and Hauck (1991) and Neuhaus and Jewell (1993) showed that in general, the parameters of $E(Y|X)$ are not the same as those of the generalized linear mixed model (1) and that the generalized estimating equations approach will provide biased estimates of generalized linear mixed model parameters. Thus, the Taylor approximation approach will also provide biased estimates of generalized linear mixed model parameters.

Neuhaus and Jewell (1993) showed that this bias can be substantial and that the parameters of the marginal model β_{PA} are approximately related to those of generalized linear mixed model β_{GLMM} by

$$\beta_{PA} \approx \beta_{GLMM}\ g'[E\{g^{-1}(b)\}]E[1/g'\{g^{-1}(b)\}] = \beta_{GLMM}\ H'(0)\ . \tag{6}$$

The direction and magnitude of the bias $H'(0)$ depends on the curvature of the link function g. For example, $0 < H'(0) < 1$ for $1/g'$ concave. Such links include the logistic, probit and complementary log-log. With logistic regression the expression simplifies and we have

$$\beta_{PA} \approx \beta_{GLMM}\ (1 - \rho_Y) \tag{7}$$

where $\rho_Y = \text{corr}\ (Y_{ij}, Y_{ik} \mid \beta_{GLMM} = 0)$.

Rodríguez and Goldman (1995) presented the results of simulation studies that illustrate the bias associated with the Taylor approximation estimators and point out that investigators are mistakenly using these estimators as estimators of within-cluster covariate effects, that is, the parameters of generalized linear mixed models. In their simulations, Rodríguez and Goldman generated hierarchical data using a mixed-effects logistic model to resemble data from a survey of maternal and child health. They generated data for children (k) within families (j) and families within communities (i). One covariate corresponded to each level of the hierarchy: X_1 (communities); X_2 (families); and X_3 (children). The response Y_{ijk} was an indicator of whether the mother had used prenatal care services with a child and the true model for the simulation was

$$\text{logit pr}(Y_{ijk} = 1|a_i, b_j, X_{ijk}) = \beta_0 + a_i + b_j + \beta_1 X_1 + \beta_2 X_2 + \beta_3 X_3$$

where $a \sim \mathrm{N}(0, {\sigma_A}^2)$, $b \sim \mathrm{N}(0, {\sigma_B}^2)$ with a independent of b. The true parameter values were $\beta_0 = \beta_1 = \beta_2 = \beta_3 = 1$ and the simulations used 100 samples each of size N=2449. The authors estimated model parameters using VARCL which implements Longford (1994) and ML3 which implements Goldstein (1991).

Table 1 presents the means of the parameter estimates over the simulations using VARCL. Rodríguez and Goldman state that ML3 gave identical results. As (7) suggests, the Taylor approximation estimators were all biased toward zero and the magnitude of the bias increased with ${\sigma_A}^2 + {\sigma_B}^2$. We calculated the intraclass correlation coefficient ρ_Y using the true parameters of the random effects distributions and numerical integration subroutines in the NAG package. The observed parameter means closely corresponded to predictions (7).

Table 1
Observed and predicted regression coefficients for the mixed-effects logistic model simulation studies of Rodríguez and Goldman (1995) and eight true variance component pairs $({\sigma_A}^2, {\sigma_B}^2)$.

True					Predicted
${\sigma_A}^2$	${\sigma_B}^2$	β_3	β_2	β_1	β_{PA} (7)
1.0	1.0	0.74	0.74	0.77	0.74
1.0	0.4	0.82	0.84	0.80	0.82
0.4	1.0	0.84	0.83	0.84	0.82
0.4	0.4	0.95	0.95	0.93	0.94
1.0	0.0	0.85	0.85	0.85	0.84
0.4	0.0	0.97	0.98	0.95	0.97
0.0	1.0	0.85	0.85	0.81	0.84
0.0	0.4	0.97	0.98	0.96	0.97

2.2 Laplace integral approximations

The Laplace integral approximation method approximates the integrand at its maximizing value by simpler functions, for which one can analytically compute the integral (De Bruijn 1981, page 60). With generalized linear mixed models, one approximates

$$\log \mathrm{L}(\beta, \mathrm{G}) = \sum_i \log \int \prod_j f(Y_{ij} = y_{ij} \mid b, X_{ij}) g(b) db \tag{8}$$

by

$$\sum_i \log \int \tilde{l}(\tilde{b}, b) db$$

where $\tilde{l}(\tilde{b}, b)$ is a Taylor series expansion of $\prod_j f(Y_{ij} = y_{ij} \mid b, X_{ij}) g(b)$ about $\tilde{b}$ which maximizes the integrand and allows analytic integration.

Several authors have proposed approaches based on Laplace's method and the assumption that $b \sim MVN[0, \Sigma(\theta)]$. Breslow and Clayton's (1993) penalized quasi-likelihood (PQL) approach uses a first order Taylor approximation to the integrand in (8) and drops terms involving the variance function $var(Y_{ij})$ and $\Sigma(\theta)$. This is the same term that Goldstein (1991) and Longford (1994) ignore when they differentiate (4). For example, with a single random effect $\theta = \sigma^2$, the PQL approach uses the approximate log likelihood

$$\sum_i \log \prod_j f(Y_{ij} = y_{ij} \mid \tilde{b}_i, X_{ij}) - \frac{\tilde{b}_i^2}{2\sigma^2} \tag{9}$$

where $\tilde{b}_i$ maximizes the integrand in (8). This PQL approach drops terms of form $[1 - \sigma^2 var(Y_{ij} \mid \tilde{b}_i)]$ from the likelihood. Since $var(Y_{ij})$ typically depends on the regression parameters β, this simplification can lead to errors in the approximation. Liu and Pierce (1993) add the terms involving $var(Y_{ij})$ back into the likelihood.

With the Laplace approximation approaches, one estimates the regression parameters β and the parameters θ of the random effects distribution by solving estimating equations obtained by differentiating an approximate log-likelihood such as (9). Wolfinger and O'Connell (1993) describe an algorithm for computing PQL estimates and implement it with a SAS macro called GLIMMIX which also computes MQL estimates.

The model fits and simulations in Breslow and Clayton (1993) suggest that the PQL approach yields attentuated estimates of β and θ. Although the authors do not mention this, the attenuation closely corresponds to what one would expect from fitting population-averaged models to mixed-effects data.

We can relate the parameters estimated by the PQL approach to those of population-averaged models by computing population-averaged covariate effects under the assumption that the responses follow a model given by a PQL likelihood such as (9). For example with logistic regression, the population-averaged covariate is the log odds ratio

$$\begin{aligned} \beta_{PA} &= \log\{Pr(Y=1|X+1)\ Pr(Y=0|X)\} \\ &\quad -\log\{Pr(Y=1|X)\ Pr(Y=0|X+1)\}\,. \end{aligned} \tag{10}$$

Using expressions for the probabilities in (10) from (9) we have

$$\begin{aligned} \beta_{PA} &= -\log[1 + exp(-\mu - \tilde{b}_{11} - \beta(X+1))] \\ &\quad +\log[1 + exp(\mu + \tilde{b}_{01} + \beta(X+1))] \\ &\quad +\log[1 + exp(-\mu - \tilde{b}_{10} - \beta X)] \\ &\quad -\log[1 + exp(\mu + \tilde{b}_{00} + \beta X)] \\ &\quad -(2\sigma^2)^{-1}[\tilde{b}_{11}^2 - \tilde{b}_{10}^2 - \tilde{b}_{01}^2 + \tilde{b}_{00}^2] = F(\beta_{PQL}) \end{aligned}$$

where $\tilde{b}_{ij}$ solves $\tilde{b}_{ij} = \sigma^2\{i - [1 + exp(-\mu - \tilde{b}_{ij} - \beta(X+j))]^{-1}\}$.

We obtain an approximate relationship between β_{PA} and β_{PQL} by expanding F in a Taylor series about $\beta_{PQL} = 0$, using implicit differentiation with the terms $\tilde{b}_{ij}$. Note that $F(0) = 0$ since $\tilde{b}_{11} = \tilde{b}_{10}$ and $\tilde{b}_{01} = \tilde{b}_{00}$ at $\beta_{PQL} = 0$. This yields

$$\begin{aligned}\beta_{PA} \;\approx\; & \beta_{PQL}\;\{1 \;+\; [1+exp(-\mu-\tilde{b}_0)]^{-1} \\ & - [1+exp(-\mu-\tilde{b}_1)]^{-1}\} = \beta_{PQL}\;(1+p_0-p_1) \qquad (11)\end{aligned}$$

where b_i solves $\tilde{b}_i = \sigma^2\{i - [1+exp(-\mu-\tilde{b}_i)]^{-1}\}$ and $logit\ p_k = \mu + \tilde{b}_k$, k=0,1. Note that $\tilde{b}_1 \geq \tilde{b}_0$ so that $p_1 \geq p_0$ and $0 \leq (1+p_0-p_1) \leq 1$. Thus, if p_0 and p_1 are both small, we would expect that β_{PQL} will be close to β_{PA}. This will be the case if the PQL variance component, σ^2 is small. In the simulations and examples of Breslow and Clayton (1993) and the examples below in Section 3, PQL gives severely attenuated estimates of σ^2 and the PQL regression coefficient estimators are very close to the population-averaged ones.

We can use the relationship between β_{PA} and β_{PQL} and (7) to yield an approximation to relate β_{PQL} and β_{GLMM}. For logistic regression, this yields

$$\beta_{PQL} \approx \beta_{GLMM}\;\{1-\rho_Y\}/\{1+p_0-p_1\}\;. \qquad (12)$$

Approximations (12) and (7) suggest that we should expect both the Taylor (GEE) and Laplace approximation methods to provide attentuated estimates of covariate effects relative to maximum likelihood with $0 \leq |\beta_{PA}| \leq |\beta_{PQL}| \leq |\beta_{GLMM}|$. We will examine the quality of the approximations (12) and (7) in the examples below.

Breslow and Lin (1995) noted the attentuation with PQL estimators and derived the following expression for bias using Taylor series approximations about $\sigma^2 = 0$

$$\hat{\beta}_{PQL} \approx \hat{\beta} \;+\; 0.5\,\sigma^2(X^T W_0 X)^{-1} X^T u \qquad (13)$$

where W_0 is diagonal with entries $var(Y_{ij}|\sigma^2 = 0)$ and $u = \partial/\partial b\, var(Y_{ij})\;|_{\sigma^2=0}$. Their bias corrected estimator subtracts the second term on the right hand side of (13) from the PQL estimator. Since both the bias expression and correction depend on Taylor approximations near no random effects, we can expect that these methods will perform poorly when the random effects have at least moderate variability. The examples below show this to be th e case. Note that (6) suggests another, potentially more accurate bias corrected estimator. We calculate this estimator by first fitting a population-averaged model to data and then calculating the factor $H'(0)$ in (6) using the numerical integration subroutines in NAG. Below we show that this approach can yield very accurate estimates of covariate effects.

3 Examples

This section compares the parameter estimates obtained from the two approximate approaches to true MLEs using model fits to two data sets. We present Breslow-Clayton PQL estimates obtained from GLIMMIX, GEE estimates using exchangeable correlation (essentially Taylor approximation estimators) and true MLEs using the mixed-effects logistic model in EGRET. We also present the bias corrected PQL estimators (13) of Breslow and Lin (1995).

3.1 Pulmonary function matched pairs data

Data for the first example come from a study of the effects of ozone exposure on respiratory morbidity (Ostro et al, 1989). The study exposed each subject to several levels of ozone and recorded the presence (Y=1) or absence (Y=0) of respiratory symptoms at each dose. We use a subsample of the data in Ostro et al (1989) consisting of 71 subjects and two ozone exposures: no exposure (X=0) and 0.16 parts per million (ppm) (X=1). Thus, the data form a set of binary matched pairs which we display in a 2×2 table corresponding to the four possible outcome pairs (Table 2). The goal of this analysis is to examine whether an individual's propensity to experience respiratory symptoms changed with exposure to ozone. Matched pairs data offer a useful illustration of methods since we know that the true MLE is the standard, closed-form, conditional likelihood estimator (Neuhaus, Kalbfleisch and Hauck 1994).

Table 3 presents the three approximate MLEs along with the true MLE. As the results of Section 2 suggest, the Taylor approximation and PQL estimators are closer to zero than the MLE. The bias corrected estimators reduce but do not eliminate the bias. The severely attentuated PQL estimate of σ^2 produces very similar values of $\tilde{b}_1$ and $\tilde{b}_0$ so that the bias factor of (11) is close to 1.0 and the PQL covariate effects estimators are close to those of the GEE approach. The predicted ratios $\hat{\beta}_{PQL}/\hat{\beta}_{ML}$ (12) and $\hat{\beta}_{GEE}/\hat{\beta}_{ML}$ (7) of 0.68 and 0.56 closely correspond to the observed ratios of 0.58 and 0.53.

Table 2
Pulmonary function matched pairs data (Ostro et al, 1989).

		Y_2 = 1	Y_2 = 0	
Y_1	1	11	3	
	0	15	42	
				71

Table 3
Parameter estimates from four approaches applied to pulmonary function data.
$\hat{\beta}$ (S.E.)

	ML EGRET	GEE (b=0)	PQL GLIMMIX	Bias Corrected (13)
β_0	-2.69	-1.40	-1.52	-1.92
	(0.79)	(0.30)	(0.34)	
Dose	1.61	0.86	0.93	1.15
	(0.63)	(0.29)	(0.40)	
σ^2	6.78		1.26	
ρ_Y	0.44	0.43		

3.2 Trachomal eye disease data

We applied the estimation procedures to data from a study of trachomal eye disease among children in Egypt. This study obtained ophthalmologic data from home eye examinations of all the children in the family. Information included indicators of whether or not the eyes displayed corneal opacity (CO), a measure of past trachomal disease, tarsal follicles (Y), a measure of current trachomal disease and demographic data such as age. Although the two measures could vary between a child's eyes, the children in this sample did not exhibit this featur e; all pairs of eyes were concordant on the two disease measures. The analysis assessed the association of past eye disease with present disease, adjusting for age. Family was the cluster and we used data on the two oldest children in each family. The sample consisted of m=74 pairs of children.

Table 4 presents the three approximate MLEs along with the true MLE. As with the matched pairs data, the Taylor approximation and PQL estimators are closer to zero than the MLE and the bias corrected estimators reduce but do not eliminate the bias. Again, the small estimated variance, σ^2, leads to very similar values of $\tilde{b}_1$ and $\tilde{b}_0$ so that the PQL covariate effects estimators are close to those of the GEE approach. Table 5 shows that the predicted ratios of estimated regression coefficients closely corresponded to the observed values.

Table 4
Parameter estimates from four approaches applied to trachomal eye disease data.
$\hat{\beta}$ (S.E.)

	ML EGRET	GEE (b=0)	PQL GLIMMIX	Bias Corrected (13)
β_0	-1.49	-1.06	-1.11	-1.27
	(0.69)	(0.49)	(0.50)	
β_{CO}	1.73	1.34	1.38	1.54
	(0.67)	(0.49)	(0.51)	
β_{AGE}	-0.19	-0.15	-0.15	-0.16
	(0.12)	(0.09)	(0.10)	
σ^2	2.13		0.66	
ρ_Y	0.25	0.26		

Table 5
Observed and predicted relationships among three approaches fit to trachoma data using (12) and (7).

		Observed	Predicted
CO	$\hat{\beta}_{PQL}/\hat{\beta}_{ML}$	0.80	0.84
	$\hat{\beta}_{GEE}/\hat{\beta}_{ML}$	0.77	0.75
AGE	$\hat{\beta}_{PQL}/\hat{\beta}_{ML}$	0.79	0.84
	$\hat{\beta}_{GEE}/\hat{\beta}_{ML}$	0.79	0.75

4 Discussion

This paper presents approximations, simulations and fits of models to data that show that the Taylor approximation approach (Goldstein 1991; Longford 1994) and the PQL approach (Breslow and Clayton 1993) can yield highly biased estimates of covariate effects and the parameters of random effects distributions. While we focus here on binary response models, estimation bias and our approach to assess its magnitude easily extend to any generalized linear mixed model whose link function is neither the identity nor the log. The bias correction proposed by Breslow and Lin (1995) slightly reduces but does not eliminate this bias. With moderate to large random effect variance, one could obtain more accurate bias corrected estimates of covariate effects using the relationship between the parameters of population-averaged and mixed models (6).

While the Taylor approximation and PQL approaches do not seem to provide accurate estimation, approaches based on the Gibbs sampler (Zeger and Karim 1991) and the EM algorithm with Laplace integral approximation (Steele 1995) do seem to provide consistent estimation of regression coefficients and the parameters of the random effects distribution. For example, Zeger and Karim (1991), Breslow and Clayton (1993) and Steele (1995) all performed nearly identical simulation studies of their methods. The Gibbs sampler and EM/Laplace methods both yielded estimated regression coefficients and random effects parameters that closely corresponded to the true values, while the PQL estimators exhibited substantial attentuation, as in the examples of this paper.

In summary, the biases exhibited by the Taylor approximation and PQL approaches indicate that these approaches require further development and modification before they should be used in practice.

5 REFERENCES

[1] Breslow, N.E. and Clayton, D.G. (1993). Approximate inference in generalized linear mixed models. *J. Amer. Statist. Assoc.* **88**, 9-25.

[2] Breslow, N.E. and Lin, X. (1995). Bias correction in generalised linear models with a single component of dispersion. *Biometrika* **82**, 81-91.

[3] de Bruijn, N.G. (1981). *Asymptotic Methods in Analysis.* Dover: New York.

[4] Goldstein, H. (1991). Nonlinear multilevel models, with an application to discrete response data. *Biometrika* **78**, 45-51.

[5] Liang, K-Y and Zeger, S.L. (1986). Longitudinal data analysis using generalised linear models. *Biometrika* **73**, 13-22.

[6] Liu, Q. and Pierce, D.A. (1993). Heterogeneity in Mantel-Haenszel-type models. *Biometrika* **80**, 543-556.

[7] Longford, N.T. (1994). Logistic regression with random coefficients. *Computational Statistics and Data Analysis* **17**, 1-15.

[8] Neuhaus, J.M., Kalbfleisch J.D., and Hauck W.W. (1991). A comparison of cluster-specific and population-averaged approaches for analyzing correlated binary data. *Int. Statist. Rev.* **59**, 25-35.

[9] Neuhaus, J.M. and Jewell, N.P. (1993). A geometric approach to assess bias due to omitted covariates in generalized linear models. *Biometrika* **80**, 807-816.

[10] Neuhaus, J.M., Kalbfleisch J.D., and Hauck W.W. (1994). Conditions for consistent estimation in mixed-effects models for binary matched pairs data. *Canadian Journal of Statistics* **22**, 139-148.

[11] Ostro, B.D., Lipsett, M.J. and Jewell, N.P. (1989). Predicting respiratory morbidity from pulmonary function tests: A reanalysis of ozone chamber studies. *J. Air Pollution Control Assoc.* **39**, 1313-1318.

[12] Rodríguez, G. and Goldman, N. (1995). An assessment of estimation procedures for multilevel models with binary responses. *J. R. Statist. Soc., Ser. A.* **158**, 73-89.

[13] Steele, B.M. (1995) *Estimation in generalized linear mixed models via the EM algorithm.* Ph.D. dissertation, University of Montana. Ann Arbor: University Microfilms International.

[14] Wolfinger, R. and O'Connell, M. (1993) Generalized linear mixed models: A pseudo-likelihood approach. *J. Statist. Comput. Simul.* **48**, 233-243.

[15] Zeger, S.L., Liang, K-Y and Albert, P.A. (1988). Models for longitudinal data: a generalized estimating equation approach. *Biometrics* **44**, 1049-1060.

[16] Zeger, S.L. and Karim, M.R. (1991) Generalized linear models with random effects; A Gibbs sampling approach. *J. Amer. Statist. Assoc.* **86**, 79-86.

Scaled Link Functions For Heterogeneous Ordinal Response Data *

Minge Xie
National Institute of Statistical Sciences
United States

Douglas G. Simpson
University of Illinois, Urbana-Champaign
United States

Raymond J. Carroll
Texas A&M University
United States

ABSTRACT This paper describes a class ordinal regression models in which the link function has scale parameters that may be estimated along with the regression parameters. One motivation is to provide a plausible model for group level categorical responses. In this case a natural class of scaled link functions is obtained by treating the group level responses as threshold averages of possible correlated latent individual level variables. We find scaled link functions also arise naturally in other circumstances. Our methodology is illustrated through environmental risk assessment data where (correlated) individual level responses and group level responses are mixed.

Key words and phrases: Ordinal regression, Aggregated observations, Marginal modeling approach, Generalized likelihood inference.

---

*The research was supported by NSF contract DMS 95-05290, and National Institute of Statistical Sciences Cooperative Agreement CR819638 and CR820897 with the U.S. EPA. R. J. Carroll's research was also supported by a grant from the National Cancer Institute (CA-57030). The authors thank Daniel Guth of the U.S. EPA for making available the data on tetrachloroethylene.

1 Introduction

Data in which the individual responses are ordinal are frequently modeled by a generalized linear model of the form

$$\Pr(Y_i \geq s|x_i) = \begin{cases} H(\beta^T x_i - \alpha_s), & \text{if } s = 1, 2, \ldots, S; \\ 1, & \text{if } s = 0; \end{cases} \tag{1}$$

where Y_i is the ordinal response of the ith individual, $i = 1, \ldots, n$, x_i is a vector of explanatory variables, and H is a general cumulative distribution function. The inverse function H^{-1} of H is called a link function (McCullagh and Nelder, 1989). Common choices for the link function H^{-1} are the inverse function of the standard normal distribution Φ^{-1}, the logit function $H^{-1}(t) = \log\{t/(1-t)\}$, and the complimentary log–log function $H^{-1}(t) = \log\{-\log(t)\}$. If the link function has the logit form, model (1) is referred to as a proportional odds ratio model (McCullagh, 1980).

Our concern is with situations in which the assumed constancy of the link function across heterogeneous observations is untenable. For example, in a toxicology risk assessment example, due to various reasons, the responses may be reported at the group (e.g., cage or chamber) level rather than at the individual (animal) level. The number of individuals in each group (cage/chamber size) is known, but the information on individual incidences is missing. With groups of unequal size, the assumption of a common scale is suspect.

We propose a scaled link method in this paper. The method is easy to implement. The scaling of the link function is equivalent to a rescaling of the regression explanatory variables (including S columns of binary variables corresponding to the severity dependent intercepts). If the scale function contains unknown parameters, then the estimation of the regression parameters is easily nested within the maximum likelihood optimization for the scale parameters.

Depending on the scaling formula selected, the observations sometimes may supply only crude information about a scaling parameter. The estimation of the scaling parameter may not be precise. We provide sensitivity studies on the use of scaling parameters. The question we try to answer is how a simpler scaling with a wrong scale parameter would affect the estimation of the other parameters based on the data at hand. This analysis technique is similar to the analysis that Hjort (1994) used to study the t model versus the normal model.

An appealing feature of the scaled link function model for group level responses is that, although the observed elements are marginal responses, the parameters of the model are defined at the individual level and are therefore comparable across groups of different sizes. Moreover, we can combine group and individual level data by treating an individual as a group of size 1. Notice the observed individual level responses within the same group are considered correlated. In addition, some high level correlated structure, for example, correlated batches which are built upon the basic model, might also exist. We use a working likelihood as an estimating criterion, and adopt generalized estimating equation (GEE) techniques (Zeger and Liang, 1986) to deal with the correlation structure.

The rest of the paper is organized as follows. Section 2 provides some derivations of scaled link function models. Section 3 provides sensitivity studies for the scaled link analysis of group level responses. Section 4 briefly reviews some results on generalized likelihood inference and generalizes our sensitivity analysis to correlated responses. In Section 5, an application of the methodology in toxicological risk assessment is discussed. Section 6 provides some further remarks.

2 Derivation and Interpretation

To model group level ordinal responses and other forms of heterogeneous data we replace (1) by a model of the form

$$\Pr(Y_i \geq s|x_i) = \begin{cases} H\{w_i\ (\beta^T x_i - \alpha_s)\}, & \text{if } s = 1, 2, \ldots, S; \\ 1, & \text{if } s = 0; \end{cases} \tag{2}$$

where the design weights w_i are scaling factors and refer to the precision of latent observations. Effectively, we replace the inverse link function $H(\,\cdot\,)$ by the scaled function $H(\,w_i\,\cdot)$. Section 2.1 provides a derivation of model (2) under a heterosdastic setting. Section 2.2 considers critical mass model in detail for group level response data. The critical mass model is a special case of Section 2.1.

2.1 Heteroscedastic latent structure for ordinal data

From a standard quantal response analysis, Model (1) has an associated latent structure. For instance, one may assume that there exist a tolerance distribution (latent underlying continuous random variable) Z and a series of ordered thresholds $-\infty = \alpha_0 < \alpha_1 < \ldots < \alpha_S < \alpha_{S+1} = +\infty$, such that observation $y = s$ occurs if and only if the unobserved latent variable Z lies in the interval of $[\alpha_s, \alpha_{s+1})$, that is, $y = \sum_{s=1}^{S} \mathbf{1}_{\{Z \geq \alpha_s\}}$, where $\mathbf{1}_{\{C\}}$ is the indicator function which equals 1 if set C is true and equals 0 if set C is false. Suppose $Z - \beta^T x$ has cumulative distribution $1 - H(-t)$, then we can find that $\Pr(Y \geq s|x)$ has the same form as (1).

We generalize this standard latent structure to a heterosdastic setting. Suppose that a latent variable Z_i follows a heteroscedastic linear model,

$$(Z_i - \beta^T x_i) w_i \,|\, x_i \;\sim\; 1 - H(-t) \tag{3}$$

but we observe only $Y_i = \sum_{s=1}^{S} \mathbf{1}_{\{Z_i \geq \alpha_s\}}$ rather than Z_i. We then have the scaled link function model (2). The weights w_i are interpreted as inverse scale factors for the latent responses.

One special case is the model (5.4) of McCullagh and Nelder (1989, p154), where $(Z_i - \beta^T x_i)/\exp(\tau^T x_i)$ was assumed to follow the standard logistic distribution. In their model, the scale w_i has the form $w_i = \exp(-\tau^T x_i)$, and the linear regression $\tau^T x_i$ plays the role of the linear predictor for the overdispersion or variance. McCullagh and Nelder (1989) suggested this model for testing the proportional odds ratio assumption against systematically increasing or systemically decreasing in score s.

Another interesting special case occurs under a hierarchical setup in which the latent variable follows a linear model with random coefficients, that is,

$$Z_i | x_i, b_i \sim N(-x_i^T b_i, 1), \quad b_i \sim N(\beta, \Gamma). \tag{4}$$

The marginal distribution of Z_i is then normal with mean $-\beta^T x_i$ and variance $1 + x_i^T \Gamma x_i$. For fully observed Z_i this is a standard growth curve model; see, for instance, Johansen (1984). Such a model might also be useful for observational data. If we observe only the $Y_i = \sum_{s=1}^{S} 1_{\{Z_i \geq -\alpha_s\}}$, then we obtain an ordinal regression model of the form (2) with $w_i = (1 + x_i^T \Gamma x_i)^{-1/2}$. In the binary case, this is a special case of the general latent model considered by Zeger et. al. (1988) and McCulloch (1994), who focused on the latent structure for modeling correlated binary outcomes. Here the observable responses are independent, but heteroscedastic.

In the preceding example the latent distribution for b_i is a way of expressing uncertainty about the linear model. The resulting link function model therefore controls the influence of extreme values of x_i. Note, in particular, that $\|w_i x_i\| \leq \lambda_{\min}^{-1/2}(\Gamma)$, where $\lambda_{\min}$ denotes the smallest eigenvalue. As a result, the maximum likelihood estimator has a bounded influence function in the sense of Hampel et. al. (1986).

2.2 Critical-mass model for ordinal group level responses

Let y_i denote the ordinal response of the ith group, $i = 1, \ldots, n$, and n_i be the group size. Suppose that the group ordinal response $y_i = s$ occurs if and only if the mean latent response of the individuals in the group falls into the threshold interval $[\alpha_s, \alpha_{s+1})$, that is $Y_i = \sum_{s=1}^{S} 1_{\{\bar{Z}_{i\cdot} \geq \alpha_s\}}$ where $\bar{Z}_{i\cdot} = n_i^{-1} \sum_{j=1}^{n_i} Z_{ij}$ and Z_{ij} is the latent response of the jth individual in the ith group.

Assume that the latent variables themselves follow a latent variable model for a given x_i,

$$Z_{ij} = \beta^T x_i + a_i + e_{ij}, \quad a_i \sim N(0, \rho), \quad e_{ij} \sim N(0, 1 - \rho) \tag{5}$$

where we have standardized the marginal variance to be 1 due to identifiable consideration, and random effects a_i and error terms e_{ij} are independent. Then we have the model,

$$P(Y_i > s | x_i) = \Phi\{w_i\,(\beta^T x_i - \alpha_s)\}$$

where

$$w_i = \left\{ \frac{n_i}{1 + (n_i - 1)\rho} \right\}^{\frac{1}{2}} \tag{6}$$

The weight function w_i^2 may be interpreted as an effective group size. If $\rho = 0$ then $w_i^2 = n_i$, whereas a positive correlation shrinks the weight towards one. In the extreme, if $\rho = 1$, then the effective group size is 1.

Identifiability of the parameter ρ requires heterogeneity of the group sizes. If the group sizes were all the same, then the weighting would simply introduce a constant scale factor in the regression parameters. If the group sizes are heterogeneous, then the weights in (6) identify β, α and ρ at the individual level, $n_i = 1$. In this way the scaled model avoids attenuation effects that would otherwise occur in the combined analysis of group responses with heterogeneous group sizes.

The above derivation extends approximately to other link functions. For instance, the inverse logistic link function, $\Psi(t) = \{1 + \exp(-t)\}^{-1}$, is near to the standard normal distribution function in absolute terms, because

$$\sup_t |\Psi(1.702\,t) - \Phi(t)| < 0.01;$$

see, e.g., Baker (1992, p16). Thus, the preceding analysis might be used as a heuristic to suggest a weight function for scaled logistic regression.

3 Wide Model versus Narrow Model Asymptotics

In the group level response model of Section 2.2, we found an effective group size of $n_i^*(\rho) = n_i^{1/2}\{1 + \rho(n_i - 1)\}^{-1/2}$. If $\rho = 1$, then $n_i^* = 1$, and group level responses are indistinguishable from the responses of individuals. From large sample theory, estimation of ρ is not a problem as long as the group size n_i varies across groups and the sample size n is large enough. But in practice, sample sizes are often not large enough to estimate ρ precisely, since the threshold observations apply only crude information about scaling.

In the example discussed in Section 5, the ρ estimate is 1 but its confidence interval $(0.1, 1]$ covers most of the ρ parameter space; see Figure 1 and Section 5 for more detail. A question that naturally arises is whether we can use ordinary regression to replace regression with scaled link functions if ρ is close to 1. Although the parameter estimates would be biased, the variances of the estimates would be decreased and the analysis simplified. This dilemma is the familiar bias-variance tradeoff. In this section, we analyze the bias-variance tradeoff for the simplified model versus the more general model. Using local asymptotics, we determine how far ρ may deviate from 1 before it becomes necessary to include the extra parameter in the model.

Write $\eta = (\alpha_1, \ldots, \alpha_S, \beta)^T$ and let z_i be its associated ith covariates. Following Hjort's (1994) general prescription, let $\mu(\eta, \rho)$ denote any parameter of interest, and let $\hat{\mu}_{wide} = \mu(\hat{\eta}, \hat{\rho})$ denote the estimate with ρ unconstrained (within its natural parameter interval $[0, 1]$), $\hat{\mu}_{narr} = \mu(\hat{\eta}_{narr}, 1)$ denote the estimate with ρ fixed at 1. We ask when the asymptotic mean square error of $\hat{\mu}_{narr}$ is smaller than or comparable to that of $\hat{\mu}_{wide}$. Of course if $\rho \neq 1$ is fixed regardless of the sample size then the answer is trivial, but such an analysis would shed little light on moderate deviations from ρ, which may not be detected with certainty in moderately sized samples. Therefore we consider sequences of the form $\rho = 1 - \delta n^{-1/2}$, where n is the sample size and δ is fixed and nonnegative. We derive the asymptotic mean square errors of the narrow and wide estimators of μ, and examine the ratio between them.

Assuming independence, the log-likelihood for model (2) is given by

$$l(\eta, \rho | y, z) = \sum_{i=1}^{n} p_i\{w_i(\rho)\eta^T z_i\} \tag{7}$$

where $p_i = p_i\{w_i(\rho)\eta^T z_i\} = f(y_i|\eta, \rho; z_i, n_i)$, the log-likelihood term for the ith observation. We write

$$\bar{\mathcal{U}}_{\eta|\rho=1} = \{n^{-1}\frac{\partial}{\partial \eta} l(\eta, \rho|y, z)\}|_{\rho=1}, \quad \bar{\mathcal{U}}_{\rho|\rho=1} = \{n^{-1}\frac{\partial}{\partial \rho} l(\eta, \rho|y, z)\}|_{\rho=1}$$

and

$$\mathcal{J}_{wide} = \lim_{n\to\infty} var_0\{n^{\frac{1}{2}} \begin{pmatrix} \bar{\mathcal{U}}_{\eta|\rho=1} \\ \bar{\mathcal{U}}_{\rho|\rho=1} \end{pmatrix}\} = \begin{pmatrix} \mathcal{J}_{\eta\eta} & \mathcal{J}_{\eta\rho} \\ \mathcal{J}_{\rho\eta} & \mathcal{J}_{\rho\rho} \end{pmatrix}, \tag{8}$$

where the variance is taken under model (2) with $\rho = 1$, and some regularity conditions are needed to ensure the existence of the limit. Also, we denote $\hat{\eta}_{narr}$ to maximize $l(\eta, 1|y, z)$, the loglikelihood function of the narrow model, and $(\hat{\eta}^T, \hat{\rho})^T$ to maximize $l(\eta, \rho|y, z)$ with $\rho = 1 - \delta n^{-\frac{1}{2}}$, the likelihood function of the wide model. We have the following theorem:

Theorem 1 Let $\mu(\eta, \rho)$ be smooth with continuous derivatives throughout the inner parameter space $(\eta, \rho) \in (-\infty, \infty) \times (0, 1)$. Assume its left derivative exists at $\rho = 1$. Under model (2) with $\rho = 1 - \delta n^{-\frac{1}{2}}$, then

$$nE\{\mu(\hat{\eta}_{narr}, 1) - \mu(\eta, 1 - \delta n^{-\frac{1}{2}})\}^2 = b^2\delta^2 + \tau^2 + o(1) \tag{9}$$

$$nE\{\mu(\hat{\eta}_{wide}, \hat{\rho}) - \mu(\eta, 1 - \delta n^{-\frac{1}{2}})\}^2 = b^2 E\{\mathbf{B}^2 1_{(\mathbf{B}<\delta)} + \delta^2 1_{(\mathbf{B}\geq\delta)}\} + \tau^2 + o(1) \tag{10}$$

where $b = \frac{\partial}{\partial\rho}\mu - (\mathcal{J}_{\eta\eta}^{-1}\mathcal{J}_{\eta\rho})^T \frac{\partial}{\partial\eta}\mu$, $\tau^2 = (\frac{\partial}{\partial\eta}\mu)^T \mathcal{J}_{\eta\eta}^{-1} \frac{\partial}{\partial\eta}\mu$, and $\mathbf{B} \sim N(0, \mathcal{J}^{\rho\rho})$ with $\mathcal{J}^{\rho\rho} = (\mathcal{J}_{\rho\rho} - \mathcal{J}_{\eta\rho}^T \mathcal{J}_{\eta\eta}^{-1} \mathcal{J}_{\eta\rho})^{-1}$.

The basic idea of proof follows Xie (1996, Section 4.5-4.6 and Appendix 2).

Define λ as the ratio of the mean square errors between the narrow model and the wide model,

$$\lambda = \frac{n\mathrm{E}\{\mu(\hat{\eta}_{narr}, 1) - \mu(\eta, 1 - \delta n^{-\frac{1}{2}})\}^2}{n\mathrm{E}\{\mu(\hat{\eta}_{wide}, \hat{\rho}) - \mu(\eta, 1 - \delta n^{-\frac{1}{2}})\}^2}. \tag{11}$$

Based on the data set at hand, we estimate how λ varies as the true ρ or δ deviates away from the value which corresponds to the narrow model.

4 Batch Correlated Observations

Batch correlated observations are common in many settings. For example in the toxicology data set considered in the next section, two levels of batch correlated structures are detected. First, the observed individual level responses within the same group are correlated. Second, these individual level responses as well as group level responses are nested within 24 studies. To handle this type of batch correlation, we use below a marginal modeling approach.

Assume that each observation satisfies marginally model (2), where $w_i = 1$ for individual level observations. We construct a working likelihood function $l(\eta, \rho)$ by multiplying their marginal likelihoods. (we actually include weights in the working log-likelihood function for individual level observations; see Simpson et al., 1996, for detail).

Write $\theta = (\eta, \rho)$. We denote the score covariance matrix and negative expected Hessian matrix by

$$\mathcal{J} = \mathrm{E}\{\mathcal{U}(\theta)\mathcal{U}(\theta)^T\} \text{ and } \mathcal{H} = -\mathrm{E}\{\frac{\partial}{\partial\theta}\mathcal{U}(\theta)\},$$

where $\mathcal{U}(\theta) = (\partial/\partial\theta)l(\theta)$ is the score function. In contrast to standard maximum likelihood theory, $\mathcal{H} \neq \mathcal{J}$ in the present context. Suppose the true parameters are in the interior of the parameter space. The parameter estimates obtained by maximizing $l(\theta)$ or setting $\mathcal{U}(\theta) = 0$ are consistent under minor regularity conditions; see for example, Li (1996). Based on the theories of Generalized Estimating Equations (GEE) (Zeger and Liang, 1986), the variance is approximated by a sandwich formula $\mathcal{H}^{-1}\mathcal{J}\mathcal{H}^{-1}$.

In order to make inference on ρ, we consider the profile likelihood analysis. The profile likelihood function $l(\rho) = l\{\hat{\eta}(\rho), \rho\}$ can be computed easily, since by setting $\tilde{z}_i = w_i(\rho)z_i$ we can $l(\rho)$ from maximizing a standard ordinal regression likelihood $l(\eta, 1|y, \tilde{x})$. Computing $-2l(\rho)$ over a grid of $[0, 1]$ provides a deviance profile as illustrated in Figure 1. If the observations are independent, a standard large sample theory ensures that $2[l(\hat{\eta}, \hat{\rho}) - l\{\hat{\eta}(\rho_0), \rho_0\}]$ has the standard χ^2 distribution where ρ_0 is the true parameter. But if the observations are batch correlated, a generalized profile likelihood theory should be used. We summarize the generalized profile likelihood theory in a following theorem. This theorem is a special case of the nonstandard asymptotic theorem of Simpson et al. (1994). For discussions on the nonstandard asymptotics, see Huber (1967), Kent (1982), Rotnitzky and Jewell (1990), and Li and McCullagh (1994).

Theorem 2 *If* $\rho = \rho_0$, *then as the batch number increases,* $2\{l(\hat{\eta}, \hat{\rho}) - l(\hat{\eta}(\rho_0), \rho_0)\}$ *converges in distribution to* μW, *where* W *is distributed as* χ_1^2 *with* 1 *degree of freedom and* $\mu = \mathcal{H}_{\rho\rho}^{-1}(\mathcal{H}^{-1}\mathcal{J}\mathcal{H}^{-1})_{\rho\rho}$.

The right corner index $\rho\rho$ indicates the diagonal matrix element associated with ρ.

We also ask whether the sensitivity analysis in last section also carries through the correlated case. Define $\mathcal{J}_{wide}$ the same as (8) and define

$$\mathcal{H}_{wide} = \lim_{n\to\infty} \mathrm{E}_0\{\frac{1}{n}\begin{pmatrix} \frac{\partial^2 \ell(\eta,\rho|y,z)}{\partial\eta\partial\eta^T}|_{\rho=1} & \frac{\partial^2 \ell(\eta,\rho|y,z)}{\partial\eta\partial\rho}|_{\rho=1} \\ \frac{\partial^2 \ell(\eta,\rho|y,z)}{\partial\rho\partial\eta^T}|_{\rho=1} & \frac{\partial^2 \ell(\eta,\rho|y,z)}{\partial^2\rho}|_{\rho=1} \end{pmatrix}\} = \begin{pmatrix} \mathcal{H}_{\eta\eta} & \mathcal{H}_{\eta\rho} \\ \mathcal{H}_{\rho\eta} & \mathcal{H}_{\rho\rho} \end{pmatrix}$$

where the expectation is taken under model (2) with $\rho = 1$, and some regularity conditions are needed to ensure the existence of the limit. Notice the n here denotes the number of independent batches instead of the total number of observations.

Parallel results of Theorem 1 can be obtained, but the right hand sides of (9) and (10) are replaced by

$$\mathrm{E}\{(b\delta + c\mathbf{B})^2\} + \tau^2 + o(1),$$

$$\mathrm{E}\{(b\mathbf{B} + c\mathbf{B})^2\mathbf{1}_{(\mathbf{B}<\delta)} + (b\delta + c\mathbf{B})^2\mathbf{1}_{(\mathbf{B}\geq\delta)}\} + \tau^2 + o(1)$$

respectively, where $b = -(\mathcal{H}_{\eta\eta}^{-1}\mathcal{H}_{\eta\rho})^T(\partial/\partial\eta)\mu + \delta\ (\partial/\partial\rho)\mu$, $c = (\mathcal{H}_{\eta\eta}^{-1}\mathcal{H}_{\eta\rho} - D_{\eta\eta}^{-1}D_{\eta\rho})^T(\partial/\partial\eta)\mu$, $\tau^2 = \{(\partial/\partial\eta)\mu\}^T D_{\eta\eta}^{-1}(\partial/\partial\eta)\mu$, and $\mathbf{B} \sim N(0, D^{\rho\rho})$ with $D^{-1} = \mathcal{H}_{wide}^{-1}\mathcal{J}_{wide}\mathcal{H}_{wide}^{-1}$.

5 Example: Analysis of Toxicology Data

The data set analyzed here contains study results from multiple studies on the effects of acute inhalation exposure to tetrachloroethylene. The responses are scored as *No-effect*, *Adverse effect* and *Severe effect*. These outcomes were determined by a toxicologist during a thorough review of the literature. Some studies only provide partial response information and censored responses are reported. We will not explore the issue of censoring in this paper; see Simpson et al. (1996b) for detailed discussions.

The data set has total of 536 observations with 380 at individual levels and 156 at group levels. They are from a total of 24 studies which range in size from 1 group to 35 groups, with median of 4 per study. For group level responses, the group size are ranging from 2 to 30 and the median size is 10. Usually the reason for group responses rather than individual incidences is that the published results are simply descriptions of lesions and tissue damage typical of the group. This leads to data in which the group size is known, and an overall group severity score can be assigned, but individual incidence information is missing.

In addition to the response, cluster and size information, we have information on the exposure concentration and duration, the species, and the gender. We fit a scaled link function model for logistic regression on $\log_{10}$(concentration) and $\log_{10}$(duration), and allow each species to have their own regression intercepts and concentration slope parameters. Of particular interest is the question of how much information group level responses provide as compared with individual outcomes. The latent correlation parameter, ρ, allows us to investigate this question.

Figure 1 shows the deviance profile function for ρ, along with the projected 95% generalized likelihood confidence interval. The cutoff value was computed following the result of Theorem 2. We see that the estimate of ρ is 1, but the confidence interval is rather wide. A naive confidence interval based on the usual χ^2 approximation is a bit narrower but suspect because of the likely correlation within studies. One conclusion we can draw from Figure 2 is that the within *group* correlation is significantly different from 0.

Figure 2 performs a sensitivity study on how a narrow model with $\rho = 1$ behaves if the true ρ grids over the range of 0 to 1. The three parameters investigated are the 10% *effective concentration level* (EC_{10}) at unit duration (1 hour) for human, rat and mice species, where the 10% effective concentration level, EC_{10}, is defined as the dose level which would leads to 10% rate of adverse or severe effect at a given duration and for a given species. Figure 2 plots the mean square error (MSE) ratio λ, defined in (11), versus the latent group correlation coefficient ρ for these three parameters. All three MSE ratios increase from below 1 to larger than 1 as ρ decreases from 1 to 0. The MSE ratio for human EC_{10} almost overlaps the ratio=1 line. It implies that no matter where the true ρ is, the use of a narrow model ($\rho = 1$) would have little effect on the performance of the estimated human one hour exposure EC_{10} in the sense of comparing MSEs. The MSE ratio for rat unit exposure EC_{10} can strike as high as 1.3, and the MSE ratio for mice unit exposure EC_{10} are mostly below 1. If we are willing to accept any MSE ratio less than 1.1, then from Figure 2 we see that ρ larger than 0.43 is sufficient to reduce to the narrow model. Observe that, according to this analysis, group level responses contain roughly the same information as a single individual level response. It implies that individual data should be obtained whenever possible.

By adopting the assumption that $\rho = 1$, we fit the data set to model

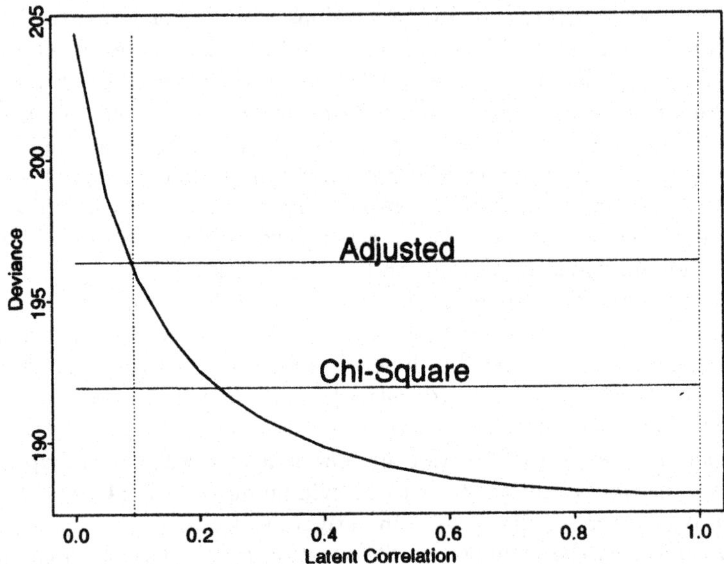

FIGURE 1. Deviance profile of latent correlation parameter for tetrachloroethylene data. Cutoff values are shown for the likelihood ratio (chi–square) and generalized likelihood (adjusted) tests.

(1), and computed the EC_{10} conditional on the duration. The solid lines in Figure 3 are effective concentration levels estimated from the fitting. These lines are called the EC_{10} lines. The dotted lines in Figures 3 (a) to (c) are their confidence bands. The slopes of concentration parameters for humans and rats are parallel, and they are both different from the mouse slope parameter. Notice that the confidence intervals for mice ED_{10} are quite large. Simpson *et al.* (1996a,b) reported the same or similar results. Their robust analysis (1996a) indicted that the problem was the lack of design points of mice at lower exposure level.

6 Discussion

If both group and individual level data are available, the latent model for the group responses provides the basis for combining these sources of information. The key is that the parameters are defined at the individual level rather than at the group level. In particular (6) implies that the individual ordinal responses follow model (2) with $w_i = 1$. Therefore the regression parameters of the group and individual response models have the same interpretation.

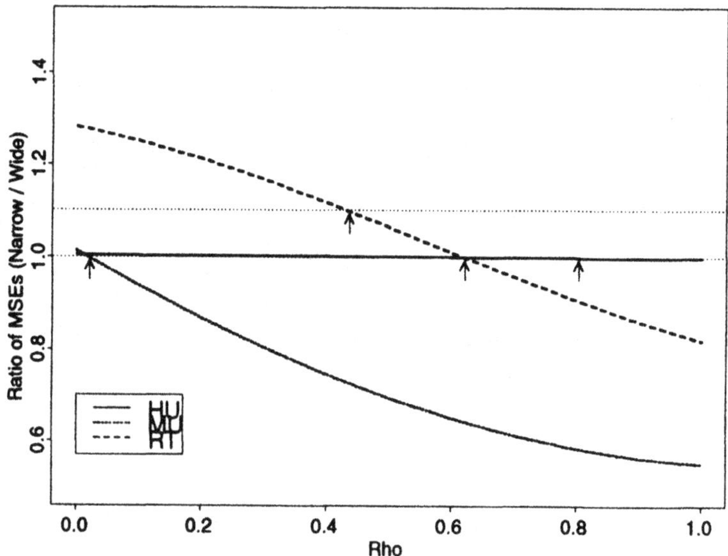

FIGURE 2. Sensitivity analysis on the one hour EC_{10}'s for humans (solid curve), mice (dotted curve), and rats (dashed curve). The x-axis is the assumed true value of ρ grid over [0,1]; the y-axis is the ratio of Mean Square Errors (MSE) as defined in (11). The three arrows on the ratio=1 line indicate the crossing points of the MSE ratios for estimated human, rat and mice EC_{10} parameters from right to left. The fourth arrow indicates the point where the MSE ratio for rat EC_{10} crosses 1.1.

In applications, however, some caution is required in combining group level and individual level responses when the individuals are also subject to group correlations. The group level responses might well appear to have a high within group (latent) correlation in part because the group level reporting itself inflates the apparent agreement among elements of the group. Thus, although the latent responses appear to be highly correlated, this need not imply that fully observed individual responses would exhibit the same high correlation. For this reason it would be a good idea to model the within group correlations separately for individual level and group level data.

The scaled models generalize the unscaled models just as weighted least squares regression generalizes ordinary least squares. The simple technique of weighting the regression variables may be useful in a variety of problems. In the group ordinal model, group size and within group correlation are natural effects on which to model the scale of the link function. In other settings it might be more natural to key on covariate information to model heterogeneity of the scale.

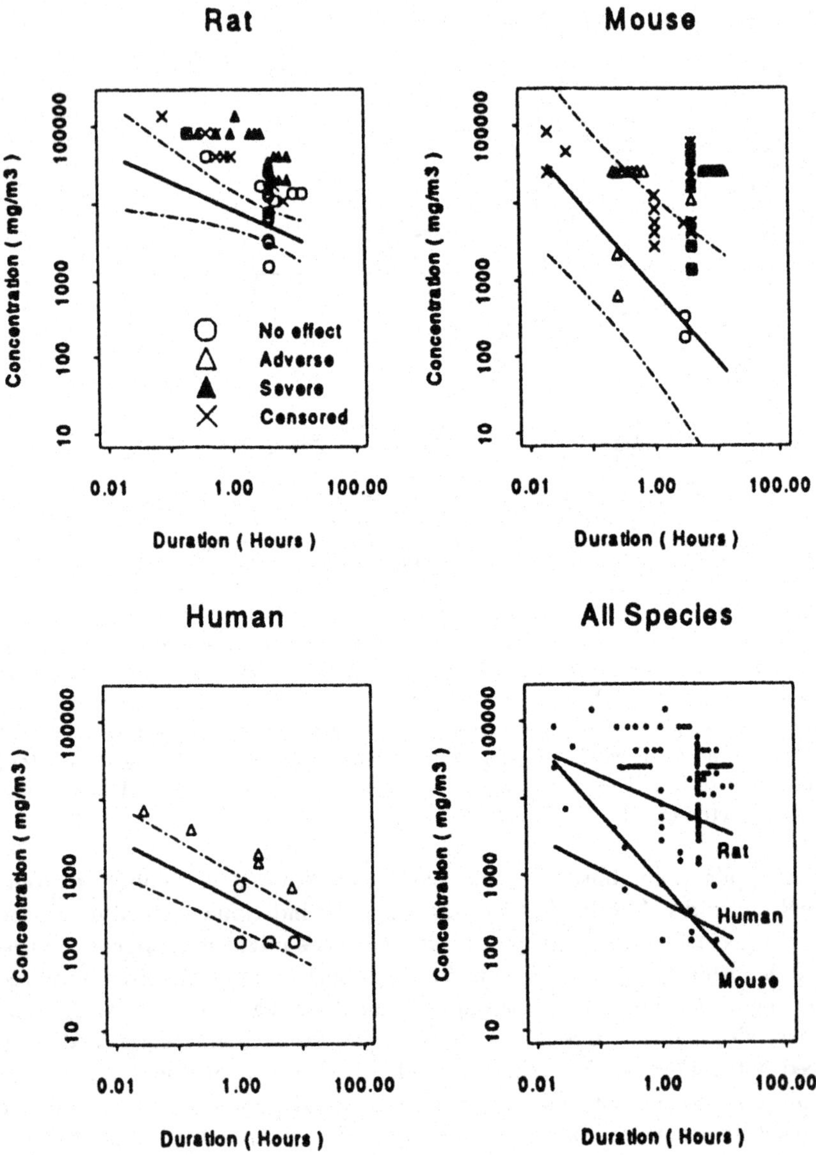

FIGURE 3. Tetrachloroethylene data showing the ordinal response versus concentration and duration for (a) rats only, (b)mice only, (c) humans only, and (d) pooled data. Lines in (a)-(c) are EC10's (solid) and their 95% confidence bounds (dotted). Lines in (d) are EC10's for humans, mice and rats.

7 REFERENCES

[1] Baker, F.B. (1992). *Item Response Theory.* Marcel Dekkar, New York.

[2] Hampel, F.R., Ronchetti, E.M., Rousseeuw, P.J., and Stahel, W.A. (1986). *Robust Statistics: The Approach Based on Influence Functions.* Wiley, New York.

[3] Hjort, N.L.(1994). The exact amount of t-ness that the normal model can tolerate , *Journal of the American Statistical Association*, 89, 665-675.

[4] Huber, P.J. (1967). The behavior of maximum likelihood estimates under nonstandard conditions. *Proceedings of the 5th Berkeley Symposium*, 1, 221-233.

[5] Johansen, S. (1984). *Functional Relations, Random Coefficients, and Nonlinear Regression with Application to Kinetic Data.* Lecture Notes in Statistics, 22, Springer-Verlag, New York.

[6] Kent, J.T. (1982). Robust properties of likelihood ratio tests. *Biometrika*, 69, 19-27.

[7] Li, B. and McCullagh, P. (1994). Potential functions and conservative estimating functions. *Annals of Statistics*, 22, 340-356.

[8] Li, B. (1996). A minimax approach to consistency and efficiency for estimating equations. To appear in *Annals of Statistics.*

[9] McCullagh, P. (1980) Regression models for ordinal data , *Journal of the Royal Statistical Society, Series B*, 42, 109-142.

[10] McCullagh, P. and Nelder,J.A. (1989). *Generalized Linear Models* (2nd edition), London: Chapman and Hall.

[11] McCulloch, C.E. (1994). Maximum likelihood variance components estimation for binary data. *Journal of the American Statistical Association*, 89, 330-335.

[12] Rotnitzky, A. and Jewell, N.P.(1990). Hypothesis testing of regression parameters in semiparametric generalized linear models for cluster correlated data, *Biometrika*, 77, 485-497.

[13] Simpson, D.G., Carroll, R.J. and Xie, M. (1994). Scaled link functions and generalized likelihood inferences for heterogeneous binary response data. Technical Report #24, National Institute of Statistical Sciences.

[14] Simpson, D.G., Carroll, R.J., Xie, M. and Guth, D.L. (1996a). Weighted logistic regression and robust analysis of diverse toxicology data. *Communications in Statistics - theorem and Method*, 25(11), 2615-2632..

[15] Simpson, D. G., Carroll, R.J., Zhou, H. and Guth, D.L. (1996b). Interval censoring and marginal analysis in ordinal regression. *Journal of Agricultural, Biological and Environmental Statistics*, 1, 354-376.

[16] Xie, M. (1996). *Regression Modeling: Latent Structure, Theories and Algorithms.* Ph.D. Dissertation, University of Illinois at Urbana-Champaign.

[17] Zeger, S.L., Liang, K.-Y. (1986). Longitudinal Data analysis for discrete and continuous outcomes, Biometrics, 42, 121-130.

[18] Zeger, S.L., Liang, K.-Y. and Albert, P.S. (1988). Models for longitudinal data: a generalized estimating equation approach. *Biometrics*, 44, 1049-1060.

Software Design for Longitudinal Data Analysis

Douglas M. Bates*
University of Wisconsin, Madison
United States

José C. Pinheiro
Bell Laboratories
United States

ABSTRACT Software for exploring and modelling longitudinal data can be made much easier to use by incorporating an object-oriented design. Current versions of S-Plus provide some object-oriented capability but experimental versions of S emphasize an even stronger commitment to object orientation. These new capabilities, combined with the development of Trellis graphics by Cleveland and Becker, caused us to reexamine the basic design of our mixed-effects modelling functions - lme and nlme. We chose to implement a groupedData class with associated constructors, modeling, and display methods. This provides powerful visualization capabilities almost automatically. In addition it dramatically simplifies the interface to the modelling code.
We describe and illustrate the use of this approach and its impact on the modeling software with special emphasis on nonlinear mixed-effects models.

Key words and phrases: Mixed-effects models, trellis graphics, nonlinear regression, self-starting models.

1 Introduction

Just as the statistical methodology for longitudinal data can be considerably more complicated than for cross-sectional data, the design of software for the exploration and modelling of longitudinal data is more complicated. As always with statistical software tradeoffs must be made between convenience for the user, sophistication of the analysis methods, and efficiency of the code. With longitudinal data additional issues of delineating experimental units or longitudinal characteristics must be considered. When so-

*This research was supported by the National Science Foundation through grant DMS-930901.

phisticated graphical techniques for data exploration or model diagnostics are also included the design problems become even greater.

For several years we have been developing classes and methods in the S language (Chambers and Hastie, 1992) for modelling longitudinal data with linear or nonlinear mixed-effects models. The nlme library is now included with versions 3.4 and higher of S-Plus from the Data Analysis Products Division of MathSoft, Inc. Its use is described in MathSoft (1996, chapter 2) and Venables and Ripley (1996, sections 6 and 9).

Although the library is useful in its current state, we have decided to change the design of the code and put a much greater emphasis on object-orientation. The primary reasons for the change are to enhance the use of trellis graphics displays; to provide a cleaner, more intuitive user interface; and to facilitate migration of the code to version 4 of the S language (Chambers, 1993). The redesign has affected several areas of the code. Here we will focus on two important areas: the use of groupedData objects to encapsulate the data and key aspects of the structure of the data, and the use of self-starting nonlinear regression models to derive starting estimates for nonlinear regression model parameters.

In §2 we describe trellis graphics displays for longitudinal data and the motivation they provide for groupedData objects. These objects are described in §3. The selfStart class of nonlinear regression models are described in §4 and our conclusions are given in §5.

2 Trellis graphics and longitudinal data

One of the most exciting recent developments in graphical display of data is the trellis approach (Cleveland, 1994; Becker, Cleveland and Shyu, 1996) to multi-panel displays of conditional plots. The approach is particularly valuable for longitudinal data that typically represent measurements of a response over time for different experimental units. We want to examine the behaviour within these units but also allow ourselves to compare behaviour between units. Trellis displays are well suited to this.

The approach is best shown with an example. Kung (1986) presents data, shown in Figure 1, on the growth of Loblolly pine trees. A common method of representing such data would be a plot with fourteen curves on it, one for each tree. Usually this type of plot becomes cluttered and difficult to read. In a trellis display like Figure 1 the measurements from different trees are plotted in separate panels but with consistent axes to facilitate comparison between panels. The panels are labelled with a strip giving an identifier, the seed source in this case, for the tree.

There are other, more subtle aspects to this plot. The order in which the panels are plotted is determined by a characteristic of the data. In this case, the panels have been ordered according to the maximum height measured

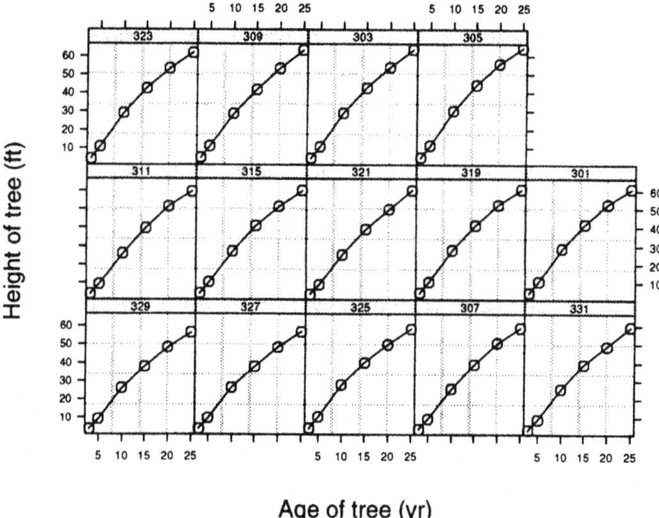

FIGURE 1. Height of Loblolly pine trees over time. Each panel is labelled with the number of the seed source for the tree.

for the tree. The shortest tree is from seed source 329 and is shown in the lower left panel. The tallest tree is from seed source 305 and is shown in the rightmost panel of the top row.

We can see a definite curvature to each of these growth curves leading us to consider models such as the asymptotic regression model

$$\theta_1 + (\theta_2 - \theta_1)\exp(-\theta_3 t), \quad \theta_3 > 0 \tag{1}$$

with parameters representing the asymptotic height, θ_1, the height at time zero, θ_2, and the rate constant, θ_3, for the growth of an individual tree. The other notable feature of these data is the consistency of the growth pattern between trees.

Often in the analysis of longitudinal data we are looking for differences in the response patterns rather than consistency - especially if the differences are related to treatments applied to or characteristics of the experimental units. Trellis displays facilitate such comparisons. For example, Figure 2 shows the Soybean data described in Davidian and Giltinan (1995, § 1.1.3, p. 7). The data were collected on eight different plots each for two genotypes of soybean in each of three growing seasons. The presentation in Figure 2 allows evaluation of the aggregate behaviour for the genotype-year combinations. The layout with genotypes determining the row and year determining the column facilitates comparisons of the response from year to year. We can see, for example, that final weights for the 'P' genotype decreased more-or-less uniformly across years while the 'F' genotype had the lowest leaf weights in 1989. We may wish to consider an interaction

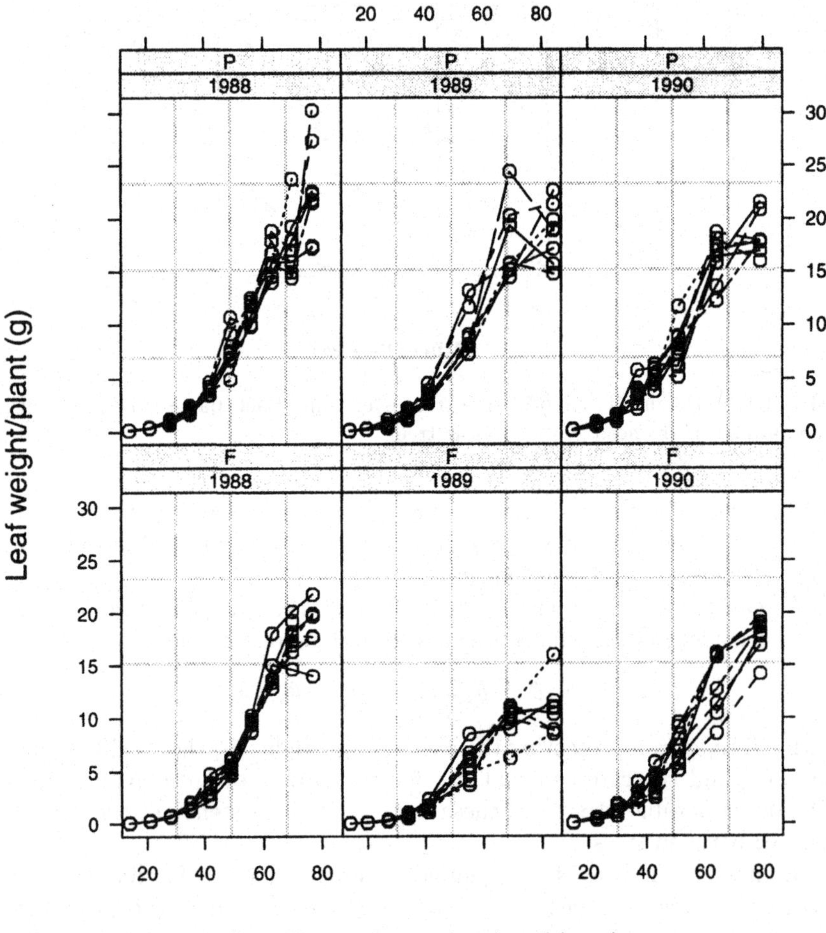

FIGURE 2. Average leaf weight per plant versus time since planting for plots of soybeans. The plots are from three different years and represent two different genotypes of soybeans.

between year and genotype when modelling these data.

The opposite arrangement, rows determined by genotype and columns determined by year (not shown), would enhance comparisons between genotypes within year. Even the arrangement in Figure 2 allows us to see that the 'P' genotype is producing heavier leaves than the 'F' genotype.

The aspect ratio of the individual panels in Figure 2 has been chosen by the "banking" method described in Cleveland (1994) to enhance comparisons of slopes.

Each of the panels in Figure 2 displays the data from eight soybean plots as overlaid lines. This makes the panels a bit too cluttered for evaluation of the behaviour of individual plots. That is best done by having one panel per plot and arranging the panels according to year and genotype (Figure 3). Here is not as easy as in Figure 2 to compare years or genotypes but this figure does reveal other characteristic of these data. We see there is considerably greater variability in the responses at the higher levels than at the lower levels. We may wish to consider modelling the variance of the response as an increasing function of the level of the response.

The ordering of the panels in Figure 3 preserves the levels of the Year and Variety (i.e. genotype) factors and applies increasing order of the maximum response within each combination of these factors.

In our terminology Year and Variety are *outer* factors for this experiment in that they do not vary within groups. (The "group" here is one plot for one year.) In contrast an *inner* factor can change within a group such as in cross-over trials where each subject is exposed to more than one treatment. For example, in the experiment described by Ludbrook (1994) and analysed in Venables and Ripley (1996) each of five rabbits was treated with the drug MDL 72222 and with a placebo. After treatment the rabbit was exposed to ascending doses of phenylbiguanide and its blood pressure was measured. The resulting data are shown in Figure 4. This figure strongly indicates that effect of MDL 72222 is to shift the curve to the right. Although different rabbits have different levels of the response the pattern of a shift to the right when treated with MDL 72222 is consistent across rabbits.

3 GroupedData objects

The data sets considered in the previous section have several characteristics in common. They consist of measurements of a continuous response at several levels of a continuous covariate, usually time or dose. Further, these measurements are grouped according to a factor. Additional covariates may be present. Some of these vary within a group (*inner* covariates) and some do not (*outer* covariates).

The choice of a data structure for this type of data will affect the ease and flexibility with which we can display the data and fit models to the

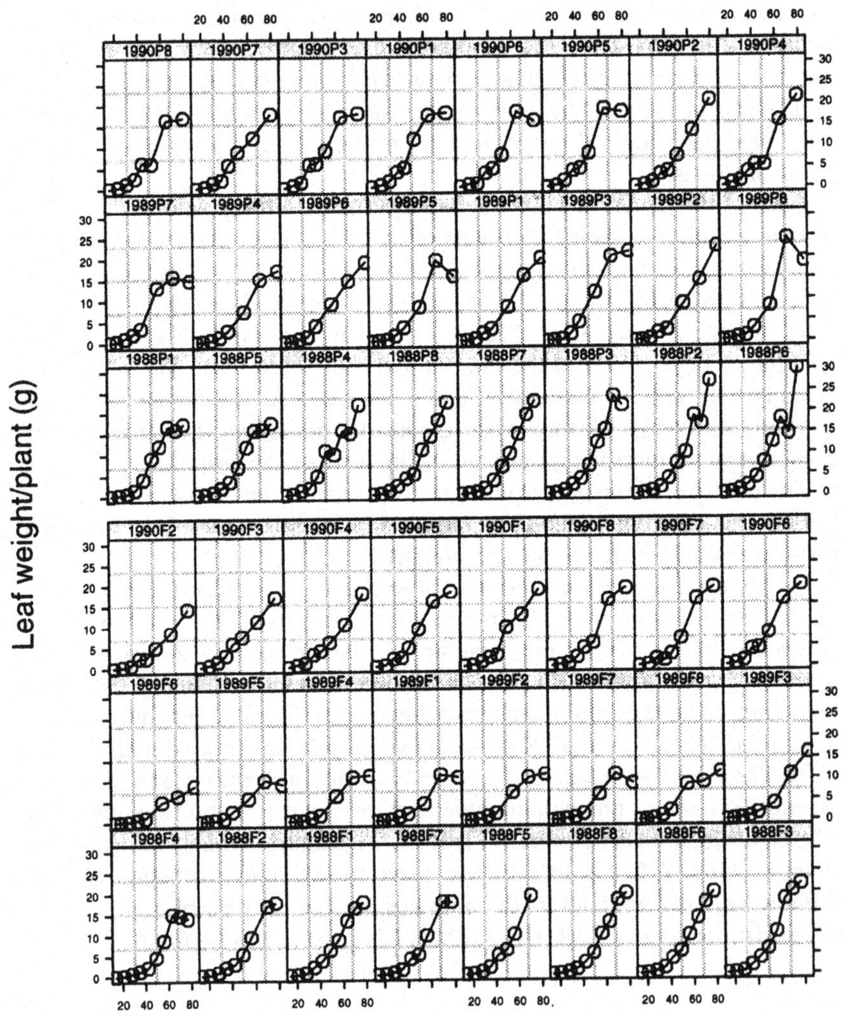

FIGURE 3. Average leaf weight per plant versus time since planting for plots of soybeans. The plots are from three different years and represent two different genotypes of soybeans. The label on a panel combines the year, the genotype, and the sequence number within that year and genotype for the experimental plot.

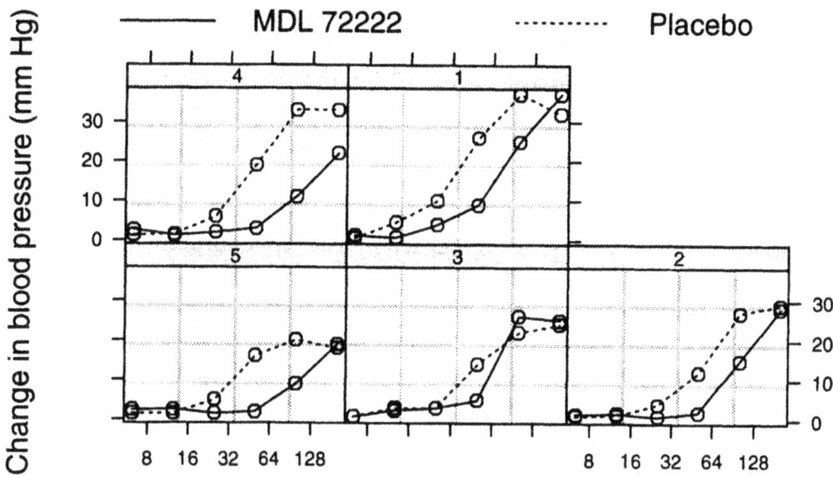

FIGURE 4. Change in blood pressure of five rabbits after ascending doses of phenylbiguanide (PBG). Each rabbit had one set of measurements made after treatment with the 5-HT_3 antagonist MDL 72222 and one set made after comparable treatment with a placebo. The dose of PBG is on a logarithmic scale.

data. We have chosen throughout to represent the data as a data.frame (i.e. a rectangular array) in S where the columns represent variables and the rows represent cases.

At a minimum the data frame must contain the response, the primary covariate, such as time, and the grouping factor, such as Seed or Plot. Additional factors or continuous covariates can be present. For example

```
> names(Loblolly)  # Loblolly pine trees
[1] "height" "age"     "Seed"
> names(Soybean)   # Soybean growth
[1] "weight"   "time"    "Plot"      "Variety" "Year"
> names(PBG)        # Blood pressure vs phenylbiganide dose
[1] "deltaBP"    "dose"      "Treatment" "Rabbit"
```

The natural trellis plots for such data depict the response versus the primary covariate in panels determined by the grouping factor. They are described by a formula of the form

```
response ~ primary | grouping
```

We found that we were writing that type of formula so frequently that it made sense to incorporate it in the data. For example

```
> formula(Loblolly)
height ~ age | Seed
```

The most convenient way of packaging the formula with the data is to create a new class of object (Chambers and Hastie, 1992, Appendix A) which we have called groupedData.

The function used to create objects of a given class is called the constructor for that class. The constructor for groupedData takes a formula and data frame as described above. By default, the grouping factor is converted to an ordered factor with the order determined by a summary function applied to the response split according to the groups. (The default summary function is the maximum.) Additionally, labels can be given for the response and the primary covariate and their units can be specified as arbitrary strings. The reason for separating the labels and the units is to allow propagation of the units to derived quantities such as the residuals from a fitted model.

For example, reading the Loblolly pine tree data from a file and converting it to a groupedData object would be accomplished by

```
> Loblolly <- groupedData(height ~ age | Seed,
+     data = read.table("Loblolly", header = T),
+     labels = list(x = "Age of tree", y = "Height of tree"),
+     units = list(x = "(yr)", y = "(ft)"))
> plot(Loblolly)       # produces Figure 1
```

This call to the constructor establishes the roles of the variables, converts the grouping factor to an ordered factor so panels in plots are ordered in a natural way and stores descriptive labels for data plots and plots of derived quantities.

When outer factors are present, as for the Soybean data, they are given as a formula such as

```
outer = ~ Variety * Year
```

Inner factors are described in a similar way. When establishing the order of the levels of the grouping factor, and hence the order of panels in a plot, re-ordering is only permitted within combinations of levels for the outer factors. That is why the panels from soybean plots of the same genotype in the same year are grouped together in Figure 3.

The plot method for the groupedData class allows an optional argument outer which can be given a logical value or a formula. A logical value of TRUE indicates that the outer formula stored with the data should be used in the plot. The right hand side of the explicit or inferred formula replaces the grouping factor in the trellis formula. The grouping factor is then used to determine which points to join with lines. For example

```
> plot(Soybean, outer = ~ Year * Variety) # produces Figure 2
> plot(Soybean, outer = T) # (not shown) Variety = rows, Year=columns
>    # Figure 3 is produced by plot with a couple of trellis arguments
>    # to enhance the layout of the panels
> plot(Soybean, layout = c(8, 6), between = list(y = c(0, 0, 0.5)))
```

An inner factor, such as Treatment in the PBG data, is used to determine which points within a panel are joined by lines.

We can see that incorporating a display formula with the data in the groupedData object makes it much easier to produce informative trellis displays. This general approach of using a data frame augmented by a formula that defines the roles of the variables is one of the powerful ideas in trellis. An alternative structure often used for longitudinal data is to represent the data as a matrix where the elements of the matrix are the responses, the rows (or columns) are determined by the groups, and the columns (or rows) are determined by the times. This can work when the data are balanced; that is, when all groups are measured at the same set of times. Any imbalance in the data makes this representation very awkward. The representation we have chosen does not encounter any problems with imbalance or with missing data. For example, the Soybean data are not balanced. The times at which the plots were sampled were different at different years. In fact, in 1988 there were different numbers of samples drawn from the plots for different genotypes.

```
> table(Soybean$Variety, Soybean$Year)
  1988 1989 1990
F   76   64   64
P   80   64   64
```

Another advantage of using a formula to describe the roles of the variables is that this information can be used within the model-fitting software to make the specification of the model easier. Even something as difficult as getting preliminary fits for a nonlinear mixed-effects model can be made as simple as

```
> Loblolly.lis <- nlsList(asymptotic, Loblolly)
```

when a self-starting nonlinear regression model has been defined as described in the next section.

4 Self-starting nonlinear regression models

The approach we have taken in nlme is to provide a variety of tools for building linear or nonlinear mixed-effects models. The final model can relate fixed effects to covariates and can include sophisticated models for random effects, for serial correlation in the within-group noise term, or for the variance of the within-group noise term. We expect, however, that the user will build the model interactively from preliminary fits rather than trying to fit an "omnibus" model from the beginning.

Of course, this iterative model building must start from somewhere. We usually consider that "somewhere" to be individual fits of a nonlinear model like the asymptotic regression model (1) for each level of the grouping factor or, when an inner factor is present, for each level of the inner factor within the grouping factor. Because we can determine the response, the primary covariate, and the grouping factor from the formula stored with the data, it is straightforward to set up the necessary nonlinear regression calls. There is, however, one part of the nonlinear regression that is always problematic; determining starting values for the parameter estimates.

When the groups of data are similar, such as the Loblolly pine trees, a single set of starting values can be applied to all the groups. However, when there are marked differences between the groups, such as the PBG data, a single set of starting values may not be adequate. An experienced analyst will often be able to find suitable starting values for each group quickly by applying a few common "tricks". For example, starting values for the asymptotic regression model can be obtained by:

1. Form an initial estimate $\theta_1^{(0)}$ of the asymptote θ_1 from a plot of the data.
2. Regress $\log(|y - \theta_1^{(0)}|)$ on t. The estimated slope is $-\theta_3^{(0)}$.
3. Use an algorithm for partially linear models (Bates and Chambers, 1992, §10.2.5) to refine estimates of θ_1, θ_2, and θ_3.

An enhancement of the final step is to use the logarithm of θ_3 instead of θ_3 in the iterative algorithm so as to enforce the positivity constraint in (1).

These steps form an algorithm for calculating starting values in a robust way. In this case, the "starting values" would also be the final parameter estimates but that isn't required.

Based upon examples like this we created a class of nonlinear regression model functions that have an auxillary function to calculate the starting values. We call these *self-starting* nonlinear regression models. The corresponding class is selfStart. Venables and Ripley (1996) describe the method we used in nlme 2.1 for communicating data to the function that calculates the starting values. This method is awkward and will be changed in nlme 3.0 but this need only concern those who will be writing the selfStart functions. The general user simply needs to know the name of the appropriate (univariate) model. It can then be used as shown in the previous section

```
> Loblolly.lis <- nlsList(asymptotic, Loblolly)
> coef(Loblolly.lis)
          Asym        R0       lrc
329  94.12877 -8.250685 -3.217588
327  94.94058 -7.757495 -3.229325
325  89.88361 -8.759223 -3.086195
307 110.69818 -8.169516 -3.390332
331 111.00287 -8.462608 -3.397574
311 109.98436 -8.558667 -3.362500
315 101.05602 -8.443651 -3.232822
321 127.13533 -7.679281 -3.575346
319 101.08717 -8.502381 -3.214016
301  95.66688 -9.078241 -3.116381
323  95.55627 -9.665035 -3.092266
309 113.51390 -7.595622 -3.352815
303 105.71443 -8.906502 -3.222905
```

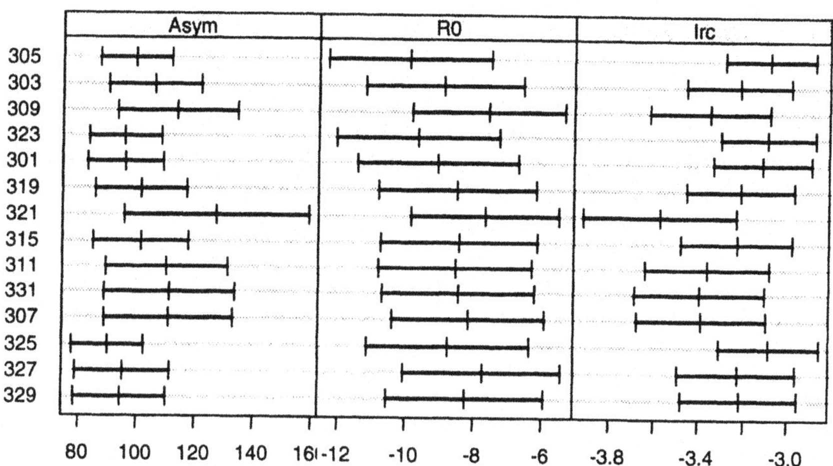

FIGURE 5. 95% confidence intervals on the parameter estimates of the asymptotic regression model fit separately to each tree in the Loblolly pine tree data

```
305  99.17167 -9.916694 -3.084837
> plot(intervals(Loblolly.lis))
```

The last call produces a trellis plot of confidence intervals on the parameter estimates as shown in Figure 5

The separate nonlinear regression fits can also be used to describe a nonlinear mixed-effects model and implicitly to provide starting estimates for the parameters

```
> Loblolly.nlme <- nlme(Loblolly.lis)
```

We can then fit alternate models say by reducing the number of random effects. Since R0, the response at time zero (written as θ_2 in (1)) seems to have the least variability between seed sources relative to the precision of the individual estimates, we eliminate it first and compare to the full model

```
> Loblolly.nlme1 <- nlme(Loblolly.lis, random= list(Asym~ ., lrc~ .))
> anova(Loblolly.nlme, Loblolly.nlme1)
               Model df    AIC    BIC  loglik
 Loblolly.nlme     1 10 242.22 266.53 -111.11
Loblolly.nlme1     2  7 238.25 255.26 -112.12

                  Test Lik.Ratio P-value
 Loblolly.nlme
Loblolly.nlme1 1 vs. 2    2.0235 0.56754
```

The model building would continue from here.

5 Conclusions

Space limitations preclude showing a thorough examination of even one of these examples. Our purpose here is simply to show the power of trellis graphics for the exploration of longitudinal data and the ease with which such displays can be created. One of the keys to the success of the statistical modelling tools described in Chambers and Hastie (1992) is the concept of the data frame and the formula language. We have extended those here to a groupedData object that incorporates both the data as a frame and a formula giving important characteristics of the data; and the selfStart class of nonlinear regression model functions.

6 References

Bates, D. M. and Chambers, J. M. (1992). *Nonlinear Models*, in Chambers and Hastie (1992), chapter 10, pp. 421–454.

Becker, R. A., Cleveland, W. S. and Shyu, M.-J. (1996). The visual design and control of trellis graphics displays, *J. of Computational and Graphical Statistics* **5**(2): 123–156.

Chambers, J. M. (1993). Classes and methods in S. II: Future directions, *Computatonal Statistics* **8**(3): 185–196.

Chambers, J. M. and Hastie, T. J. (eds) (1992). *Statistical Models in S*, Wadsworth, Belmont, CA.

Cleveland, W. S. (1994). *Visualizing Data*, Hobart Press.

Davidian, M. and Giltinan, D. M. (1995). *Nonlinear Models for Repeated Measurement Data*, 1st edn, Chapman & Hall, London.

Kung, F. H. (1986). Fitting logistic growth curve with predetermined carrying capacity, *ASA Proceedings of the Statistical Computing Section* pp. 340–343.

Ludbrook, J. (1994). Repeated measurements and multiple comparisons in cardiovascular research, *Cardiovascular Research* **28**: 303–311.

MathSoft (1996). *Version 3.4 for Unix Supplement*, Data Analysis Products, MathSoft Inc., Seattle, WA.

Venables, W. N. and Ripley, B. D. (1996). Complements to Modern Applied Statistics with S-Plus. Supplement to the current edition of MASS covering new features.
URL: *http://www.stats.ox.ac.uk/pub/MASS/Compl.ps.gz*

Asymptotic Properties of Nonlinear Mixed-Effects Models

Eugene Demidenko*
Dartmouth Medical School
United States

ABSTRACT The asymptotic properties of four estimators for nonlinear mixed-effects models are investigated: maximum likelihood estimator (MLE), an estimator based on the first-order approximation to the expectation function (Vonesh and Carter (1992)), the two-stage, and the Lindstrom-Bates (1990) estimators. Two asymptotic situations are considered: (i) when $N \to \infty$ and n_i is finite and (ii) $N \to \infty$ and $\min n_i \to \infty$, where N is the number of individuals and n_i is the number of observations on the ith individual. For a simple one-parameter balanced exponential model only the MLE is consistent when the numbers of observations per individual, $\{n_i\}$ are finite. The estimator based on the first-order approximation is always inconsistent, i.e., has a systematic bias. The asymptotic bias for the other three estimators is evaluated when $N \to \infty$ and $n_i = const$. When $N \to \infty$ and $\min n_i \to \infty$, the MLE, Lindstrom-Bates and two-stage estimators are equivalent. The bias for the two-stage estimator based on a second order approximation is evaluated for the general nonlinear mixed-effects model, and a bias-corrected version of this estimator is proposed.

Key words and phrases: Random effects, maximum likelihood, repeated measures, longitudinal data.

1 Introduction

The nonlinear mixed-effects (NLME) model has received substantial attention in the literature. Recently published monographs by Davidian and Giltinan (1995), and Vonesh and Chinchilli (1997) provide a comprehensive source of up-to-date knowledge on the subject. It is well known that maximum likelihood estimation for nonlinear mixed-effects models leads

*Author address: Eugene Demidenko, Dartmouth Medical School, HB 7927, Hanover, NH 03755-3861

maximum likelihood estimation for nonlinear mixed-effects models leads to a cumbersome integration problem, because random parameters appear inside the nonlinear expectation function. To avoid this problem several other estimators have been proposed. For instance, Pocock et al. (1981) suggested an intuitively appealing two-stage estimator. Another approach based on the first-order approximation to extract the random effects from the expectation regression function, was originally proposed by Sheiner and Beal (1980) and developed by Vonesh and Carter (1992). Another method using a first-order approximation was suggested by Lindstrom and Bates (1990); however they approximate nonlinear functions around means and random effects. Wolfinger (1993) showed that the Lindstrom-Bates estimator can be obtained using Laplace's approximation to the likelihood function. Recently, Pinheiro and Bates (1995) compared several estimators for nonlinear mixed-effects models via statistical simulations.

Little is known about the statistical properties of estimators for nonlinear mixed-effects models even in large samples, and this question is open (Davidian and Giltinan, 1995). Unlike for linear models, it is impossible to state any general statistical properties for nonlinear models in finite samples even when variance parameters are known. Therefore, the only way to make any general statements on the NLME model estimation is to consider asymptotic properties of estimators, i.e., when the number of observations goes to infinity. In mixed-effects models the following two asymptotic situations can be distinguished (Vonesh and Carter 1992):

1. The number of individuals, N tends to infinity and the number of observations per individual, n_i remains finite, i.e., uniformly bounded.

2. The number of individuals N tends to infinity along with $\min n_i$.

For linear models the first condition is sufficient to guarantee the consistency, asymptotic normality and efficiency (Vonesh and Carter 1987, Stukel and Demidenko 1997). For instance, for the NLME model, Vonesh and Carter (1992) proved that their four-step estimator is normally distributed and asymptotically efficient when N tends to infinity along with $\min_i n_i$ if the original model is replaced by its first-order approximation, 'pseudo-model'. However, it is important to realize that the approximate pseudo NLME model does not coincide with the original one, and their results cannot be extended to the originally formulated nonlinear model with random effects within the nonlinear regression function.

The goal of the present paper is to establish asymptotic properties of the above estimators in the two asymptotic situations.

The structure of the paper is as follows. In section 2 the general nonlinear mixed-effects model and the four estimators are introduced: the maximum likelihood estimator (MLE), the Vonesh-Carter, the two-stage and the Lindstrom-Bates estimators. In section 3, a simple one-parameter exponential nonlinear mixed-effects model is investigated. An attractive feature of this model is that the first-order approximation and the two-stage estimators admit a closed form solution. The exact asymptotic bias when $N \to \infty$ and $n_i = n = const$ is calculated for all estimators. In section 4 we formulate the result on the equivalence of the ML, two-stage and Lindstrom-Bates estimators in the first asymptotic situation. A bias-corrected version of the two-stage estimator is proposed in section 5.

Proofs of mathematical results are not presented here due to the paper length limitation. Interested readers can send requests to the author to obtain an extended version of the paper along with full proofs.

2 The NLME model and four estimators

In this section the general nonlinear mixed-effects model is formulated and four estimators are introduced: the maximum likelihood, Vonesh-Carter, the two-stage and Lindstrom-Bates estimators.

2.1 The NLME model

The general nonlinear mixed-effects model is written in two stages (Sheiner and Beal 1985, Lindstrom and Bates 1990, Davidian and Giltiman 1995, Vonesh and Chinchilli 1997). The first stage consists of N within-individual nonlinear regression models with random parameters $\mathbf{a}_i$,

$$\mathbf{y}_i = \mathbf{f}_i(\mathbf{a}_i) + \boldsymbol{\epsilon}_i, \quad i = 1, ..., N \tag{1}$$

where $\mathbf{y}_i$ is the $n_i \times 1$ vector dependent variable, $\mathbf{f}_i$ is a known nonlinear $n_i \times 1$ vector function, $\mathbf{f}_i(\mathbf{a}_i) = (f(\mathbf{a}_i; \mathbf{x}_{i1}), f(\mathbf{a}_i; \mathbf{x}_{i2}), ..., f(\mathbf{a}_i; \mathbf{x}_{i,n_i}))'$, $\mathbf{x}_{ij}$ is a vector of covariates; $\mathbf{a}_i$ is an unobservable $m \times 1$ vector of random parameters with unknown $m \times m$ covariance matrix $\sigma^2\boldsymbol{\Omega}$; $\boldsymbol{\epsilon}_i$ is the $n_i \times 1$ error vector with $E(\boldsymbol{\epsilon}_i) = \mathbf{0}$ and $cov(\boldsymbol{\epsilon}_i) = \sigma^2\mathbf{I}$; N is the number of individuals, and n_i is the number of observations on the ith individual. The second stage is a linear model

$$\mathbf{a}_i = \mathbf{Z}_i\boldsymbol{\beta} + \mathbf{b}_i \tag{2}$$

where $\mathbf{Z}_i$ is the $m \times k$ design matrix, and $\boldsymbol{\beta}$ is the $k \times 1$ vector of population parameters of interest; and $\mathbf{b}_i$ are the random effects, $E(\mathbf{b}_i) = \mathbf{0}$, $cov(\mathbf{b}_i) = \sigma^2\boldsymbol{\Omega}$. The random effect $\mathbf{b}_i$ and common error term $\boldsymbol{\epsilon}_i$ are assumed independent to each other and between individuals. Also, it is assumed that matrix $\sum \mathbf{Z}_i'\mathbf{Z}_i$ has full rank, $\sigma^2 > 0$ and matrix $\boldsymbol{\Omega}$ is positive definite. The vector $\boldsymbol{\theta} = (\sigma^2, vech'(\boldsymbol{\Omega}))'$ has dimension $1 + m(m+1)/2$ and is called the variance parameter. Also, the random terms $\boldsymbol{\epsilon}_i$ and $\mathbf{b}_i$ are assumed to have normal distributions. Four estimators of $\boldsymbol{\beta}$ are considered in the following subsections. They all coincide for the linear mixed-effects model with known variance parameters. However, they all differ and have different statistical properties when applied to the general NLME model.

2.2 Maximum likelihood estimator

Unlike in the linear mixed-effects model, there is no closed form solution to the MLE of NLME model even when variance parameters σ^2 and $\mathbf{\Omega}$ are known. Moreover, the presence of an integral in marginal distribution of $\mathbf{y}_i$ makes the maximum likelihood procedure cumbersome especially for multidimensional random effects.

As follows from maximum likelihood theory, the MLE is consistent and asymptotically normally distributed and efficient when $N \to \infty$ and the $\{n_i\}$ are bounded. Thus, the asymptotic variance based on the information matrix is the milestone for efficiency comparisons to other estimators. Recently such comparisons have performed for the logistic regression model with random intercept term (Neuhaus and Lesperance 1996). Unfortunately, the calculation of the information matrix for NLME models again leads to an intractable integration problem. However, for NLME model it is possible to come up with a lower bound for the variance of the $\widehat{\boldsymbol{\beta}}$. Thus, our current aim is to find such a bound for the asymptotic variance of the MLE. We use the following result which provides an upper bound for the information matrix, and can be considered as a generalization of a result by Schervish (1995).

Lemma 1 *Let* $\mathbf{Y}$ *and* $\mathbf{A}$ *be two random vector variables.* $\mathbf{A}$ *is unobservable with marginal density* $f_2(\mathbf{a};\boldsymbol{\tau})$ *where* $\boldsymbol{\tau}$ *is parameter vector.* $\mathbf{Y}$ *is observable and the conditional density of* $\mathbf{Y} \mid \mathbf{A}$ *is* $f_1(\mathbf{y},\mathbf{a})$. *Therefore the marginal density of* $\mathbf{Y}$ *is* $f(\mathbf{y};\boldsymbol{\tau}) = \int f_1(\mathbf{y},\mathbf{a}) f_2(\mathbf{a};\boldsymbol{\tau}) d\mathbf{a}$. *Then,*

$$\mathcal{J}_{\mathbf{Y}} \leq \mathcal{J}_{\mathbf{A}}, \tag{3}$$

so that the matrix $\mathcal{J}_{\mathbf{A}} - \mathcal{J}_{\mathbf{Y}}$ *is positive semidefinite, where* $\mathcal{J}_{\mathbf{Y}}$ *is the Fisher information about* $\boldsymbol{\tau}$ *based on* $\mathbf{Y}$ *and* $\mathcal{J}_{\mathbf{A}}$ *is the information based on* $\mathbf{A}$.

Applying this Lemma to the model (1,2) we come to the following absolute lower bound for the asymptotic covariance of the MLE:

$$cov(\widehat{\boldsymbol{\beta}}_{ML}) \geq \sigma^2 \left(\sum_{i=1}^{N} \mathbf{Z}_i' \mathbf{\Omega}^{-1} \mathbf{Z}_i \right)^{-1}. \tag{4}$$

We notice that this inequality remains true whether or not the variance parameters are known. Also, it is interesting to note that the lower bound (4) depends neither on the first stage model nor on the number of observations per individual, n_i. As it is follows from section 5 this inequality turns into an equality when $N \to \infty$ and $\min n_i \to \infty$.

Formula (4) has an interesting interpretation: it corresponds to a hypothetical situation when the $\mathbf{a}_i$ are observable. Indeed, in that case the best estimator, as follows from (2), would be a generalized least squares estimator with the covariance matrix coinciding with the right-hand side of (4).

2.3 Vonesh-Carter estimator

To circumvent the integration problem, Vonesh and Carter (1992) suggested to replace the NLME model by another nonlinear model with linear random effects derived as the first-order approximation to (1) around $E(\mathbf{a}_i) = \mathbf{Z}_i\boldsymbol{\beta}$. Thus, instead of (1,2) a pseudo NLME model is considered:

$$\mathbf{y}_i = \mathbf{f}_i(\mathbf{Z}_i\boldsymbol{\beta}) + \mathbf{R}_i(\mathbf{Z}_i\boldsymbol{\beta})\mathbf{b}_i + \epsilon_i, \tag{5}$$

where $\mathbf{R}_i = \partial\mathbf{f}_i/\partial\mathbf{a}_i$ and $\mathbf{b}_i \sim N(\mathbf{0},\sigma^2\boldsymbol{\Omega})$. A four-step estimation procedure based on (5) was suggested by Vonesh and Carter when the variance parameters are unknown. They proved that for model (5), the four-step VC-estimator is asymptotically equivalent to the MLE when both $N \to \infty$ and $\min n_i \to \infty$. However, it is important to remember that the model (5) does not coincide with the original model (1,2) and, consequently, the properties of this estimator do not necessarily remain true for the original model. Moreover, as is shown in section 3, the VC-estimator is not consistent for model (1) in either of the two asymptotic situations.

2.4 Two-stage estimator

Several authors (e.g., Pocock et al. 1981) proposed a two-stage (TS) procedure to estimate parameters $\boldsymbol{\beta}$: (i) estimate $\mathbf{a}_i$ individually from (1) by nonlinear least squares, (ii) substitute them into the second stage model and apply generalized least squares. Thus, at the first step, N individual nonlinear regression problems are solved to obtain $\widehat{\boldsymbol{\alpha}}_i^{LS}$. The conditional approximate covariance matrix for $\widehat{\boldsymbol{\alpha}}_i^{LS}$, based on the standard theory of nonlinear regression, is $\mathbf{V}_i = \widehat{\sigma}^2(\mathbf{R}_i'\mathbf{R}_i)^{-1}$, where $\mathbf{R}_i$ is the $n_i \times m$ derivative matrix of $\mathbf{f}_i$ at $\widehat{\boldsymbol{\alpha}}_i^{LS}$ and $\widehat{\sigma}^2$ is the pooled variance estimate. Next, generalized least squares (GLS) is applied to model (2) to obtain the two-stage (TS) estimator $\widehat{\boldsymbol{\beta}}_{TS}$. If the estimation of (1) fails for some i due to nonconvergence it is not included in the second-stage model. The number of successful individual regressions must be large enough to make GLS applicable. An estimate of $\boldsymbol{\Omega}$ can be obtained as $\sum(\mathbf{d}_i\mathbf{d}_i' - \mathbf{V}_i)/N$ where $\mathbf{d}_i$ is the OLS-residual vector for (2). Another approach is to apply maximum likelihood procedure to (2), known as global TS (Davidian and Giltinan 1995). Stukel and Demidenko (1997) have shown that the TS-estimator for linear mixed-effects model is consistent, asymptotically normally distributed and efficient when $N \to \infty$ and $\{n_i\}$ are fixed, even in a more general setting.

2.5 Lindstrom-Bates estimator

Lindstrom and Bates (1990) suggested approximating the nonlinear function $\mathbf{f}_i$ not around $E(\mathbf{a}_i) = \mathbf{Z}_i\boldsymbol{\beta}$, as Vonesh and Carter did, but around

$E(\mathbf{a}_i) + \widehat{\mathbf{b}}_i$ where $\widehat{\mathbf{b}}_i$ is an 'estimate' of $\mathbf{b}_i$. The suggested procedure consists of two steps:

1. Penalized nonlinear least squares: $\sum(\| \mathbf{y}_i - \mathbf{f}_i(\mathbf{Z}_i\boldsymbol{\beta}+\boldsymbol{\tau}_i) \|^2 + \boldsymbol{\tau}_i'\boldsymbol{\Omega}^{-1}\boldsymbol{\tau}_i)$ is minimized with respect to $\boldsymbol{\tau}_1, ..., \boldsymbol{\tau}_N$ and $\boldsymbol{\beta}$, given $\boldsymbol{\Omega}$.

2. Linear mixed-effects. Given 'estimates' of the random effects $\widehat{\boldsymbol{\tau}}_i$ and $\widehat{\boldsymbol{\beta}}$, derived in the previous step, apply the linear mixed-effects maximum likelihood estimation procedure based on the approximate linear mixed-effects model

$$\mathbf{w}_i \sim N(\mathbf{R}_i\mathbf{Z}_i\boldsymbol{\beta}, \sigma^2(\mathbf{I} + \mathbf{R}_i\boldsymbol{\Omega}\mathbf{R}_i'))$$

with pseudo-observations $\mathbf{w}_i = \mathbf{y}_i - \mathbf{f}_i(\mathbf{Z}_i\widehat{\boldsymbol{\beta}} + \widehat{\mathbf{b}}_i) + \mathbf{R}_i\widehat{\mathbf{b}}_i + \mathbf{R}_i\mathbf{Z}_i\widehat{\boldsymbol{\beta}}$ where $\mathbf{R}_i$ is the derivative of $\mathbf{f}_i$ at $\mathbf{a}_i = \mathbf{Z}_i\widehat{\boldsymbol{\beta}} + \widehat{\mathbf{b}}_i$.

The algorithm alternates between these two steps until convergence. Wolfinger (1993) pointed out that the two steps agree at convergence. He also showed that this procedure can be derived by applying Laplace's approximation to the log-likelihood function.

3 The one-parameter exponential model

In this section a simple example of a nonlinear mixed-effects model is considered, a one-parameter exponential model with random parameter. The simplicity of this model allows us to find a closed form solution and calculate the bias directly or find a good approximation for all four estimators considered in the previous section. On the other hand, this model reflects all the features of more complicated nonlinear mixed-effects models such as bias or possible nonexistence of estimates experienced in practice (Demidenko 1995). Based on this model, we show that all estimators, except the MLE, are inconsistent when the $\{n_i\}$ are finite and $N \to \infty$. In the next section this model will be applied to illustrate the asymptotic mean square error (MSE) calculation and efficiency comparison.

The following one-parameter balanced exponential model is considered

$$y_{ij} = e^{a_i} + \epsilon_{ij}, \quad \epsilon_{ij} \sim N(0, \sigma^2), \qquad i = 1, ..., N,\ j = 1, ..., n \tag{6}$$

with second stage model

$$a_i = \beta + b_i \quad \delta_i \sim N(0, \sigma^2\omega^2), \tag{7}$$

where the ϵ_{ij} and b_i are independent. It implies that $\overline{y}_i = \sum y_{ij}/n$, $i = 1, ..., N$ are independent and identically distributed (iid). To simplify, only β, the parameter of interest, is assumed to be unknown in this section, i.e., parameters $\sigma^2 > 0$ and $\omega^2 > 0$ are known. In this section we determine the asymptotic bias as a function of n, for three estimators when $N \to \infty$ and $n_i = n$ are fixed. It should be noted that for finite n some estimators may not exist with a nonzero probability even for large N. Therefore, we have to take this into account when comparing estimators.

3.1 The maximum likelihood estimator

The likelihood function for the model defined by (6,7) does not admit a closed form solution because it contains an integral. If I_β denotes the information then the asymptotic variance $var_{as}(\sqrt{N}\widehat{\beta}_{ML}) = I_\beta^{-1} \geq \sigma^2\omega^2$, as follows from (4). Recall that $\widehat{\beta}_{ML}$ is consistent and asymptotically normally distributed when $N \to \infty$ and n is fixed. As will be shown later, the asymptotic variance of the MLE attains its absolute lower bound $\sigma^2\omega^2$ when $n \to \infty$. We shall compare I_β^{-1}, which depends on n, to MSE of different estimates in section 5.

3.2 Vonesh-Carter estimator

Following the idea of Vonesh and Carter we substitute (6,7) by the pseudo NLME model,

$$y_{ij} = e^{\beta} + \eta_{ij} \tag{8}$$

where $\eta_{ij} = e^{\beta}b_i + \epsilon_{ij}$. Letting $\boldsymbol{\eta}_i = (\eta_{i1}, \eta_{i2}, ..., \eta_{in})'$ and $\mathbf{1} = (1, 1, ..., 1)'$, the covariance matrix of the random vector $\boldsymbol{\eta}_i$ can be written as $cov(\boldsymbol{\eta}_i) = \sigma^2\mathbf{V}(\beta)$ where $\mathbf{V}(\beta) = \mathbf{I}+e^{2\beta}\omega^2\mathbf{1}\mathbf{1}'$. Let an initial estimate of β be β_*. Then the VC-estimator is the solution to a nonlinear regression problem with the weight matrix $\mathbf{V}_* = \mathbf{V}(\beta_*)$. After some algebra one can show that the VC-estimator for (6,7) is

$$\widehat{\beta}_{VC} = \ln\left(\frac{1}{Nn}\sum_{i,j} y_{ij}\right). \tag{9}$$

It is interesting to notice that for this model the VC-estimator does not depend on the initial estimate β_*. Using the law of large numbers we calculate its asymptotic limit: $\lim \widehat{\beta}_{VC} = \ln e^{\beta+\sigma^2\omega^2/2} = \beta + .5\sigma^2\omega^2$ when $n \to \infty$. Therefore, the VC-estimator is inconsistent and has a systematic positive bias $.5\sigma^2\omega^2$ even if $n \to \infty$. The probability that the VC-estimator exists goes to 1 when $N \to \infty$ regardless of n because $\sum y_{ij}/Nn$ converges to $e^{\beta+\sigma^2\omega^2/2} > 0$ with probability 1.

3.3 Two-stage estimator

Individual least squares estimation of (6) leads to $\widehat{a}_i = \ln \overline{y}_i$. Given 'estimate' of a_i, one can apply generalized least squares and come to the TS-estimator, $\widehat{\beta}_{TS} = N^{-1}\sum \ln \overline{y}_i$. Again, by the law of large numbers $\lim \widehat{\beta}_{TS} = E \ln\left(e^{\beta+b_1} + \overline{\varepsilon}_1\right)$ with probability 1 when $N \to \infty$, where $\overline{\varepsilon}_1 \sim N\left(0, \sigma^2/n\right)$, $b_1 \sim N(0, \sigma^2\omega^2)$, and $\overline{\varepsilon}_1, b_1$ are independent. The TS-estimator has a systematic negative bias for fixed n. This follows from the inequality $\ln(a + x) < \ln(a) + x/a$ for $x \neq 0, a > 0, a + x > 0$. The bias for the TS-estimator can be calculated exactly as a two-dimensional integral or approximately based on the following general second-order approximation formula

$$Er(u,v) = r(0,0) + \frac{1}{2}var(u)\left.\frac{\partial^2 r}{\partial u^2}\right|_{u=0,v=0} + \frac{1}{2}var(v)\left.\frac{\partial^2 r}{\partial v^2}\right|_{u=0,v=0} \qquad (10)$$

where $r = r(u,v)$ is any function of independent random variables u and v, and $E(u) = E(v) = 0$. Applying this formula we obtain $\lim \widehat{\beta}_{TS} - \beta \simeq -(2n)^{-1}\sigma^2 e^{-2\beta}$. As we see, the bias is negative and has the order of $1/n$. Also, the bias does not depend on the variance of the random effects, ω^2. In particular, if σ^2 is close to zero one can expect almost unbiased estimation using the two-stage method.

There is one well-known drawback of the TS-estimator: it may not exist when n is fixed and particularly small. Indeed, formula for $\widehat{\beta}_{TS}$ fails when $\overline{y}_i \leq 0$ for the exponential model. Since $\overline{y}_i$ is a continuous variable with the range $(-\infty, \infty)$ and all $\overline{y}_i$ are iid, $\Pr(\overline{y}_i > 0) = \Pr(\overline{y}_1 > 0) = q_n < 1$ and $\Pr(\widehat{\beta}_{TS}$ does not exist$) = 1 - q_n^N \to 1$, because q_n is constant for fixed n. Therefore, the standard TS-estimator does not exist with probability 1 for fixed n! In fact, it may not exist even if $n \to \infty$. To obtain existence with probability 1 we must satisfy the following limit: $N \ln q_n \to 0$. Since $q_n \to 0$ when $n \to \infty$ it means that n must be large enough. However, there is a remedy: if $\overline{y}_i \leq 0$, we simply do not include the corresponding term in the sum of $\ln \overline{y}_i$. Then the corrected TS-estimator exists with probability one. The approximate formula for the bias (10) works for $\widetilde{\beta}_{TS}$ as well.

3.4 The Lindstrom-Bates estimator

Since σ^2 and ω^2 are known, we implement only the penalized nonlinear least squares step. The Lindstrom-Bates (LB)-estimator, $\widehat{\beta}_{LB}$ is the solution to $N+1$ estimating equations $e^{2(\beta+\tau_i)} - e^{\beta+\tau_i}\overline{y}_i + (n\omega^2)^{-1}\tau_i = 0$ and $N^{-1}\sum(e^{2(\beta+\tau_i)} - e^{\beta+\tau_i}\overline{y}_i) = 0$ where $i = 1, ..., N$. It is easy to see, the estimating equation for the LB-estimator can be reduced to $N^{-1}\sum \widehat{\tau}(\beta, \overline{y}_i) = 0$ where $\widehat{\tau}(\beta, \overline{y}_i)$ is the solution to the first N estimating equations as a function of β and $\overline{y}_i$. The LB-estimator is also inconsistent when $n = const$. To determine the exact systematic bias the following fact will be used. Let $u_1, u_2, ...u_N$ be iid random variables with a distribution dependent on a parameter β; the true parameter is denoted by β_0. Let the estimating equation for $\widehat{\beta}_N$ be $\frac{1}{N}\sum_{i=1}^N S(u_i;\beta) = 0$. Then $\lim_{N\to\infty} \widehat{\beta}_N = \beta_*$ where β_* is the solution to the equation $\overline{S}(\beta, \beta_0) := E_{\beta_0}S(u_1;\beta) = 0$ (e.g., Huber 1981). Based on this fact, in order to compute the bias of $\widehat{\beta}_{LB}$ we introduce function $\overline{S}(\beta, \beta_0) = E_{\beta_0}\widehat{\tau}(\beta, \overline{y})$ where $\widehat{\tau}(\beta, \overline{y})$ is the solution to the nonlinear equation $e^{2(\beta+\tau)} - e^{\beta+\tau}\overline{y} + (n\omega^2)^{-1}\tau = 0$. Then the asymptotic limit of $\widehat{\beta}_{LB}$, when $N \to \infty$ and n is fixed, is the root of the equation $\overline{S}(\beta, \beta_0) = 0$.

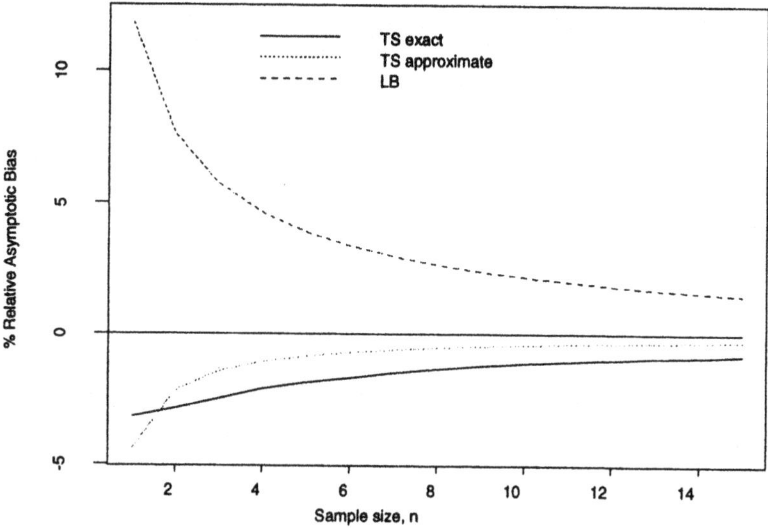

FIGURE 1. The asymptotic relative bias of the TS and LB - estimates when $N \to \infty$ and $n = 1, 2, ..., 15$ for one-parameter balanced exponential model (6,7) with $\beta = 0.7$, $\sigma = 0.5$, $\omega = 1.5$.

In Figure 1 we compare the relative asymptotic bias $(\widehat{\beta} - \beta_0)/\beta_0 \cdot 100\%$ for the TS and LB-estimators for $\sigma = 0.1$, $\omega = 2$, $\beta_0 = 0.5$ when $N \to \infty$ and n is fixed. The VC-estimator is not shown since its bias $.5\sigma^2\omega^2$ is constant with relative bias 40%. As we can see the approximation formula for bias in TS-estimator represents the true bias quite well. One can expect that this approximation will result a lower bias because it does not take into account the variance of random effects. The probability of nonexistence of the TS-estimator is low: for $n = 1$ we have $1 - q = 0.0182$, and for $n = 15$ the TS-estimator does not exist with probability 0.0003. It is interesting to observe that the bias of the LB-estimator for this model is positive and larger in absolute value than of the TS-estimator.

4 The equivalence of the ML, LB and TS estimators when $N \to \infty$ and $\min n_i \to \infty$

The VC-estimator is dropped from asymptotic consideration because it is not consistent even when $\min n_i \to \infty$, as was shown in the previous section.

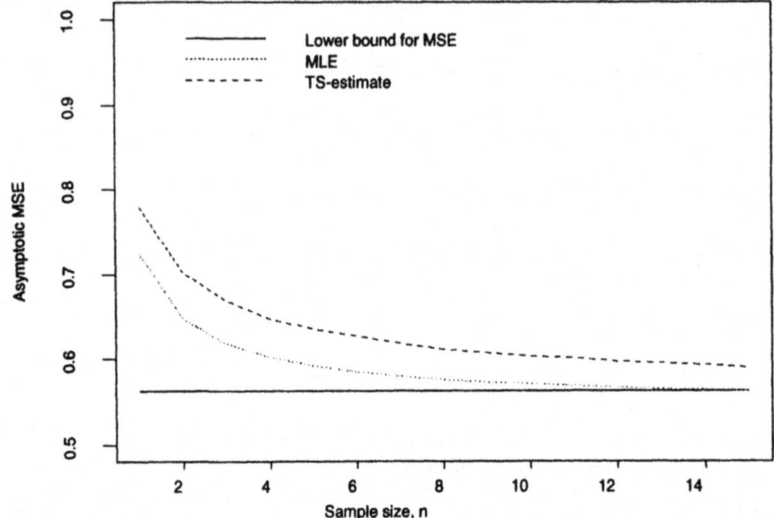

FIGURE 2. The asymptotic MSE of the MLE and the TS-estimate for the model (6,7). The lower bound for the MSE is $\sigma^2\omega^2$, the asymptotic variance of the MLE when $n \to \infty$.

Theorem 2 *Under mild asymptotic assumptions the maximum likelihood, the two-stage and Lindstrom-Bates estimators are asymptotically equivalent when $N \to \infty$ and $\min n_i \to \infty$.*

It follows from the proof that when $N \to \infty$ and $\min n_i \to \infty$ all three estimators: the ML, LB and TS have the same asymptotic distribution and are equivalent to the following simplified TS-estimator

$$\widehat{\beta} = (\sum \mathbf{Z}_i'\widehat{\mathbf{\Omega}}_1^{-1}\mathbf{Z}_i^{-1})^{-1} \sum \mathbf{Z}_i'\widehat{\mathbf{\Omega}}_1^{-1}\widehat{\alpha}_i^{LS}$$

where $\widehat{\mathbf{\Omega}}_1$ is any consistent estimate of $\mathbf{\Omega}$.

To assess the quality of the ML and TS-estimators for fixed n, we compute the asymptotic MSE for the univariate balanced exponential model (6,7). The LB-estimator is dropped from the analysis because it is asymptotically equivalent to the TS-estimator. The lower bound for the MSE, as follows from (4), is $\sigma^2\omega^2$. The exact asymptotic MSE for the TS-estimator is calculated as a two-dimensional integral. Recall, the MSE for the MLE is equal to I_β^{-1} where I_β is the information.

In Figure 2 the asymptotic MSE is shown for various values of n with parameters defined in the previous section. The MSE for the MLE is less than for the TS-estimator, as one could expect from maximum likelihood theory. When $n \to \infty$ the MSE approaches its absolute lower bound $\sigma^2\omega^2$.

5 Bias-corrected two-stage estimator

It is clear that the bias of the TS-estimator is driven by the fact that for fixed n_i the individual LS-estimates $\widehat{\boldsymbol{\alpha}}_i^{LS}$ are biased (this fact was also pointed out by Vonesh and Carter 1992). Moreover, if $n_i \to \infty$ when $N \to \infty$, then without loss of information we can substitute $\boldsymbol{\alpha}_i$ by $\widehat{\boldsymbol{\alpha}}_i^{LS}$ and assume the $\{\boldsymbol{\alpha}_i\}$ are observable. Therefore, to find a bias correction to the TS-estimator we have to evaluate $E(\widehat{\boldsymbol{\alpha}}_i^{LS}|\mathbf{a}_i) - \mathbf{a}_i$. Omitting i, the normal equation for the individual LS-estimator can be written as $\mathbf{R}'(\boldsymbol{\alpha})(\mathbf{f}(\mathbf{Z}\boldsymbol{\beta}+\mathbf{b})+\boldsymbol{\varepsilon}-\mathbf{f}(\boldsymbol{\alpha}))=\mathbf{0}$. The solution to this equation, $\widehat{\boldsymbol{\alpha}}^{LS}$ is an implicit function of $\boldsymbol{\varepsilon}$ and $\mathbf{b}$. We aim to evaluate the bias by the second order approximation of $\widehat{\boldsymbol{\alpha}}^{LS}$ as a function of $\mathbf{b}$ and $\boldsymbol{\varepsilon}$ in the neighborhood $\boldsymbol{\varepsilon}=\mathbf{0}$ and $\mathbf{b}=\mathbf{0}$. Therefore, our approximation will be better for smaller variances σ^2 and $\boldsymbol{\Omega}$. The approximation formula for the bias is similar to (10) that was used for the one-parameter exponential model. Since $\boldsymbol{\varepsilon}$ and $\mathbf{b}$ are independent, the cross-derivative vanishes and we only need to calculate the second derivatives of $\widehat{\boldsymbol{\alpha}}^{LS}$ with respect to $\boldsymbol{\varepsilon}$ and $\mathbf{b}$ at zero. Notice that for $\boldsymbol{\varepsilon}=\mathbf{0}$ and $\mathbf{b}=\mathbf{0}$ we have $\widehat{\boldsymbol{\alpha}}^{LS}=\mathbf{Z}\boldsymbol{\beta}$. Omitting tedious calculations, we obtain that the second derivative of $\widehat{\boldsymbol{\alpha}}^{LS}$ with respect to random effects at zero is zero, as in section 3. Further, in order to find the bias for $\widehat{\boldsymbol{\alpha}}^{LS}$ driven by the error term $\boldsymbol{\varepsilon}$ we adopt the theory on bias in nonlinear estimation based on the second-order approximation developed by Box (1971). The formula he derived for bias is $\widehat{\boldsymbol{\alpha}}^{LS} - E\widehat{\boldsymbol{\alpha}}^{LS} \simeq \mathbf{c}_i := -.5\sigma^2(\mathbf{R}'\mathbf{R})^{-1}\mathbf{R}\mathbf{d}$ where $\mathbf{d}$ is the $n \times 1$ vector with the jth element $tr((\mathbf{R}'\mathbf{R})^{-1}\mathbf{H}_j)$ and $\mathbf{H}_j$ is the Hessian matrix of f_j. Since the effect of random effects on the bias is zero, this formula for the bias represents the overall effect of random terms $\boldsymbol{\varepsilon}$ and $\mathbf{b}$, at least when the variances of $\boldsymbol{\varepsilon}$ and $\mathbf{b}$ are small. Finally, the bias-corrected version of the TS-estimator has the form

$$\widehat{\boldsymbol{\beta}}_{TS}^{c} = \left[\sum \mathbf{Z}_i'(\mathbf{V}_i+\widehat{\boldsymbol{\Omega}})^{-1}\mathbf{Z}_i\right]^{-1}\left[\sum \mathbf{Z}_i'(\mathbf{V}_i+\widehat{\boldsymbol{\Omega}})^{-1}\left(\widehat{\boldsymbol{\alpha}}_i^{LS}+\mathbf{c}_i\right)\right]$$

where $\mathbf{c}_i$ is the estimated bias and $\widehat{\boldsymbol{\Omega}}$ any consistent estimate. One can expect this correction to work well for small σ^2 and $\boldsymbol{\Omega}$.

6 Discussion

Methods of estimation for nonlinear mixed-effects models based on a straightforward linear approximation are not consistent regardless of the number of observations per individual. This may be explained in the following way. Let $E(y|a) = f(a)$ be a simple statistical model with a random variable $a \sim N(\beta, \tau^2)$ inside a nonlinear function f. We aim to extract an intrinsic nonlinear random variable a using a first-order approximation, substituting $f(a)$ by $f(\beta) + (a-\beta)f'(\beta)$. However, these two models have different means. For instance, assuming that f is convex, i.e., $f'' > 0$, we have $Ef(a) > E(f(\beta) + (a - \beta)f'(\beta)) = f(\beta)$ with a positive difference of order $.5\tau^2 f''(\beta)$. Since the approximate model has a systematic, unremovable bias, it is not surprising that all estimators based on this approximation are inconsistent. Similar arguments can be used to show that higher order approximations encounter the same problem (e.g., Solomon and Cox 1992). Therefore, applying any Taylor series expansion can reduce the bias but not eliminate it completely when $N \to \infty$ and the n_i are bounded.

Furthermore, neither the two-stage, nor the Lindstrom and Bates procedure are consistent when the number of observations per individual is finite. Therefore, is there a reason to use a cumbersome procedure like LB if it asymptotically equivalent to a much simpler two-stage procedure? The TS-procedure was criticized (e.g., Vonesh and Carter 1992) for the fact that it requires a large number of observations per individual. However, for the NLME model, the same requirement is needed for LB-procedure. Comparisons of the TS and VC estimators to the LB -estimator based on statistical simulations confirm the basic conclusions of the asymptotic analysis in the present paper (Stukel and Demidenko 1997). Further work should be done to investigate statistical properties of the bias-corrected TS-estimator suggested in this paper.

The maximum likelihood method does not require a large number of observations per individual. Therefore, in practice we would recommend using it, especially when n_i are relatively small. The number of random effects is a critical point for the integration problem. In particular, when there is only one random effect the integration problem is not complex. Pinheiro and Bates (1995) came to the conclusion that the Lindstrom-Bates estimator might be a good starting point for the maximum likelihood procedure. Keeping in mind the increased power of computers we cannot excuse ourselves from avoiding "computationally intensive" methods: in most cases, the cost of collecting data exceeds the costs of developing, programming, and running computationally intensive procedures.

The asymptotic issues are of particular importance when experiments can be designed. Given the ability to increase the number of individuals and the number of observations on individuals, which is more important N or n_i? Hopefully, this paper can shed some light on this question. However, one should remember that applying asymptotic properties to finite sample sizes could be misleading.

ACKNOWLEDGMENTS

I thank Therese Stukel, Edward Vonesh, and Jose Pinheiro for helpful comments. This work was supported by National Cancer Institute grants CA52192 and CA50597.

7 REFERENCES

[1] Box, M.J. (1971). Bias in nonlinear estimation. *Journal of the Royal Statistical Society, ser. B* **33,** 171-190.

[2] Davidian, M. and Gallant, A.R. (1992). Smooth nonparametric maximum likelihood estimation for population pharmacokinetics, with application to quinidine. *Journal of Pharmacokinetics and Biopharmaceutics* **20**, 529-556.

[3] Davidian, M. and Giltinan, D.M. (1995). *Nonlinear Models for Repeated Measurement Data.* London: Chapman and Hall.

[4] Demidenko, E. (1995). On the existence of the least squares estimate in nonlinear growth curve models of exponential type. *Communications in Statistics - Theory and Methods* **25,** 159-182.

[5] Huber, P.J. (1981). *Robust Statistics.* New York: Wiley.

[6] Lindstrom, M.J. and Bates, D.M. (1990). Nonlinear mixed-effects models for repeated measures. *Biometrics* **46**, 673-687.

[7] Neuhaus, J.M. and Lesperance, M.L. (1996). Estimation efficiency in a binary mixed-effects model setting. *Biometrika* **83,** 441-446.

[8] Pinheiro, J.C. and Bates, D.M. (1995). Approximations to the log-likelihood function in the nonlinear mixed-effects model. *Journal of Computational and Graphical Statistics* **4,** 12-35.

[9] Pocock, S.J., Cook, D.G. and Beresford, S.A.A. (1981). Regression of area mortality rates on explanatory variables: what weighting is appropriate? *Applied Statistics* **30,** 286-295.

[10] Rao, C.R.(1973). *Linear Statistical Inference and its Applications. Second Edition.* New York: Wiley.

[11] Schervish, M.J. (1995). *Theory of Statistics.* New York: Springer-Verlag.

[12] Sheiner, L.B. and Beal, S.L. (1980). Evaluation of methods for estimating population pharmacokinetic parameters. *Journal of Pharmacokinetics and Biopharmaceutics* **8**, 553-571.

[13] Sheiner, L.B. and Beal, S.L. (1985). Pharmacokinetic parameter estimates from several least squares procedures: superiority of extended least squares. *Journal of Pharmacokinetics and Biopharmaceutics* **13**, 185-201.

[14] Solomon, P.J. and Cox, D.R. (1992). Nonlinear component of variance models. *Biometrika* **79**, 1-11.

[15] Stiratelli, R., Laird, N.M. and Ware, J.H. (1984). Random-effects models for serial observations with binary response, *Biometrics* **40,** 961-971.

[16] Stukel, T. and Demidenko, E. (1997). Efficient estimation for general linear growth curve models. *Biometrics* **53,** 340-348.

[17] Stukel, T. and Demidenko, E. (1997). Comparison of methods for general nonlinear mixed-effects models. *Modelling Longitudinal and Spatially Correlated Data: Methods, Applications, and Future Directions.* Springer Lecture Notes in Statistics. New York: Springer-Verlag.

[18] Vonesh, E.F. and Carter R.L. (1987). Efficient inference for random-coefficient growth curve models with unbalanced data. *Biometrics* **43,** 617-628.

[19] Vonesh, E.F. and Carter R.L. (1992). Mixed-effects nonlinear regression for unbalanced repeated measures. *Biometrics* **48,** 1-17.

[20] Vonesh, E.F. (1992). Non-linear models for the analysis of longitudinal data. *Statistics in Medicine* **11,** 1929-1954.

[21] Vonesh, E.F. (1996). A note on the use of Laplace's approximation for nonlinear mixed-effects models. *Biometrika* **83,** 447-452.

[22] Vonesh, E.F. and Chinchilli, V.M. (1997). *Linear and Nonlinear Models for the Analysis of Repeated Measurements.* New York: Marcel Dekker.

[23] Wolfinger, R. (1993). Laplace's approximation for nonlinear mixed-effects models. *Biometrika* **80,** 791-795.

Structured Antedependence Models for Longitudinal Data

Dale L. Zimmerman*
University of Iowa
United States

Vicente Núñez-Antón†
Universidad del País Vasco
Spain

ABSTRACT Antedependence (AD) models can be a useful class of models for the covariance struçture of continuous longitudinal data. Like stationary autoregressive (AR) models, AD models allow for serial correlation within subjects but are more general in the sense that they do not stipulate that the variance is constant nor that correlations between measurements equidistant in time are equal. Thus, AD models are more parsimonious class of models for nonstationary data than the completely unstructured model of the classical multivariate approach.
For some nonstationary longitudinal data, a highly structured AD model may be more useful than an unstructured AD model. For example, if the variances increase over time, as is common in growth studies, or if measurements equidistant in time become more highly correlated as the study progresses (due, e.g., to a "learning" effect), then a model that incorporates these structural forms of nonstationarity is likely to be more useful. We introduce and illustrate the utility of some structured AD models. Properties of these models and estimation of model parameters by maximum likelihood are considered. An example is given in which a structured AD model is superior to both a stationary AR model and an unstructured AD model.

Keywords and phrases Antedependence models; longitudinal data; repeated measures; structured covariance matrices.

---

*Department of Statistics and Actuarial Science, University of Iowa, Iowa City, Iowa 52242 U.S.A.

†Núñez-Antón's work was supported by Dirección General de Enseñanza Superior del Ministerio Español de Educación y Cultura under research grant PB95-0346.

1 Introduction

Consider Table 1, which displays a matrix of sample variances, along the main diagonal, and sample correlations, off the main diagonal, corresponding to data from a longitudinal study reported by Kenward (1987). In this study the weights of cattle receiving a treatment for intestinal parasites were recorded on 11 occasions, the first 10 of which were evenly separated by two-week intervals; more details pertaining to these data are given later. The matrix exhibits several interesting features. First, the variances are not constant, but instead tend to increase over time. Second, the correlations are all positive and decrease more-or-less monotonically within columns. Third, and most interestingly, correlations within each subdiagonal (each diagonal below the main diagonal) are not constant, but instead tend to increase over time.

How might this covariance structure be modeled? A variety of models for the covariance structure of longitudinal data have been proposed [Jennrich and Schluchter (1986), Lee (1988), Diggle (1988), Jones and Boadi-Boateng (1991), Muñoz, Carey, Schouten, Segal, and Rosner (1992)], but most are inappropriate here. For example, the oft-used compound-symmetry model is unsuitable, owing to the widely disparate sample variances and the attenuation in sample correlations within columns. We might momentarily entertain stationary autoregressive (AR) models or other stationary time series models, but these models do not comport with the nonstationarity manifested in the sample variances and same-lag (within-subdiagonal) sample correlations. Moreover, although an inverse square-root transformation stabilizes the variances of these data, the nonstationary behavior of the correlations persists after transformation.

As an alternative to highly structured models, we might consider the general multivariate (MV) model, in which no structure is imposed upon the covariance matrix (beyond that needed for positive definiteness). However, in light of the discernible covariance structure here, this would be a substantially overparameterized model. Diggle (1988) notes that such overparametrization leads to inefficient estimation of mean response profiles and potentially poor assessment of those estimates' standard errors. Moreover, in situations where there are more measurement times than subjects (which is not the case here), the sample covariance matrix is not invertible and hence some useful inference procedures (e.g. Hotelling's T^2-test) are precluded.

A family of models flexible enough to accommodate the structural covariance features of these data, but considerably more parsimonious than the MV model, are antedependence (AD) models. AD models are generalizations of AR models that allow the variances and same-lag correlations to vary over time. As originally conceived (Gabriel, 1962) and subsequently used (Byrne and Arnold, 1983; Kenward, 1987), an sth-order AD model places no restrictions on how the variances and same-lag correlations (up

TABLE 1. Sample variances, along the main diagonal, and correlations, off the main diagonal, corresponding to the "Treatment A" cattle in the longitudinal study reported by Kenward (1987).

106										
.82	155									
.76	.91	165								
.66	.84	.93	185							
.64	.80	.88	.94	243						
.59	.74	.85	.91	.94	284					
.52	.63	.75	.83	.87	.93	306				
.53	.67	.77	.84	.89	.94	.93	341			
.52	.60	.71	.77	.84	.90	.93	.97	389		
.48	.58	.70	.73	.80	.87	.88	.94	.96	470	
.48	.55	.68	.71	.77	.83	.86	.92	.96	.98	445

to lag s) change over time and so in this sense it is unstructured (though it possesses more structure than the MV model). In cases such as the one exhibited here, however, it may be sensible to confer some additional structure upon the model, e.g., variances that increase as a linear function of time and/or lag-one correlations that increase monotonically.

The purpose of this paper is to introduce and illustrate the usefulness of some structured AD models for longitudinal data. The practical value of our models lies in their ability to describe actual covariance structures more accurately than previously proposed structured models while avoiding the overparametrization of general (unstructured) AD models. Section 2 briefly reviews general AD models and their properties. Section 3 introduces some structured families of AD models. Maximum likelihood estimation of model parameters in a general longitudinal setting and testing of hypotheses about those parameters are described in section 4. The application of these methods to a particular structured AD model is illustrated, using Kenward's data, in section 5. Section 6 states conclusions and describes some extensions.

2 General Antedependence Models

A set of random variables $Y_1, Y_2, \ldots, Y_T$ (indexed by time) whose joint distribution is multivariate normal is said to be sth-order antedependent if Y_t and Y_{t+k+1} are independent given $Y_{t+1}, Y_{t+2}, \ldots, Y_{t+k}$ for $t = 1, \ldots, T-k-1$ and for all $k \geq s$ (Gabriel, 1962). Equivalently, a T-variate normal random vector $\mathbf{Y} \equiv (Y_1, \ldots, Y_T)'$ with mean $\boldsymbol{\mu} \equiv (\mu_1, \ldots, \mu_T)'$ follows an

AD(s) model if

$$
\begin{aligned}
Y_1 &= \mu_1 + \epsilon_1, \\
Y_t &= \mu_t + \sum_{k=1}^{s^*} \phi_{kt}(Y_{t-k} - \mu_{t-k}) + \epsilon_t \qquad (t = 2, \ldots, T) \qquad (1)
\end{aligned}
$$

where $s^* = \min(s, t-1)$, the ϵ_t's are independent normal random variables with zero means and possibly time-dependent variances $\sigma_t^2 > 0$, and the ϕ_{kt}'s are such that the covariance matrix is positive definite.

AD models have several important properties. They are nested, i.e. if $\mathbf{Y}$ follows an AD(s) model then it follows an AD($s+1$) model as well. Furthermore, particular cases of the general AD model are equivalent to the MV and AR(s) models. More specifically, the unstructured AD($T-1$) model and the MV model are identical, and the AR(s) model is a special case of the AD(s) model in which: (a) $\phi_{kt} \equiv \phi_k$ for $k = 1, \ldots, s$ and $t = s+1, \ldots, T$; (b) the s roots of the AR(s) characteristic equation

$$
1 - \phi_1 x - \phi_2 x^2 - \cdots - \phi_s x^s = 0
$$

all exceed unity in modulus; (c) $\sigma_{s+1}^2 = \sigma_{s+2}^2 = \cdots = \sigma_T^2 > 0$; and (d) the "initial values" $\{\phi_{kt}\colon k = 1, \ldots, t-1;\ t = 2, \ldots, s\}$ and $\sigma_1^2, \sigma_2^2, \ldots, \sigma_s^2$ are chosen appropriately.

Like stationary AR models, AD models allow for serial correlation within subjects but they are more general in the sense that they do not stipulate that the variances are constant nor that correlations between measurements equidistant in time are equal. The general AD(s) model requires more parameters than the AR(s) model and (except when $s = T-1$) fewer parameters than the MV model. More precisely, we see from (1) that the covariance matrix of an unstructured AD(s) model is specified by $q \equiv (s+1)(2T-s)/2$ parameters, while the AR(s) and MV models are specified by, respectively, $s+1$ and $T(T+1)/2$ covariance parameters.

Let $\boldsymbol{\Sigma} = \{\sigma_{tu}\}$ denote the covariance matrix of an AD(s) vector $\mathbf{Y}$; observe that σ_{tt} and σ_t^2 represent different quantities. The elements of $\boldsymbol{\Sigma}$ are functions of the q autoregressive and variance parameters in (1) and can be evaluated recursively using analogues of the Yule-Walker equations. Consider, for example, the case $s = 2$. Subtracting μ_t from both sides of (1), then multiplying both sides by $(Y_{t-k} - \mu_{t-k})$ and finally taking expectations, we obtain

$$
\begin{aligned}
\sigma_{11} &= \sigma_1^2, \\
\sigma_{21} &= \phi_{12}\sigma_1^2, \\
\sigma_{22} &= \phi_{12}^2\sigma_1^2 + \sigma_2^2, \\
\sigma_{t,t-k} &= \phi_{1t}\sigma_{t-1,t-k} + \phi_{2t}\sigma_{t-2,t-k} + \sigma_t^2 I_{\{k=0\}} \\
&\quad (k = 0, 1, \ldots, t-1;\ t = 3, \ldots, T).
\end{aligned}
$$

Equation (1) is an *autoregressive* specification of the general AD(s) model, i.e. a specification in terms of the q autoregressive coefficients $\{\phi_{kt}: k = 1,\ldots,s^*; t = 2,\ldots,T\}$ and innovation variances $\{\sigma_t^2: t = 1,\ldots,T\}$. The AD($s$) model can be specified equivalently in two other ways: (1) in terms of the q elements along the main diagonal and first s subdiagonals of Σ, which we call a *covariance matrix* specification; and (2) in terms of the q elements along the main diagonal and first s subdiagonals (and superdiagonals) of Σ^{-1}, which we call a *concentration matrix* specification. In fact, all elements of the inverse of an AD(s) covariance matrix except those on the main diagonal and first s subdiagonals (and first s superdiagonals) are equal to zero (Gabriel, 1962). Thus, AD models are a particular subclass of graphical models.

Gabriel (1962), Byrne and Arnold (1983), and Kenward (1987) have proposed the application of unstructured AD models to the particular setting of longitudinal studies, and such a possibility is also noted in the recent books of Jones (1993) and Diggle, Liang, and Zeger (1994). Several relevant inference problems have been considered. Gabriel (1962) derives the likelihood ratio test for determining the order, s, of the model. For the case $s = 1$ and under the assumption of data balanced on time, Byrne and Arnold (1983) obtain explicit expressions for the maximum likelihood estimators of $\boldsymbol{\mu}$ and Σ and derive the likelihood ratio test for $\boldsymbol{\mu} = \mathbf{0}$. For the general case, Kenward (1987) expresses likelihood ratio test statistics for linear hypotheses about $\boldsymbol{\mu}$ in terms of residual sums of squares from appropriate analyses of covariance.

3 Structured Antedependence Models

We have noted that the unstructured AD model often is considerably more parsimonious than the general MV model and hence may be useful for longitudinal data exhibiting nonstationary serial correlation. For some nonstationary longitudinal data, however, an even more parsimonious structured AD model may be more useful. For example, if variances increase over time, as is common in growth studies, or if measurements equidistant in time become more highly correlated as the study progresses (due, e.g., to a "learning" effect), then a model that incorporates these structural forms of nonstationarity is likely to be more useful. Such a model will have greater applicability if it is also a function of continuous, rather than discrete, time as this will permit the accommodation of unequally spaced or missing observations. Accordingly, we subsequently denote the measurement times corresponding to an arbitrary subject as $0 \leq t_1 < t_2 < \cdots < t_T$.

Recall that there are three equivalent specifications of the unstructured AD(s) model. Structure may be imposed upon any of these specifications, according to whichever seems most appropriate, useful, or interpretable in a particular situation. Zimmerman, Núñez-Antón, and El-Barmi (1997) introduce some structured AD(1) models that are specified in terms of the variances and lag-one correlations of the responses (a covariance matrix specification). Their family of models is

$$\begin{aligned}\rho_{i,i-1} &\equiv \frac{\sigma_{i,i-1}}{\sqrt{\sigma_{ii}\sigma_{i-1,i-1}}} = \rho^{f(t_i;\lambda)-f(t_{i-1};\lambda)} \quad (i = 2,\dots,T),\\ \sigma_{ii} &= \sigma^2 g(t_i;\psi) \quad (i = 1,\dots,T)\end{aligned} \tag{2}$$

where $0 < \rho < 1$, $\sigma^2 > 0$, $f(\cdot)$ and $g(\cdot)$ are specified functions (the latter positive-valued), and $\boldsymbol{\lambda}$ and $\boldsymbol{\psi}$ are vectors of relatively few parameters. Special cases of (2) in which

$$f(t;\lambda) = \begin{cases} (t^\lambda - 1)/\lambda & \text{if } \lambda \neq 0 \\ \log t & \text{if } \lambda = 0 \end{cases} \tag{3}$$

and $g(t)$ was either a quadratic function or a step function were fitted successfully to data from two longitudinal studies. According to (2) and (3), if measurement times are equally spaced then the lag-one correlations are a monotone function of t: they increase if $\lambda < 1$ and decrease if $\lambda > 1$. When $\lambda = 1$ and $g(t) \equiv 1$, the continuous-time analogue of the AR(1) model is obtained.

A natural extension of (2) to a covariance-specified AD(s) model ($s \geq 2$) is given by

$$\begin{aligned}\rho_{i,i-k} \equiv \frac{\sigma_{i,i-k}}{\sqrt{\sigma_{ii}\sigma_{i-k,i-k}}} &= \rho_k^{f(t_i;\lambda_k)-f(t_{i-k};\lambda_k)}\\ &(i = k+1,\dots,T;\ k = 1,\dots,s),\\ \sigma_{ii} = \sigma^2 g(t_i;\psi) &\quad (i = 1,\dots,T)\end{aligned} \tag{4}$$

where $\rho_1,\dots,\rho_s$ are all positive and such that $\boldsymbol{\Sigma}$ is positive definite, and all other quantities are defined as in (2). A potentially useful special case of this model is that in which f is given by (3), which, when measurement times are equally spaced, prescribes that the lag k correlations are monotone increasing if $\lambda_k < 1$, monotone decreasing if $\lambda_k > 1$, or constant if $\lambda_k = 1$ ($k = 1,\dots,s$).

Structured autoregressive or concentration matrix specifications of an AD(s) model may also be considered. An example of the former that bears a superficial resemblance to (4) is given by

$$\begin{aligned}\phi_{k,i} &= \phi_k^{f(t_i;\lambda_k)-f(t_{i-k};\lambda_k)} \quad (i = s+1,\dots,T;\ k = 1,\dots,s),\\ \sigma_i^2 &= \sigma^2 g(t_i;\psi) \quad (i = s+1,\dots,T)\end{aligned} \tag{5}$$

where $\phi_1,\dots,\phi_s$ are positive and all other quantities are defined as in (2). (Note that this model does not impose any structure on the autoregressive coefficients and innovation variances corresponding to the first s measurement times. It has been our experience that keeping these "initial" quantities unstructured results in a better-fitting model than requiring them to adhere to the structural relationship that applies to these quantities at later times.) An example of the latter, which again bears a resemblance to (4), is given by

$$\gamma_{i,i-k} \equiv \frac{-\sigma^{i,i-k}}{\sqrt{\sigma^{ii}\sigma^{i-k,i-k}}} = \gamma_k^{f(t_i;\lambda_k)-f(t_{i-k};\lambda_k)}$$
$$(i = k+1,\ldots,T;\ k = 1,\ldots,s),$$
$$\pi_i \equiv 1/\sigma^{ii} = \sigma^2 g(t_i;\psi) \qquad (i = 1,\ldots,T) \tag{6}$$

where $\sigma^{i,i-k}$ is the $(i,i-k)$th element of Σ^{-1}, and $\gamma_1,\ldots,\gamma_s$ are positive and again all other quantities are defined as in (2). It is well known (e.g. Whittaker, 1990, Corollaries 5.8.1 and 5.8.2) that $\gamma_{i,i-k}$ is the partial correlation coefficient between Y_i and Y_{i-k} conditioned on the rest of the measurements and that π_i is the partial variance of Y_i conditioned on the rest of the measurements. Thus, (6) specifies a structured AD(s) model in terms of partial correlations and partial variances.

Particular cases of (5) and (6) in which f is given by (3) may be useful in practice. If measurement times are equally spaced, then such special cases prescribe monotonicity for the autoregressive coefficients or partial correlations, respectively. Note, however, that the monotonicity of either set of quantities, by itself, neither implies nor is implied by the monotonicity of the variances and/or the same-lag correlations. Indeed, the range of possible covariance structures engendered by (5) and (6) is not altogether transparent. Figures 1 and 2 depict covariance structures corresponding to some second-order cases of (5) and first-order cases of (6), respectively. For each case, the diagonal elements of the covariance matrix (the variances) and the first column (less its first element) and the first one or two subdiagonals of the correlation matrix (the lag-one or lag-two correlations) are displayed. For all cases of both models, $t = 1, 2, \ldots, 10$, $g(t) \equiv 1$, $\sigma^2 = 1$, and $f(t;\lambda_k) = t^{\lambda_k}$; note that, since $\lambda_k \neq 0$ for all cases, this choice of $f(t;\lambda_k)$ is merely a simpler parametrization of (3). Furthermore, in all cases of (5) shown here, $\phi_1 = \phi_2 = 0.5$, $\sigma_{11} = \sigma_{22} = 1.92$, and $\sigma_{12} = 1.28$. These choices, together with those for f, σ^2, and g, yield a stationary AR(2) model when $\lambda_1 = \lambda_2 = 1$. In all cases of (6), $\gamma_1 = 0.5$.

Figures 1 and 2 indicate that generally, the larger the value(s) of λ_1 (and λ_2) in these models, the smaller the variances and correlations. Moreover, for the cases of model (5) the variances, lag-one correlations, and lag-two correlations are monotone nondecreasing or nonincreasing over time, depending on whether $\lambda_1 > 1$ or $\lambda_1 < 1$. For the cases of model (6), the variances and lag-one correlations are not monotone: they are symmetric about the main diagonal's midpoint or first sub-diagonal's midpoint, respectively, when $\lambda_1 = 1$ but become increasingly skewed to the right as λ_1 increases.

4 Estimation and Testing

We now briefly consider inference for structured AD models in a general longitudinal data-model situation. Suppose that the jth of n subjects has been observed T_j times and let $\mathbf{Y}_j$ denote the $T_j \times 1$ vector of these responses. Suppose further that $\mathbf{Y}_j$ follows the linear model

$$\mathbf{Y}_j = \mathbf{X}_j\boldsymbol{\beta} + \mathbf{e}_j \qquad (j = 1, \ldots, n) \tag{7}$$

where $\mathbf{X}_j$ is a $T_j \times m$ design matrix of rank m for subject j; the $\mathbf{e}_j$'s are independent multivariate normal random vectors with mean $\mathbf{0}$ and a structured AD(s) covariance matrix $\boldsymbol{\Sigma}_j = \boldsymbol{\Sigma}_j(\boldsymbol{\theta})$; and $\boldsymbol{\beta}$ and $\boldsymbol{\theta}$ are vectors of unknown parameters with parameter space $\{(\boldsymbol{\beta}, \boldsymbol{\theta})\colon \boldsymbol{\beta} \in R^m, \boldsymbol{\theta} \in \Theta\}$ where Θ is the set of $\boldsymbol{\theta}$-values for which $\boldsymbol{\Sigma}_j$ is positive definite for all j. The specific parameters in $\boldsymbol{\theta}$ depend on: (a) the order s of the AD model; (b) which of the three specifications is used; and (c) the choices of $f(\cdot)$ and $g(\cdot)$. We assume that these quantities or choices have been determined or made on the basis of preliminary analyses or other considerations.

Applying well-known results, under model (7) a maximum likelihood (ML) estimate of $\boldsymbol{\theta}$ is a value $\hat{\boldsymbol{\theta}}$ that maximizes

$$\begin{aligned} L^*(\boldsymbol{\theta}; \mathbf{Y}_1, \ldots, \mathbf{Y}_n) &= -\frac{1}{2}\sum_{j=1}^{n} \log|\boldsymbol{\Sigma}_j(\boldsymbol{\theta})| - \frac{1}{2}\sum_{j=1}^{n} \mathbf{Y}_j'\boldsymbol{\Sigma}_j^{-1}(\boldsymbol{\theta})\mathbf{Y}_j \\ &\quad + \frac{1}{2}\hat{\boldsymbol{\beta}}'(\boldsymbol{\theta})\sum_{j=1}^{n} \mathbf{X}_j'\boldsymbol{\Sigma}_j^{-1}(\boldsymbol{\theta})\mathbf{Y}_j, \end{aligned}$$

where $\hat{\boldsymbol{\beta}}(\boldsymbol{\theta}) = [\sum_{j=1}^{n} \mathbf{X}_j'\boldsymbol{\Sigma}_j^{-1}(\boldsymbol{\theta})\mathbf{X}_j]^{-1}[\sum_{j=1}^{n} \mathbf{X}_j'\boldsymbol{\Sigma}_j^{-1}(\boldsymbol{\theta})\mathbf{Y}_j]$ and a ML estimate of $\boldsymbol{\beta}$ is $\hat{\boldsymbol{\beta}} = \hat{\boldsymbol{\beta}}(\hat{\boldsymbol{\theta}})$. An explicit expression for $\hat{\boldsymbol{\theta}}$ generally does not exist and hence it must be obtained by maximizing L^* numerically, using any of a variety of optimization algorithms.

Nested hypotheses about model parameters can be tested in standard ways. Let L_1 denote the maximized log-likelihood for model (7) and let L_0 denote the maximized log-likelihood for a submodel that imposes c independent constraints on the parameters. We can test the null hypothesis that the submodel holds by comparing $2(L_1 - L_0)$ to a chosen percentage point of the chi-squared distribution with c degrees of freedom. Alternatively, models can be compared using penalized likelihood criteria. Both approaches are illustrated in the next section.

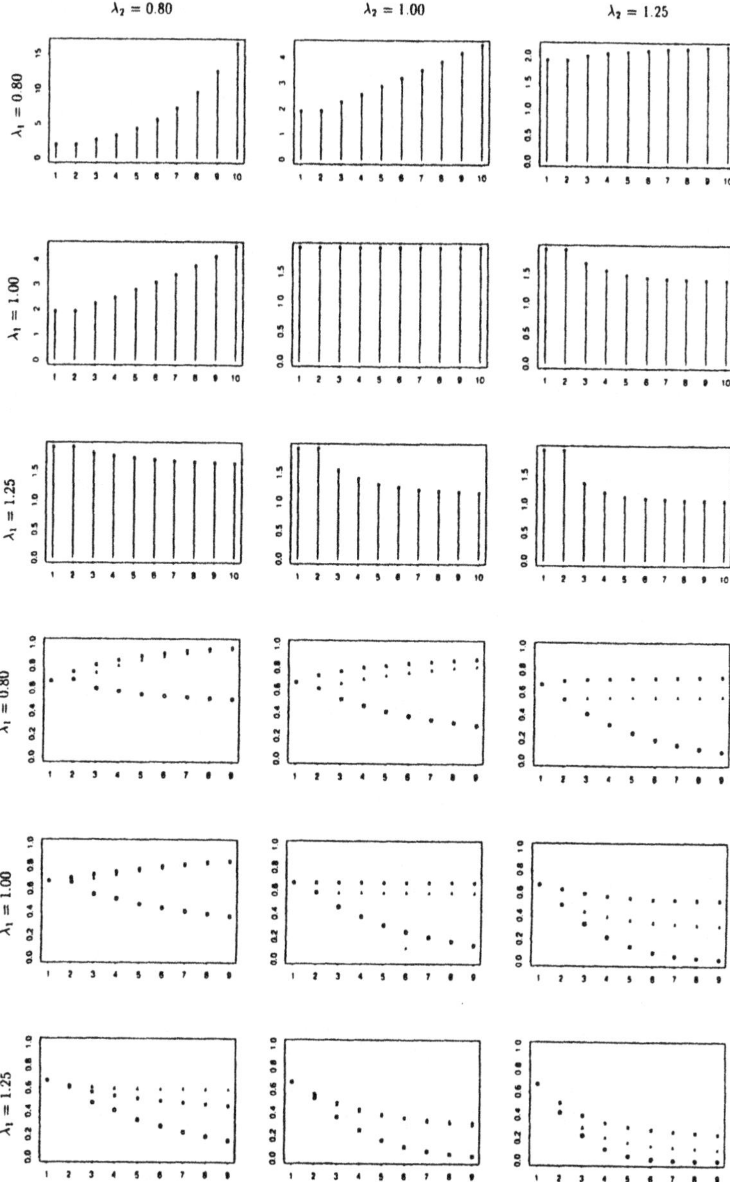

FIGURE 1. Variances (top three rows of plots) and selected correlations (remaining rows) plotted against time for nine cases of model (5). Lag-one and lag-two correlations are denoted by squares and triangles, respectively, and the first row of the correlation matrix (omitting its first element) by open circles.

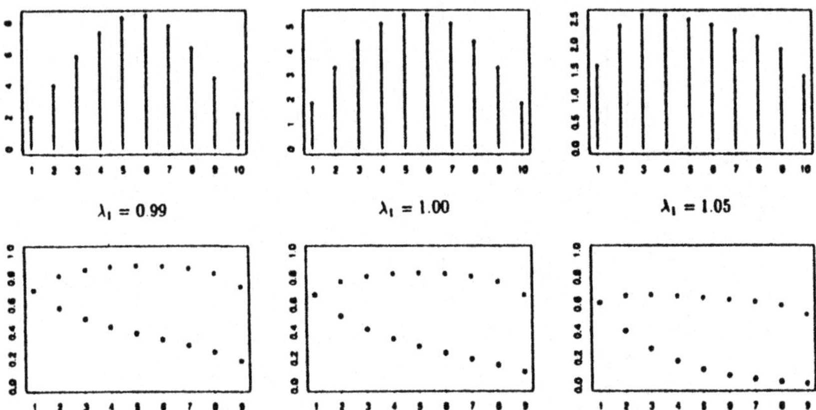

FIGURE 2. Variances (top) and selected correlations (bottom) plotted against time for three cases of model (6). Lag-one correlations are denoted by squares and the first row of the correlation matrix (omitting its first element) by open circles.

5 Example

Kenward (1987) describes an experiment in which cattle receiving two treatments, A and B say, for intestinal parasites were weighed 11 times over a 133-day period. Thirty animals received treatment A and thirty received treatment B. The first 10 measurements on each animal were made at two-week intervals and the final measurement was made after a one-week interval. Measurement times were common across animals and rescaled to $t = 0, 1, \ldots, 8, 9, 9.5$, and no observations were missing. We use these data to illustrate the utility of a structured AD model.

The hypothesis of equality of the two within treatment-group covariance matrices was tested by the classical likelihood ratio test and rejected ($P = .02$). Consequently, we considered each treatment group's covariance structure separately, and for brevity we report here the results for group A only. Gabriel's (1962) test for the order of antedependence indicated that an AD(2) model would suffice. Examination of the sample variances and same-lag correlations (Table 1) revealed clear structural features, as we noted in the introductory section. On the other hand, the inverse of the covariance matrix did not possess discernible structure on its main diagonal or first two subdiagonals. Therefore, we limited our consideration of structured AD models for these data to the covariance matrix and autoregressive specifications. Good-fitting models of both types were found, but for the sake of brevity we present results for the autoregressive specification only.

Based on the preliminary examination of the quantities in Table 1, model (7) with common mean vector $\boldsymbol{\mu}$ and an AD(2) covariance structure given

TABLE 2. Fitted variances, along the main diagonal, and correlations, off the main diagonal, corresponding to the "Treatment A" cattle in the longitudinal study reported by Kenward (1987).

100										
.82	148									
.76	.91	178								
.71	.85	.93	209							
.67	.80	.87	.94	240						
.63	.76	.82	.89	.94	272					
.60	.72	.78	.84	.90	.95	302				
.57	.69	.75	.81	.86	.91	.95	333			
.55	.66	.72	.77	.83	.87	.92	.96	364		
.53	.64	.69	.75	.79	.84	.88	.92	.96	395	
.52	.62	.67	.73	.77	.82	.86	.90	.93	.97	463

by a special case of (5) appeared to be potentially useful and hence was fitted to the data. For this case of (5) we took $f(t;\lambda_k) = t^{\lambda_k}$ $(k = 1,2)$ and $g(t) \equiv 1$. Thus, in this case the log-likelihood function, L^*, was a function of the 8×1 parameter vector $\boldsymbol{\theta} = (\sigma_{11}, \sigma_{22}, \sigma_{12}, \phi_1, \lambda_1, \phi_2, \lambda_2, \sigma^2)'$. Note that if an unstructured AD(2) model were adopted, then L^* would be a function of 30 parameters. These plus the 11 parameters in the mean vector are clearly too many to be estimated efficiently from the 30 available observations, hence the need for more parsimonious models.

Following Diggle (1988), L^* was maximized using the Nelder-Mead simplex algorithm (Nelder and Mead, 1965), with a step size of .01 for each variable. The procedure was repeated with several different starting values in order to allay concern that the procedure terminated at a local, but not a global, maximum. In every case the maximization procedure yielded the estimate

$$\hat{\boldsymbol{\theta}} = (100.0, 148.3, 100.1, 0.96, 0.83, 0.23, 1.07, 29.9)'.$$

The fitted variances and correlations corresponding to this estimate are displayed in Table 2. Note the rather good agreement with Table 1.

To compare the fit of our structured AD model to those of other models, we used Schwarz's (1978) *BIC*, a penalized likelihood criterion. In a general covariance model selection problem,

$$BIC_i = -\frac{2}{n} L_{\max,i} + p_i \frac{\log n}{n}$$

where i indexes the models under consideration, n is the sample size, $L_{\max,i}$ is the maximized log-likelihood for model i, and p_i is the number of un-

TABLE 3. Values of L_{max}, p, and BIC for each of several models.

Model	L_{max}	p	BIC
Unstructured AD(2)	-1035.98	30	72.47
Structured AD(2)	-1054.13	8	71.18
Stationary AR(2)	-1062.89	3	71.20
Structured AD(2) with $\lambda_1 = \lambda_2 = 1$	-1054.20	6	70.96

known variance and covariance parameters in model i. Smaller values of BIC are associated with better-fitting models. Table 3 shows the values of $L_{max,i}$, p_i, and BIC_i for an unstructured AD(2) model, our structured AD(2) model, and the stationary AR(2) model. As measured by BIC, the structured AD(2) model has a slight edge over the AR(2) model, and both are superior to the unstructured AD(2) model.

Finally, we conducted a likelihood ratio test of $H_0 : \lambda_1 = \lambda_2 = 1$ versus H_a : not H_0. Observe that H_0 corresponds to autoregressive coefficients that do not vary over time; nevertheless the corresponding covariance structure may be nonstationary since σ_{11}, σ_{22} and σ_{12} are arbitrary (provided that they yield a positive definite $\boldsymbol{\Sigma}$). The test indicated no evidence against H_0 ($P = 0.98$). The fitted variances and correlations corresponding to this reduced model did not differ appreciably from those given in Table 2, but this model's BIC was somewhat smaller than those of the original structured model and the stationary AR(2) model; see Table 3. Moreover, another likelihood ratio test soundly rejected ($P < .001$) the stationary AR(2) model in favor of the reduced AD(2) model. Hence, the reduced model would be our covariance model of choice for subsequent analyses, e.g. for testing hypotheses concerning $\boldsymbol{\mu}$.

6 Discussion

We have presented some families of structured AD models for the analysis of longitudinal data. These families allow for parsimonious modeling of nonstationary covariance structure, which in turn provides more efficient estimators of the mean structure than is possible with an unstructured AD model or the general multivariate model. As such, they are similar in spirit to the parsimonious models proposed by Jennrich and Schluchter (1986), Diggle (1988), Jones and Boadi-Boateng (1991), and Muñoz et al. (1992), but unlike these models ours do not presuppose stationarity of the covariance structure.

AD models represent one generalization of AR models for dealing with nonstationarity in the covariance structure. Another is the ARI(s, d), i.e. the autoregressive integrated model of order (s, d), or even more generally the ARIMA(s, d, u), i.e. the autoregressive integrated moving average model of order (s, d, u). These models may be worthy competitors to a structured AD(s) model in some instances. However, parsimonious ARI and ARIMA models appear to be less flexible because the variances in these models can only increase with t and the correlations likewise may not be capable of emulating the behavior exhibited by the sample correlations in some situations.

Nonconstant variances and nonconstant same-lag correlations can sometimes be modeled with a random effects (or random coefficients) model (Jones, 1990). However, there are problems with using such a model for this purpose (Lindsey, 1993), and it will generally be much more informative to model nonstationary serial correlation more directly with an AD or ARIMA model. This is not to say that a model with random coefficients *and* antedependent serial correlation should not be considered. Lindsey (1993, p. 118) argues that a model with both of these features would usually contain too many parameters to be useful, but his argument pertains to unstructured antedependence and would not apply to highly structured versions of antedependence.

In addition to accommodating variation in average response between subjects (through random effects) and serial correlation (through structured antedependence), we could allow for measurement-error variation (or, equivalently, imperfect correlation between repeated measurements arbitrarily close in time) by adding independent and identically distributed normal error terms to the model. Such a model, which would extend Diggle's (1988) general model so as to accommodate nonconstant variances and/or nonconstant same-lag correlations, was not necessary in our example, however.

Finally, we note that our structured approach can be extended without difficulty to variable-order AD models (Macchiavelli and Arnold, 1994), in which the order of antedependence depends on t.

7 References

[1] Byrne, P. J. and Arnold, S. F. (1983). Inference about multivariate means for a nonstationary autoregressive model. *Journal of the American Statistical Association* 78, 850-855.

[2] Diggle, P. J. (1988). An approach to the analysis of repeated measurements. *Biometrics* 44, 959-971.

[3] Diggle, P. J., Liang, K. Y. and Zeger, S. L. (1994). *Analysis of Longitudinal Data.* Oxford University Press, New York.

[4] Gabriel, K. R. (1962). Ante-dependence analysis of an ordered set of variables. *Annals of Mathematical Statistics* 33, 201-212.

[5] Jennrich, R. L. and Schluchter, M. D. (1986). Unbalanced repeated-measures models with structured covariance matrices. *Biometrics* 42, 805-820.

[6] Jones, R. H. (1990). Serial correlation or random subject effects? *Communications in Statistics - Simulation and Computation* 19, 1105-1123.

[7] Jones, R. H. (1993). *Longitudinal Data with Serial Correlation: A State-Space Approach.* Chapman and Hall, London.

[8] Jones, R. H. and Boadi-Boateng, F. (1991). Unequally spaced longitudinal data with AR(1) serial correlation. *Biometrics* 47, 161-175.

[9] Kenward, M. G. (1987). A method for comparing profiles of repeated measurements. *Applied Statistics* 36, 296-308.

[10] Lee, J. C. (1988). Prediction and estimation of growth curves with special covariance structures. *Journal of the American Statistical Association* 83, 432-440.

[11] Lindsey, J. K. (1993). *Models for Repeated Measurements.* Oxford University Press, Oxford.

[12] Macchiavelli, R. E. and Arnold, S. F. (1994). Variable order antedependence models. *Communications in Statistics – Theory and Methods* 23, 2683-2699.

[13] Muñoz, A., Carey, V., Schouten, J. P., Segal, M., and Rosner, B. (1992). A parametric family of correlation structures for the analysis of longitudinal data. *Biometrics* 48, 733-742.

[14] Nelder, J. A. and Mead, R. (1965). A simplex method for function minimization. *The Computer Journal* 7, 308-313.

[15] Schwarz, G. (1978). Estimating the dimension of a model. *Annals of Statistics* 16, 461-464.

[16] Whittaker, J. (1990). *Graphical Models in Applied Multivariate Statistics.* Wiley, Chichester.

[17] Zimmerman, D. L., Núñez-Antón, V., and El-Barmi, H. (1997). Computational aspects of likelihood-based estimation of first-order antedependence models. *Journal of Statistical Computation and Simulation*, forthcoming.

Effect of Confounding and Other Misspecification in Models for Longitudinal Data

Mari Palta, Chin-Yu Lin, and Wei-Hsiung Chao*
University of Wisconsin—Madison
United States

ABSTRACT Confounding, measurement error and selection bias are major concerns in observational studies. In a study of sleep disorders motivating our research, it was suspected that one or more of these problems were the cause of inconsistencies between regression coefficients obtained by different methods. We discuss such possibilities by examining the effect of omitted confounding variables on the generalized estimating equation (GEE) approach and on conditional logistic regression. Assuming that a covariate z_{ij} is unmeasured or otherwise omitted, we specify a structure with normally distributed $\mathbf{x}_i$ and $\mathbf{z}_i$ that allows their relationship to be different within and between individuals. This may arise, for example, from differences between persons entering the study at different ages or from time trends. The structure may also be interpreted as describing certain types of measurement error and selection bias.

We find that fitting a model which includes $\bar{x}_{i.}$ yields the correct mean structure, hence the same limit with any working correlation for GEE. However, fitting a model without $\bar{x}_{i.}$, using exchangeable working correlation in certain situations yields different results for different assumed correlations. When the working correlation approaches 1, the coefficient of x_{ij} approaches the one in the model with $\bar{x}_{i.}$. This latter coefficient, for the logit link, can be converted into the one for conditional logistic regression by a scale change.

Key words and phrases: misspecification, generalized linear models, GEE, conditional logistic regression, confounding, omitted covariates

---

*Mari Palta is Professor, Department of Preventive Medicine, University of Wisconsin, Madison, WI 53705. Chin-Yu Lin is a graduate student, Department of Statistics, Madison, WI 53706. Wei-Hsiung Chao is Assistant Research Fellow, Institute of Statistical Science, Academia Sinica, Taipei, Taiwan 11529. This work was supported by grants P01 HL42242 from the National heart Lung and Blood Institute and R01 CA53786 from the National Cancer Institute.

1 Introduction

Longitudinal data play an important role in many areas of health research, including epidemiology. Recently, estimating regression coefficients for such data by generalized estimating equations (GEE) has become popular. This is partly due to the assurance of estimation consistency as long as the mean structure is correctly specified, even if the variance structure is not (Liang and Zeger, 1986). Especially in observational studies, however, questions arise whether the mean structure is indeed correct and what the consequences might be otherwise. For example, interest may be focused on possible omission of confounding covariates from the model. Neuhaus and Jewell (1993) addressed this issue for non-longitudinal, generalized linear models.

We formulate a model for confounding in a longitudinal generalized linear model framework. Our model also describes certain forms of measurement error and selection bias, and leads to situations where consistency of GEE estimators may not hold, and to unexpected discrepancies between estimators. We derive approximate formulas for asymptotic expectation of regression coefficients obtained by different working correlation matrices in GEE. These are compared to those from conditional logistic regression.

In a study of sleep disorders (Young et al.,1993) we consider how the above forms of bias and misspecification may explain contradictory findings. A sample of 3,102 Wisconsin State employees received questionnaires 4 years apart. GEE estimation using an independence working correlation indicated that the proportion of individuals feeling excessive daytime sleepiness "at least sometimes" decreases with age, while conditional logistic regression indicated an increase.

2 Model for confounding

Consider the generalized linear model for the binary response y_{ij}

$$\mathrm{u}_{ij} = \mathrm{E}(y_{ij}|\alpha_i, \boldsymbol{x}_i, \boldsymbol{z}_i), \qquad h(\mathrm{u}_{ij}) = \alpha_i + \beta x_{ij} + \gamma z_{ij}, \tag{1}$$
$$\mathrm{Var}(y_{ij}|\boldsymbol{x}_i, \boldsymbol{z}_i) = g(\alpha_i + \beta x_{ij} + \gamma z_{ij}),$$

where i=1,...,n are individuals, j=1,...,k are time points, h is a link function, and α_i are random intercepts assumed to be normally distributed with mean α and variance σ_α^2 independently of each other and of x_{ij} and z_{ij}. Now assume that z_{ij} is unmeasured or otherwise omitted from model (1). To examine the effects of this omission in the longitudinal setting, we use the covariate structure proposed by Palta and Yao (1991)

$$\begin{pmatrix} x_{ij} \\ z_{ij} \end{pmatrix} = \begin{pmatrix} \mu_{x_i} \\ \mu_{z_i} \end{pmatrix} + \begin{pmatrix} e_{x_{ij}} \\ e_{z_{ij}} \end{pmatrix}, \tag{2}$$

where μ_{x_i} and μ_{z_i} are the means of x and z for subject i over the time period,

$$\begin{pmatrix} \mu_{x_i} \\ \mu_{z_i} \end{pmatrix} \overset{iid}{\sim} \mathrm{N}(\mathbf{0}, \mathbf{D}_1), \quad \begin{pmatrix} e_{x_{ij}} \\ e_{z_{ij}} \end{pmatrix} \overset{iid}{\sim} \mathrm{N}(\mathbf{0}, \mathbf{D}_2),$$

$$\mathbf{D}_1 = \sigma_1^2 \begin{bmatrix} 1 & R_1\sqrt{C_1} \\ R_1\sqrt{C_1} & C_1 \end{bmatrix}, \text{ and } \mathbf{D}_2 = \sigma_2^2 \begin{bmatrix} 1 & R_2\sqrt{C_2} \\ R_2\sqrt{C_2} & C_2 \end{bmatrix}. \quad (3)$$

The vectors (μ_{x_i}, μ_{z_i}) and $(e_{x_{ij}}, e_{z_{ij}})$ are assumed to be independent.

As they reflect the underlying across and within individual spread of x, σ_1^2 and σ_2^2 describe the study design. Alternatively, these parameters can be viewed as determining the within individual correlation of x. The parameters C_1 and C_2 scale z relative to x, and allow z to differ from x in its within individual correlation. Finally, the parameters R_1 and R_2 allow for different degree of confounding by z within and between individuals, as may be the case for cohort and period effects (see e.g. Dwyer, 1992).

For example, Newschaffer et al. (1992) considered decline in cholesterol with age among the aged, and found both cohort and period effects. Hypothetically, our scenario could apply as follows. Assume that x is age, and z is intake of saturated fat. If dietary habits set in childhood promote lower fat intake in older generations, R_1 is less than 0. If, intake also increased with time due to availability of fat-rich, pre-processed foods R_2 is greater than 0.

By well-known relationships for the multivariate normal distribution (Andersen, 1984), the conditional distributions of $z_{ij}|\boldsymbol{x}_i$ and $z_{ij}|x_{ij}$ are

$$\begin{aligned} z_{ij}|\boldsymbol{x}_i \;&\sim\; \mathrm{N}\Big(R_2\sqrt{C_2}x_{ij} + r_k\Delta\bar{x}_i. \\ &\quad \sigma_1^2C_1 + \sigma_2^2C_2 - (R_2\sqrt{C_2} + r_k\Delta)^2\sigma_1^2/r_k - \sigma_2^2R_2^2C_2(1-1/k)\Big), \quad (4) \\ z_{ij}|x_{ij} \;&\sim\; \mathrm{N}\left(\frac{\sigma_1^2R_1\sqrt{C_1} + \sigma_2^2R_2\sqrt{C_2}}{\sigma_1^2+\sigma_2^2}x_{ij},\right. \\ &\quad \left.\sigma_1^2C_1 + \sigma_2^2C_2 - \frac{(\sigma_1^2R_1\sqrt{C_1} + \sigma_2^2R_2\sqrt{C_2})^2}{\sigma_1^2+\sigma_2^2}\right), \quad (5) \end{aligned}$$

where $\Delta = R_1\sqrt{C_1} - R_2\sqrt{C_2}$, and $r_k = \sigma_1^2/(\sigma_1^2 + \sigma_2^2/k)$.

3 Alternative interpretations of above model

The above structure may be re-interpreted as presenting certain forms of measurement error or selection bias. The term involving z_{ij} in (1) may be viewed as modeling an error in either y_{ij} or x_{ij}. In the latter case, when $R_1 = 0$ and $R_2 = 0$ (1) fulfills the assumptions of the simplest Berkson type measurement error model (Carroll, et al, 1995). This may arise, for example if x_{ij} is an intended dose of a drug, but random (unknown) errors are made in its administration. Invoking a latent variable model as in Palta and Lin (1996), shows this to be equivalent to viewing a continuous variable ν_{ij} underlying y_{ij} to be measured with error at the intended dosages. When $R_2 \neq 0$ and/or $R_1 \neq 0$, a situation of dependent measurement error arises.

A well known example (see Kleinbaum et al., 1982) can be interpreted in a similar way. In studying the association of endometrial cancer and estrogen supplementation in post-menopausal women, let ν_{ij} be a latent true malignancy level, which is measured with error. Denote by y_{ij} the resulting diagnosis of cancer. Suppose that x_{ij} is estrogen dose and z_{ij} is the amount of bleeding which may be related to estrogen dose (i.e. $R_2 \neq 0$ and/or $R_1 \neq 0$). Increased bleeding may lead to greater medical attention and hence detection of previously undiscovered cancer. Therefore, bleeding could be seen here as destroying a typical measurement error model assumption of independence between error in measuring ν_{ij} and the covariate x_{ij}.

Usually, however, the above endometrial cancer example is cast as a form of selection bias, where individuals with a positive response (in say a case-control study framework) have higher probability of study inclusion when bleeding (hence estrogen) is present. To directly visualize (1) as a selection bias model, assume for simplicity of making the point, that $z_{ij} = z_i$. Now the individual intercept term becomes $\alpha_i + \gamma z_i$, and compared to the situation when $\gamma \neq 0$, certain individuals have been randomly over- or under-sampled. When $R_1 = 0$, we have a usual generalized mixed effects model. When $R_1 \neq 0$ the sampling distribution of the intercept depends on the exposure x_{ij}.

4 Correct mean structure under the above model

Under the above model with probit or logit link, Chao and Palta (1995) derived the correct mean structure for GEE estimation when data on z_{ij} are unavailable :

$$\begin{aligned} h(E(y_{ij}|\boldsymbol{x}_i)) &= \frac{\alpha + (\beta + \gamma R_2\sqrt{C_2})x_{ij} + \gamma r_k \Delta \overline{x}_{i.}}{\sqrt{1 + c^2\sigma_\alpha^2 + c^2\gamma^2\sigma^2_{z_{ij}|\boldsymbol{x}_i}}} \\ &= \alpha^* + \beta^* x_{ij} + \gamma^* \overline{x}_{i.}, \end{aligned} \tag{6}$$

where $c = 1$ for probit link, and $c = 16\sqrt{3}/15\pi$ for logit link. If the true link function is logit, the first equality is approximate.

5 Implications of ignoring confounder

We first consider the implications of confounding for GEE estimation when we fit the model without $\overline{x}_{i.}$. Denote the estimated parameter vector by

$\widehat{\boldsymbol{\beta}} = (\widehat{\alpha}^*, \widehat{\beta}^*)'$. The estimate of $\boldsymbol{\beta}$ is obtained by solving the generalized estimating equation

$$S(\boldsymbol{\beta}) = \sum_{i=1}^{n} \frac{\partial \mathbf{u}_i'}{\partial \boldsymbol{\beta}} \boldsymbol{V}_i^{-1}(\boldsymbol{\beta})(\boldsymbol{Y}_i - \mathbf{u}_i) = 0,$$

where $\mathbf{u}_i = (\ \mathrm{E}(y_{i1}|x_{i1}), ..., \mathrm{E}(y_{ik}|x_{ik})\ )'$, $\boldsymbol{Y}_i = (y_{i1}, ..., y_{ik})'$, $\boldsymbol{V}_i = \boldsymbol{A}_i^{\frac{1}{2}} \boldsymbol{R} \boldsymbol{A}_i^{\frac{1}{2}'}$, $\boldsymbol{A}_i$ is a diagonal matrix with the variances of $y_{ij}, j = 1, ..., k$ in the diagonal, and $\boldsymbol{R}$ is the working correlation matrix. We assume the probit or logit link. Consider the first-order Taylor expansion of $S(\boldsymbol{\beta})$ at $\boldsymbol{\beta}$=0. The generalized estimation equation is approximately

$$\sum_{i=1}^{n} \boldsymbol{x}_i' \boldsymbol{R}^{-1}(\boldsymbol{Y}_i - \frac{1}{2}\ 1 - d\ \boldsymbol{x}_i \boldsymbol{\beta}) = 0,$$

where $d = 0.25$ for the logit and $d = \phi(0)$ for the probit link, and ϕ is the density of the standard normal distribution. Assuming $\boldsymbol{R}$ is compound symmetry with correlation $\rho \neq 0$, Palta and Yao (1991) showed that

$$\widehat{\beta}^*(\rho) = \frac{1}{d}\ \frac{(1-\rho)(\frac{n}{n-1})kS_B^2\widetilde{\beta} + (1-\rho+k\rho)(\frac{k-1}{n})\sum_{i=1}^{n} S_{W_i}^2 b_i}{(1-\rho)(\frac{n}{n-1})kS_B^2 + (1-\rho+k\rho)(\frac{k-1}{n})\sum_{i=1}^{n} S_{W_i}^2},$$

where

$$S_B^2 = \frac{\sum_{i=1}^{n}(\overline{x}_{i.} - \overline{x}_{..})^2}{n-1}, \qquad S_{W_i}^2 = \frac{\sum_{i=1}^{n}(x_{ij} - \overline{x}_{i.})^2}{k-1},$$

$$\widetilde{\beta} = \frac{\sum_{i=1}^{n}(\overline{x}_{i.} - \overline{x}_{..})(\overline{y}_{i.} - \overline{y}_{..})}{\sum_{i=1}^{n}(\overline{x}_{i.} - \overline{x}_{..})^2}, \quad \text{and } b_i = \frac{\sum_{i=1}^{n}(x_{ij} - \overline{x}_{i.})(y_{ij} - \overline{y}_{i.})}{\sum_{i=1}^{n}(x_{ij} - \overline{x}_{i.})^2}.$$

Since

$$E\left(y_{ij}|\boldsymbol{x}_i\right) = h^{-1}(\alpha^* + \beta^* x_{ij} + \gamma^* \overline{x}_{i.}) \approx \frac{1}{2} + d\ (\alpha^* + \beta^* x_{ij} + \gamma^* \overline{x}_{i.}), \tag{7}$$

$\mathrm{E}(\widetilde{\beta}) \approx d\ (\beta^* + \gamma^*)$ and $\mathrm{E}(b_i) \approx d\ \beta^*$. Using the fact that S_B^2 and $S_{W_i}^2$ are unbiased variance estimates of $\sigma_1^2 + \sigma_2^2/k$ and σ_2^2 respectively,

$$\widehat{\beta}^*(\rho) \quad \overset{approx}{\longrightarrow} \quad \beta(\rho) = \frac{\beta + \gamma R_2 \sqrt{C_2} + \gamma \Delta \frac{(1-\rho)\sigma_1^2}{(1-\rho)\sigma_1^2 + (\rho k - 2\rho + 1)\sigma_2^2}}{\sqrt{1 + c^2\sigma_\alpha^2 + c^2\gamma^2\sigma_{Z_{ij}|\boldsymbol{x}_i}^2}}, \tag{8}$$

where $c = 1$ for the probit and $c = 16\sqrt{3}/15\pi$ for the logit link. Algebraic considerations show that the approximation in equation (7) can be expected to be valid only when the response probability is not extreme (between 0.105 and 0.895 for the probit link).

Pepe and Anderson (1994) pointed out that in the situation when

$$E\left(y_{ij}|\boldsymbol{x}_i\right) \neq E\left(y_{ij}|x_{ij}\right), \quad j = 1, ..., k, \tag{9}$$

consistent estimators of $E(y_{ij}|x_{ij})$ can be obtained only when the independence correlation is applied. Therefore, as

$$E(y_{ij}|x_{ij}) \quad = \quad \Phi(\frac{\alpha + (\beta + \gamma R_2\sqrt{C_2} + \gamma\Delta\frac{\sigma_1^2}{\sigma_1^2+\sigma_2^2})x_{ij}}{\sqrt{1 + c^2\sigma_\alpha^2 + c^2\gamma^2\sigma^2_{Z_{ij}|x_{ij}}}}), \tag{10}$$

for $\rho = 0$, i.e. the GEE estimators obtained with an independence working correlation,

$$\widehat{\beta}^*(0) \quad \longrightarrow \quad \frac{\beta + \gamma R_2\sqrt{C_2} + \gamma\Delta\frac{\sigma_1^2}{\sigma_1^2+\sigma_2^2}}{\sqrt{1 + c^2\sigma_\alpha^2 + c^2\gamma^2\sigma^2_{Z_{ij}|x_{ij}}}}. \tag{11}$$

Our results for $\rho \neq 0$ showing the coefficient in (8) not to be equal to the limiting value in (11), illustrate that under (9), estimators may not be consistent. It is of interest to note that the choice $\rho = 0$ gives weight to between individual and time point level confounding in accordance with the study design features σ_1^2 and σ_2^2. Increasing ρ gives decreasing weight to between individual confounding. We also observe that when ρ approaches 1, the limiting value in (8) approaches the coefficient of x_{ij} in (6).

We now investigate the implications of confounding for estimation by conditional logistic regression (see e.g. Conaway, 1989 for a general formulation). The model specified in Section 2 can be reformulated as

$$\begin{aligned} & h\left(E\left(y_{ij}|\alpha_i, \boldsymbol{x}_i, z_{ij}\right)\right) \\ = \quad & (\alpha_i + \gamma\mu_{z_i} + \gamma v_i) + (\beta + \gamma R_2\sqrt{C_2})x_{ij} - \gamma r_k R_2\sqrt{C_2}\overline{x}_{i.} + \gamma w_{ij}, \\ = \quad & \alpha_i^* + (\beta + \gamma R_2\sqrt{C_2})x_{ij} - \gamma r_k R_2\sqrt{C_2}\overline{x}_{i.} + \gamma w_{ij}, \end{aligned} \tag{12}$$

where v_i and w_{ij} are normally distributed with mean zero and variance $r_k\sigma_2^2R_2^2C_2/k$ and $\sigma_2^2C_2(1 - R_2^2)$ respectively, independently of each other and the other variables, and where $\alpha_i^* = \alpha_i + \gamma\mu_{z_i} + \gamma v_i$. The first equality follows by the fact that

$$\mathbf{e}_{z_i}|\mathbf{x}_i \sim \mathrm{N}\left(R_2\sqrt{C_2}\mathbf{x}_i - r_kR_2\sqrt{C_2}\overline{x}_{i.}\mathbf{1}, \sigma_2^2C_2(1 - R_2^2)\mathbf{I} + \frac{\sigma_2^2}{k}r_kR_2^2C_2\mathbf{1}\mathbf{1}'\right),$$

and that for the normal distribution, $e_{z_{ij}} = \mu_{e_{z_{ij}}|\boldsymbol{x}_i} + v_i + w_{ij}$. Suppose the true link is logit. Since z_{ij} is omitted, the actual model fit in the conditional logistic regression is

$$\mathrm{logit}\left(\mathrm{E}(y_{ij}|\alpha_i^*, \boldsymbol{x}_i)\right) \approx \frac{\alpha_i^* + (\beta + \gamma R_2\sqrt{C_2})x_{ij} - \gamma r_k R_2\sqrt{C_2}\overline{x}_{i.}}{\sqrt{1 + c^2\gamma^2\sigma_2^2C_2(1 - R_2^2)}},$$

where $c = 16\sqrt{3}/15\pi$. The subject effects (α_i^*) are removed from fitting by the conditioning procedure. Thus, the estimate of β obtained by conditional logistic regression converges to

$$\beta_{CL} = \frac{\beta + \gamma R_2 \sqrt{C_2}}{\sqrt{1 + c^2 \gamma^2 \sigma_2^2 C_2 (1 - R_2^2)}}. \tag{13}$$

The coefficient (13) differs from the coefficient of x_{ij} in (6) by a different denominator attenuation factor. This is because the random errors associated with the two models are on different scales. Therefore, when subject effects are present, the coefficient β^* in (6) is equal to β_{CL} multiplied by $1/\sqrt{1 + c^2\Sigma}$, where $\Sigma = \sigma_{\alpha^*}^2/[1 + c^2\gamma^2\sigma_2^2(1 - R_2^2)]$. Σ can be estimated by maximum likelihood [available software: MIXOR (Hedeker and Gibbons, 1994)]. Related topics are discussed in Palta and Lin (1996). We note that the conditional logistic regression coefficient is subject only to time point level confounding. Also, the random variation terms α_i^* need not be normally distributed for conditional logistic estimation. By the well-known approximate relationship between the logistic and normal distributions (Johnson and Kotz, 1970, P.6), the conditional logistic approach can also be applied to estimate probit coefficients.

6 Monte Carlo results

We investigated the accuracy of formula (8) by Monte Carlo studies. Data were generated from a latent structure as described by Chao et al. (1997). Due to the large number of parameters involved, we show only a few illustrative scenarios, in Figure 1. The panels in Figure 1 indicate the relationship of the approximate asymptotic limit (8), given as the solid line to the working correlation ranging from 0 to 0.99. The means of estimators obtained from (the same) 200 iterations of each scenario fit at various fixed compound symmetry correlations are shown as dots. Also shown (at $\rho = 1$) is the mean estimator of β^* in (6). As expected, these are close.

Situations (a) and (b) show scenarios illustrative of the presence of both between and within individual confounding with the latter being stronger. The parameters were set at $\alpha = 0.3$, $\gamma = 1$, $\sigma_1^2 = 1$, $\sigma_2^2 = 0.3$, $R_1 = R_2 = 0.32$, $C_1 = 0.1$, $C_2 = 0.2$, $n = 200$ and $k = 5$. The two levels of β were 0.1 and 0.5 and allow decreasing strength of the confounder, defined by $\gamma = 1$ relative to the primary risk factor x. Scenarios (c) and (e) differ in having higher β, set as 1 and 2, respectively. The performance of the approximation at first appears moderate for (c) and (e). However, as the asymptotic expectation at $\rho = 0$ does not require an approximation (consistency holds in this case), one may suspect that the sample size is insufficient. The same two scenarios with sample size $n = 400$ are shown in (d) and (f) with better fit. Scenarios (g) and (h) illustrate the relationship of ρ to to the estimated regression coefficient for pure between and within individual confounding, respectively. Parameters are the same as

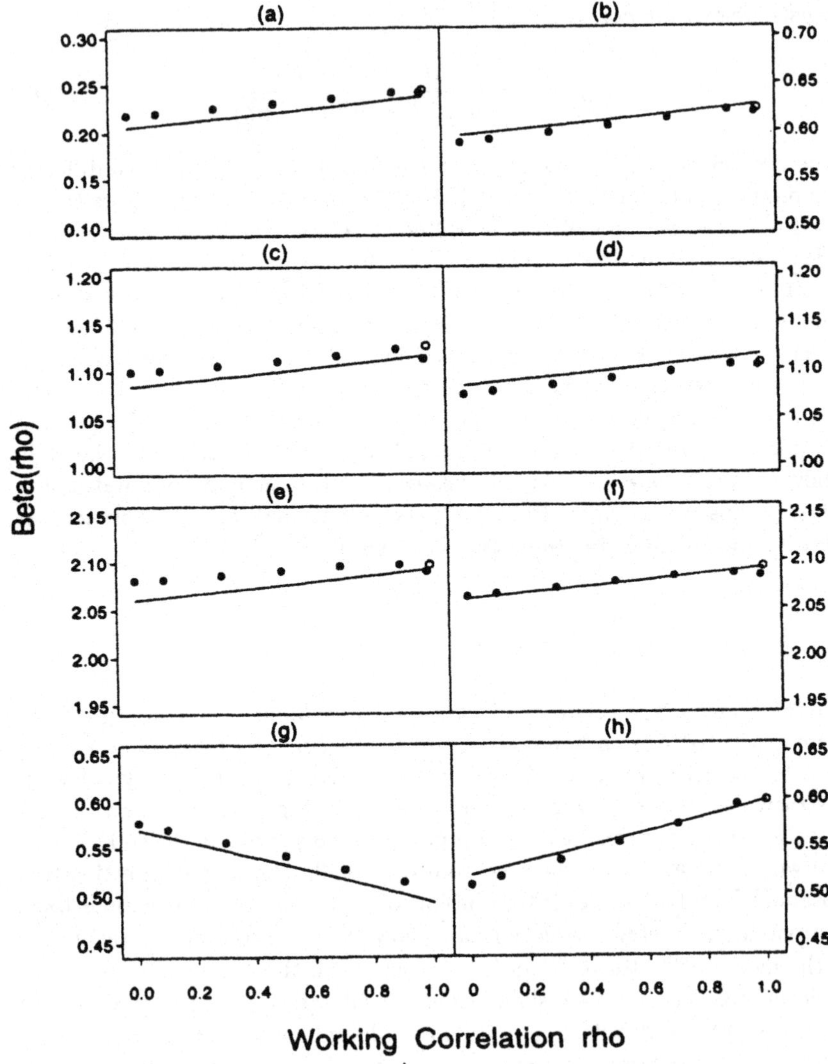

FIGURE 1. Monte Carlo estimates and the asymptotic limits obtained from GEE approach with missing confounders.

in scenario (b), except that $R_1 = 0.32$, $R_2 = 0$ $C_1 = 0.1$, $C_2 = 0$ in (g) and $R_1 = 0$, $R_2 = 0.32$ $C_1 = 0$, $C_2 = 0.1$ in (h). These figures point to the the disappearance of bias with between individual confounding when ρ approaches 1 and the increase in bias with larger ρ and within individual confounding, respectively.

TABLE 1. Regression coefficients (standard error) for models of feeling excessive daytime sleepiness "at least sometimes" fit by different methods.

Method		Gender (0=M, 1=F)	Age (yrs)	Body mass index (kg/m^2)
Conditional Logistic			0.052 (0.019)	0.041 (0.030)
Conditional Logistic (converted)			0.033 (0.012)	0.026 (0.019)
GEE	$\rho = 0$	0.169 (0.061)	–0.017 (0.004)	0.028 (0.006)
	$\rho = 0.42$ estim.	0.176 (0.061)	–0.013 (0.004)	0.029 (0.005)
	$\rho = 0.90$	0.210 (0.062)	0.006 (0.006)	0.031 (0.009)
	$\rho = 0.95$	0.220 (0.064)	0.014 (0.007)	0.031 (0.011)
	$\rho = 0.975$	0.223 (0.065)	0.020 (0.009)	0.029 (0.014)
	$\rho = 0.99$	0.207 (0.073)	0.026 (0.010)	0.027 (0.016)
	with $\bar{x}_{i.}$	0.164 (0.062)	0.030 (0.010)	0.027 (0.006)
	coefficient of $x_{i.}$ is –0.049 (0.011).			

7 Sleep survey results

The methodologic questions considered in this paper arose from a cohort study of sleep disorders among persons who were age 30–60 years and state employees in Wisconsin at the time of a baseline survey during 1989–1992 (Young et al., 1993). A total of 3,102 individuals answered this as well as a followup survey in 1994. We analyze responses to the question "Please indicate to what extent you have each of the following sleep problems......Feeling of excessive daytime sleepiness" dichotomizing the responses into "never or rarely" versus "at least sometimes". Table 1 shows the results from different regression analyses of this item on age, adjusting for body mass index (BMI) and gender (0=male, 1=female). In the GEE model which included mean age across the two surveys for each individual, its coefficient (–.049) was highly significant ($p < .0001$), indicating lack of fit. Confounding by cross-sectional (cohort) or longitudinal (period) effects, dependent measurement error and selection bias are therefore all possibilities.(Another possibility, non-linearity was ruled out).

The negative sign of the coefficient of mean age indicates that any cohort effects would be such as to decrease feeling of sleepiness with age. Possibilities include differences in life style leaving younger persons sleep deprived. Selection bias may have arisen from individuals in the work force who are tired taking early retirement or otherwise resigning. A recent report (Bliwise, 1996) indicates that admission of tiredness is more likely among contemporary men than it was among men in the pre World War II era. Older individuals may have retained some of this attitude, leading to generation related measurement error in the response. Considering period effects, increased tiredness may be due to changing working conditions at the state between surveys, or increasing work pressures with longer employment.

Numerically, the coefficients conform well to expectations based on our formulas. Conditional logistic regression and GEE with mean age included give coefficients which are in the same direction. As noted in Section 5, the estimators obtained by the conditional logistic approach can be converted to the same scale as the ones obtained by the GEE method. MIXOR yields $\widehat{\Sigma} = 4.576$. The converted estimates are shown in the second row in Table 1. Results for increasing ρ in the model fit with GEE, without mean age, show a positive coefficient for age, as well. The coefficients do not quite reach the same magnitude as those in the last row, presumably because of the approximations involved in the formulas that imply they should, and also because actually fitting a GEE model with such high working correlations involves near singularity.

8 Discussion

Our results show that when confounding is present, different analytic approaches to longitudinal data may yield different results. As the extent of confounding may differ on the between and within individual levels, it is critical whether the analysis gives more weight to within or between individual information. Investigation of the asymptotic expectation of GEE estimators with compound symmetry working correlations shows that increasing the working correlation gives more weight to the within individual component, hence is more sensitive to within individual confounding. We also show the approximate equivalence of using high working correlation, including $\overline{x}_{i.}$ in the model and conditional logistic regression, with our assumptions of confounding structure.

Interestingly, our model for confounding has connections with models for measurement error, latent variable models and selection bias. Differentiating between these possibilities is difficult and requires knowledge of subject matter and data collection. Nonetheless, the presence of unexpected discrepancies between estimators serves as a useful indicator of model violations.

REFERENCES

Andersen, T.W. (1984). *Multivariate Statistical Analysis*, 2nd ed. John Wiley & Sons , New York.

Bliwise, D.L. (1996). Historical change in the report of daytime fatigue. *Sleep*, in press.

Carroll, R.J., Ruppert, D., and Stefanski, L.A. (1995). *Measurement Error in Nonlinear Models.* Chapman & Hall, New York.

Chao, W.-H. and Palta, M. (1995). Effect of Omitted Confounders on the Analysis of Correlated Binary Data. *1995 Proceedings of the Epidemiology Section.* American Statistical Association, Alexandria, VA, pp 60-65.

Chao, W.-H., Palta, M. and Young, T. (1997). Effect of Omitted Confounders on the Analysis of Correlated Binary Data. *Biometrics* In press.

Conaway, M.R. (1989). Analysis of repeated categorical measurements with conditional likelihood methods.*Journal of the American Statistical Association* **84** , 53-62.

Dwyer, J.H., Feinleib, M., Lippert, P, and Hoffmeister, H. (1992). *Statistical Models for Longitudinal Studies of Health.* Oxford University Press, New York.

Hedeker, D. and Gibbons, R.D. (1994). A Random-Effects Ordinal Regression Model for Multi-Level Analysis. *Biometrics* **50**, 993-953.

Johnson, N. L. and Kotz, S. (1970). *Distributions in Statistics, Continuous Univariate Distributions.* Vol 2. Houghton-Mifflin, Boston.

Kleinbaum D.G., Kupper, L.L., and Morgenstern, H. (1982). *Epidemiologic Research.* Lifetime Learning Publications, elmont, CA, p 198.

Liang, K.Y., and Zeger, S.L. (1986). Longitudinal Data Analysis Using Generalized Linear Models. *Biometrika* **73**, 13-22.

Neuhaus, J. M., and Jewell, N. P. (1993). A geometric approach to assess bias due to omitted covariates in generalized linear models. *Biometrika* **80**, 807–815.

Newschaffer, C. J., Bush, T. L., and Hale W. E. (1992). Aging and total cholesterol levels: Cohort, period and survivorship effects. *American Journal of Epidemiology* **136**, 23–34.

Palta, M., and Lin, C.-Y. (1996). Latent variables, measurement error and methods for analyzing longitudinal binary and ordinal data. *Technical Report # 106* University of Wisconsin Department of Biostatistics, Madison WI.

Palta, M., and Yao, T.-J. (1991). Analysis of Longitudinal Data with Unmeasured Confounders. *Biometrics* **47**, 1355–1369.

Pepe, M. S. and Anderson, G. L. (1994). A cautionary note on inference for marginal regression models with longitudinal data and general correlated response data. *Communication in Statistics, Part B–Simulation and Computation* **23**, 939–951.

Young, T., Palta, M., Dempsey, J., Skatrud, J., Weber, S., and Badr, S. (1993). The occurrence of sleep-disordered breathing among middle-aged adults. *New England Journal of Medicine* **328**, 1230–1235.

Zeger, S.L., Liang, K.Y., and Albert, P.S. (1988). Models for Longitudinal Data: A Generalized Estimating Equation Approach. *Biometrics* **44**, 1049-1060.

The Linear Mixed Model. A Critical Investigation in the Context of Longitudinal Data.

Geert Verbeke* and Emmanuel Lesaffre

Biostatistical Centre for Clinical Trials, Leuven Belgium

ABSTRACT : In this paper, we investigate the impact of certain model assumptions of the linear mixed model, in the context of longitudinal data. We first discuss the robustness of ML-inferences with respect to the normality assumption for the random effects, and we extend the model by introducing heterogeneity in the random-effects population. Further, we extend the sample semi-variogram to investigate the residual covariance structure when random effects other than intercepts are included in the model. All results are illustrated using data on prostate cancer, taken from the Baltimore Longitudinal Study of Aging.

Key words and phrases: Linear mixed model, Misspecification, Sandwich estimator, Empirical Bayes, Finite mixtures, Serial correlation, Semi-variogram.

1 Introduction

In medical science, studies are often designed to investigate changes in a specific parameter which is measured repeatedly over time in the participating subjects. Such longitudinal studies are most appropriate for the investigation of individual changes over time and for the study of effects of aging and other factors likely to influence change. Data from designed longitudinal experiments can often be analysed with classical multivariate analysis of variance techniques. However, such methods impose model assumptions that are usually not met in observational studies, since the circumstances under which the measurements are collected cannot always

---

*Corresponding author address: Geert Verbeke, Biostatistical Centre for Clinical Trials, Kapucijnenvoer 35, B-3000 Leuven, Belgium

fully be controlled. Individuals may enter the study and withdraw from the study at any time, for different reasons. Further, individuals may be observed a different number of times, at different periods of time, and the intervals between observations may be different as well.

A frequently used alternative model for such highly unbalanced longitudinal data is the linear mixed-effects model (Laird and Ware 1982) which assumes that the $n_i \times 1$ vector $\boldsymbol{y}_i$ of responses for the ith individual can be modeled as $\boldsymbol{y}_i = X_i\boldsymbol{\alpha} + Z_i\boldsymbol{b}_i + \boldsymbol{e}_i$, $i = 1, \ldots, N$, where X_i and Z_i are $n_i \times p$ and $n_i \times q$ full rank covariate matrices, and $\boldsymbol{\alpha}$ is a vector of unknown parameters, called fixed effects, describing the population mean. Further, $\boldsymbol{b}_i$ is a vector of subject-specific regression coefficients, called random effects, assumed to be independent of the error terms $\boldsymbol{e}_i$. Very often, it is assumed that $\boldsymbol{b}_i \sim N(\boldsymbol{0}, D)$ and $\boldsymbol{e}_i \sim N(\boldsymbol{0}, \sigma^2 I_{n_i})$, in which case $\boldsymbol{y}_i$ is marginally normally distributed with mean $X_i\boldsymbol{\alpha}$ and covariance matrix $\text{Var}(\boldsymbol{y}_i) = Z_i D Z_i' + \sigma^2 I = V_i = W_i^{-1}$. The parameters in this marginal distribution are then estimated using maximum likelihood (ML) or restricted maximum likelihood (REML) methods, and empirical Bayes (EB) estimates for the random effects are obtained by replacing the parameters in the posterior means $E(\boldsymbol{b}_i|\boldsymbol{y}_i)$ by their estimated values, yielding $\widehat{\boldsymbol{b}_i} = \widehat{D} Z_i' \widehat{W_i}(\boldsymbol{y}_i - X_i\widehat{\boldsymbol{\alpha}})$.

The aim of this paper is to develop methods for checking the underlying assumptions and to investigate the robustness with respect to deviations from some of these assumptions. In Section 2.1, we will investigate the large sample behaviour of the MLE's of the fixed effects $\boldsymbol{\alpha}$ and the variance components D and σ^2 when the random effects are incorrectly assumed to be normally distributed. Further, extensive simulations will be used in Section 2.2 to study the performance of these asymptotic results in small or moderate samples. In Section 3.1 it will be shown that the normality assumption for the random effects can seriously influence their EB estimates, and that this assumption is often very difficult to check. We will hereby concentrate on the detection of a mixture in the random-effects distribution. This is of importance in models where the systematic part has been misspecified due to the omission of a categorical covariate. For instance, studies on the evolution of the blood pressure of patients treated with an antihypertensive drug often report 'responders' and 'non-responders'. In order to accomodate such clustered random effects, we will extend the model to the so-called 'heterogeneity model' in Section 3.2. In Section 4, we will extend the sample semi-variogram of Diggle (1988) to models with random effects other than intercepts, as an informal check for the assumed covariance matrix of the residual components $\boldsymbol{e}_i$. Finally, all our results will be illustrated in Section 5 using data on prostate cancer, taken from the Baltimore Longitudinal Study of Aging.

2 Robustness of MLE's with respect to non-normality of the random effects

In this section, we will investigate how much the MLE's of $\boldsymbol{\alpha}$, D and σ^2 are affected by the normality assumption of the random effects $\boldsymbol{b}_i$. So far, only the paper by Butler and Louis (1992) addressed this problem. Using simulations and the analysis of a real dataset, they have shown that wrongly specifying the random-effects distribution of univariate random effects has little effect on the fixed-effects estimates as well as on the estimates of the residual variance and the variance of the random effects. No evidence was found for any inconsistencies among these estimators. However, it was shown that the standard errors of all parameter estimators need correction in order to get valid inferences. We will now extend this result to the case of multivariate random effects, deriving asymptotic properties for the MLE's $\widehat{\boldsymbol{\alpha}}_N$, $\widehat{D}_N$ and $\widehat{\sigma}^2_N$, and we will investigate how these asymptotics perform in small or moderate samples.

2.1 *Asymptotics*

Let $\boldsymbol{\theta}$ denote the vector of all parameters in our marginal linear mixed model, and let Θ be the corresponding parameter space. Further, let $A_N(\boldsymbol{\theta})$ be minus the matrix of second-order derivatives of the log-likelihood function with respect to the elements of $\boldsymbol{\theta}$, and let $B_N(\boldsymbol{\theta})$ be the matrix with cross-products of first-order derivatives of the log-likelihood function, also with respect to $\boldsymbol{\theta}$. Their estimated versions, obtained by replacing $\boldsymbol{\theta}$ by its MLE are denoted by $\widehat{A}_N$ and $\widehat{B}_N$ respectively. The following theorem can then be proven (see Verbeke and Lesaffre 1996b) :

Theorem 1 *Under general regularity conditions, $\widehat{\boldsymbol{\theta}}_N$ is asymptotically normally distributed with mean $\boldsymbol{\theta}$ and with asymptotic covariance matrix $\widehat{A}_N^{-1}\ \widehat{B}_N\ \widehat{A}_N^{-1}/N$, as $N \rightarrow \infty$.*

Because $\widehat{\boldsymbol{\alpha}}_N = (\sum_i X_i'\widehat{V}_i^{-1}X_i)^{-1} \sum_i X_i'\widehat{V}_i^{-1}\boldsymbol{y}_i$, one often approximates the covariance matrix for $\widehat{\boldsymbol{\alpha}}_N$ by $(\sum_i X_i'\widehat{V}_i^{-1}X_i)^{-1}$ (see e.g. procedure MIXED in SAS 1996) which can easily be seen to equal $\widehat{A}_{N,11}^{-1}/N$, where $\widehat{A}_{N,11}$ is the leading block in $\widehat{A}_N$ which corresponds to the fixed effects. Hence, we have that the asymptotic covariance matrix suggested by Theorem 1 adds extra variability to this 'naive' estimate, by taking into account the estimation of the variance components, but it also corrects for possible misspecification of the random-effects distribution.

In order to investigate the effect of this last correction, we can compare the variance of any linear combination $\boldsymbol{\lambda}'\widehat{\boldsymbol{\theta}}$ obtained from Theorem 1 (=corrected) with its variance obtained from classical maximum likelihood theory (=uncorrected). Their ratio equals $\boldsymbol{\lambda}'\widehat{A}_N^{-1}\widehat{B}_N\widehat{A}_N^{-1}\boldsymbol{\lambda}/\boldsymbol{\lambda}'\widehat{A}_N^{-1}\boldsymbol{\lambda}$ and is always between $\lambda_{\min}$ and $\lambda_{\max}$, the smallest and largest eigenvalue of $\widehat{B}_N \widehat{A}_N^{-1}$. Therefore $\lambda_{\min} \approx \lambda_{\max} \approx 1$ may indicate that the random effects are approximately normally distributed.

Note also that $\widehat{A}_N^{-1} \widehat{B}_N \widehat{A}_N^{-1} / N$ is of the same form as the so-called "information sandwich" estimator for the asymptotic covariance matrix of fixed effects, estimated with quasi-likelihood methods (see e.g. Liang and Zeger 1986). However, our asymptotic result relates to both the fixed effects and the parameters in the "working correlation" model. Further, our model is incorrectly specified only through the random-effects distribution; the covariance structure is assumed to be correct.

2.2 Finite sample results

In order to compare the performance of the uncorrected and corrected standard errors in finite samples, Verbeke and Lesaffre (1996b) have set up an extensive simulation study. For several sample sizes, 2000 datasets were simulated with random intercepts and slopes sampled from a bivariate normal, a symmetric mixture of two bivariate normals, an asymmetric mixture of two bivariate normals, a bivariate lognormal, and a bivariate discrete distribution with 4 support points. Each simulated data set was then analysed using a linear mixed model assuming normality for the random effects. Corrected and uncorrected standard errors for all parameters in the marginal model were compared, and coverage probabilities of confidence intervals constructed with these standard errors were calculated.

In general, one can conclude that, for the fixed effects, the corrected and uncorrected standard errors are very similar. This is in agreement with the results of Sharples and Breslow (1992) who showed that, for correlated binary data, the sandwich estimator for the covariance matrix of fixed effects is almost as efficient as the uncorrected model-based estimator when the assumed form of the covariance matrix is correct, even under the correct model.

For the random components on the other hand, and more specifically for the elements in D, this is only true under the correct model (normal random effects). When the random effects are not normally distributed the corrected standard errors were clearly superior to the uncorrected ones, but occasionally still not performing very well. In some cases, the correction enlarges the standard errors to get confidence levels closer to the nominal level. For example, in up to 99.95% of the samples with lognormally distributed random effects, the uncorrected confidence interval for the random-intercepts variance was smaller than the corrected one, and therefore contained the correct parameter value less often. Further, $\lambda_{\max}$ was larger than 10 in 1217 out of the 2000 datasets, while $\lambda_{\min}$ was smaller than 0.2 in only 72 of the 2000 cases. In other cases, the correction results in smaller standard errors, protecting against conservative confidence intervals. In one situation for example, all 2000 simulated samples with discrete random effects had an uncorrected confidence interval for the random-intercepts variance which was larger than the corrected one, leading to confidence confidence levels much larger than 95%. We also found that in this case, λ_{max} was always smaller than 1.6 while λ_{min} was smaller than 0.2 in 70.8% of the datasets.

Although the corrected standard errors are good estimates for the variability of the parameter estimators, they may still yield incorrect confidence intervals for small samples, due to biased estimation of the parameters. This is especially the case for the random components in the model. An extension of our asymptotic results to REML estimates might therefore be useful.

3 Robustness of EB estimates with respect to non-normality of the random effects

In this section, we will investigate how much the normality-assumption for the random effects $\boldsymbol{b}_i$ influences their EB estimates $\widehat{\boldsymbol{b}_i}$. Note that our results from Section 2 justify assuming that the parameters in the marginal model are known.

3.1 The impact of the normality assumption on the random-effects estimates

The impact of the normality assumption on the EB estimates $\widehat{\boldsymbol{b}_i}$ can be well illustrated for the case where the correct random-effects distribution is a mixture of two multivariate normal distributions with common covariance matrix, $p\ N(\boldsymbol{\mu}_1, D)\ +\ (1-p)\ N(\boldsymbol{\mu}_2, D)$. It is then readily seen that $\widehat{\boldsymbol{b}_i}$, obtained under normality, again follows a mixture of two normals, with proportions p and $(1-p)$, and with mean and covariance depending on the covariates Z_i. However, as shown by Verbeke and Lesaffre (1996a), this new mixture will be unimodal if the eigenvalues of $\sigma^2(Z_i'Z_i)^{-1}$ are sufficiently large, independently of the modality of the original mixture for $\boldsymbol{b}_i$. This means that the detection of a mixture in the random-effects distribution, should not be based on the $\widehat{\boldsymbol{b}_i}$ when the residual variance is large, or when there is not much spread in the random effects covariates Z_i (e.g. when the $\boldsymbol{b}_i$ represent random intercepts). This is also in agreement with Strenio, Weisberg and Bryk (1983) where it was shown that the $\widehat{\boldsymbol{b}_i}$ are shrunk towards the population mean, and that this shrinkage is more severe in cases where measurements are not very precise (large σ^2).

In practice, the estimates $\widehat{\boldsymbol{b}_i}$ are frequently used to highlight special profiles or to look for (groups of) individuals evolving differently in time. Examples can be found in Waternaux, Laird and Ware (1989) and in De Gruttola, Lange and Dafni (1991). It is therefore important to investigate to what extent the $\widehat{\boldsymbol{b}_i}$ distribution represents the true random effects distribution. First, histograms of the $\widehat{\boldsymbol{b}_i}$ are only fully interpretable when the Z_i are the same for all individuals, since otherwise the $\widehat{\boldsymbol{b}_i}$ are no longer identically distributed. Further, since $\widehat{\boldsymbol{b}_i}$ depends on $\boldsymbol{b}_i$ as well as on $\boldsymbol{e}_i$, the weighted QQ-plots introduced by Lange and Ryan (1989) can, strictly speaking, not distinguish between wrong distributional assumptions for the random effects or for the error terms.

3.2 The heterogeneity model

To accomodate clustered $\boldsymbol{b}_i$'s, Verbeke and Lesaffre (1996a) extended the linear mixed model by assuming that the random effects are sampled from a mixture of g normal distributions with means $\boldsymbol{\mu}_j$ and common covariance matrix D, i.e. $\boldsymbol{b}_i \sim \sum_{j=1}^{g} p_j N(\boldsymbol{\mu}_j, D)$. Each component of the mixture then represents a cluster containing a proportion p_j from the population, $\sum_{j=1}^{g} p_j = 1$. In order to assure that $E(\boldsymbol{y}_i) = X_i\boldsymbol{\alpha}$, the additional constraint $E(\boldsymbol{b}_i) = \sum_{j=1}^{g} p_j \boldsymbol{\mu}_j = \boldsymbol{0}$ is needed. Note how this extended model can be seen as a hierarchical Bayes model where, given $\boldsymbol{\mu}$, $\boldsymbol{b}_i \sim N(\boldsymbol{\mu}, D)$, and where $\boldsymbol{\mu}$ equals $\boldsymbol{\mu}_j$ with probability p_j, $j = 1, \ldots, g$. We will therefore call this model the 'heterogeneity' model, and the classical linear mixed model then becomes our 'homogeneity' model. The vector $\boldsymbol{\psi}$ of all parameters in the marginal model can now be estimated using the EM algorithm.

Let $p_{ij}(\boldsymbol{\psi})$ now denote the posterior probability for the ith individual to belong to the jth component of the mixture, we then have that $E(\boldsymbol{b}_i|\boldsymbol{y}_i, \boldsymbol{\psi})$ equals $DZ_i'W_i(\boldsymbol{y}_i - X_i\boldsymbol{\alpha}) + A_i \sum_{j=1}^{g} p_{ij}(\boldsymbol{\psi})\boldsymbol{\mu}_j$, where $A_i = I - DZ_i'W_iZ_i$. The second term can now be seen as a correction of the EB estimate under normality, toward the component means of the mixture, proportional to the posterior probability of belonging to each of these components.

Further, classification of profiles no longer has to be based on the random-effects estimates. It is very common in mixture models to assign the ith case to the component for which it has the largest posterior probability, i.e. to the j(i)th component defined by $p_{i,j(i)}(\widehat{\boldsymbol{\psi}}) = \max_{1 \leq j \leq g} p_{ij}(\widehat{\boldsymbol{\psi}})$. Note however, that there is no reason why this posterior classification should correspond to any prior classification of the subjects, as will be illustrated in the example in Section 5.

Finally, one main issue in formulating a heterogeneity model is the choice of the appropriate number g of mixture components. It is known from analogous but simpler settings that, due to boundary problems, the null distribution of the likelihood ratio statistic for testing $H_0 : g = g_0$ versus $H_a : g = g_a > g_0$ does not necessarily converge to a χ^2 distribution. Verbeke and Lesaffre (1996a) therefore proposed to simulate this null distribution or to use some omnibus goodness-of-fit test to find the smallest value for g such that the resulting model fits the data well.

4 The detection of residual serial correlation

So far, we have assumed the residual components in $\boldsymbol{e}_i$ to be independent, all having the same variance. A more general covariance structure, considered by Diggle, Liang and Zeger (1994) assumes that $\boldsymbol{e}_i$ is the sum of two independent components $\boldsymbol{\varepsilon}_{1i}$ and $\boldsymbol{\varepsilon}_{2i}$, where $\boldsymbol{\varepsilon}_{1i}$ incorporates the fact that part of an individual's observed profile may be a response to time-varying stochastic processes operating within that individual. This type of random variation results in a correlation between serial measurements on the same subject, called serial correlation, which is usually a decreasing function of the time separation between these measurements. Finally, $\boldsymbol{\varepsilon}_{2i}$ represents the usual measurement-error component, $\boldsymbol{\varepsilon}_{2i} \sim N(0, \sigma^2 I_{n_i})$. Mansour, Nordheim and Rutledge (1985), Diem and Liukkonen (1988), Diggle (1988), Chi and Reinsel (1989) and Núñez-Antón and Woodworth (1994) all discuss covariance structures for longitudinal data, which are special cases of the above general covariance structure. In this section, we will discuss an informal method which allows us to decide whether serial correlation should be added to our original linear mixed model, and how its covariance matrix should then be modelled. We will assume that if serial correlation is present, it satisfies $\boldsymbol{\varepsilon}_{1i} \sim N(0, H_i)$ where H_i has (j,k)-element $\tau^2\, g(|t_{ij} - t_{ik}|)$ for some unknown constant τ and unknown positive decreasing function $g(\cdot)$ with $g(0) = 1$. Frequently used functions are the exponential and Gaussian serial correlation functions $g(u) = \exp(-\phi\, u)$ and $g(u) = \exp(-\phi\, u^2)$, for some unknown parameter $\phi > 0$.

Similar to the sample semi-variogram approach of Diggle (1988), we start by selecting a so-called preliminary mean structure $X_i^* \boldsymbol{\alpha}^*$ for $\boldsymbol{y}_i$ (possibly saturated) and by calculating OLS residuals $\boldsymbol{r}_i = \boldsymbol{y}_i - X_i^* \widehat{\boldsymbol{\alpha}}^*_{\text{OLS}}$, ignoring the longitudinal character of the data. Further, since Diggle, Liang and Zeger (1994) suggest that, in practice, the effect of $\boldsymbol{\varepsilon}_{1i}$ may often be dominated by the random effects, we remove this $\boldsymbol{b}_i$-effect by calculating transformed residuals $\boldsymbol{\Re}_i = A_i' \boldsymbol{r}_i \approx A_i' \boldsymbol{\varepsilon}_{1i} + A_i' \boldsymbol{\varepsilon}_{2i}$, where the matrices A_i have columns orthogonal to the columns of the Z_i. The transformed residuals $\boldsymbol{\Re}_i$ satisfy (see Verbeke, Lesaffre and Brant 1996)

$$\begin{aligned} &\frac{1}{2}\, E(\Re_{ij} \;-\; \Re_{ik})^2 \\ &= \;\sigma^2 \;+\; \tau^2 \;+\; \tau^2 \sum_{r<s} (A_{irj} - A_{irk})\,(A_{isj} - A_{isk})\; g(u_{irs}), \qquad (1) \end{aligned}$$

where A_{irs} denotes the (r,s)-element of the matrix A_i, and where $u_{irs} = |t_{ir} - t_{is}|$ is the time-lag between the rth and the sth measurement for the ith subject.

When we have balanced data, then only a small number of values u_{irs} can occur, which we denote by $u_0, \ldots, u_M$. We can then make a scatterplot of the OLS estimates for $\tau^2 g(u_t)$ obtained from model (1) versus u_t, $t = 0, \ldots, M$ to get a general impression of the shape of the unknown serial correlation function $g(\cdot)$. When the data are highly unbalanced, we then use linear interpolation to approximate $g(u_{irs})$ in (1) by a linear combination of $g(u_t)$ and $g(u_{t+1})$, where u_t and u_{t+1} are elements of a set of prespecified points $u_0, \ldots, u_M$, such that $u_t \leq u_{irs} \leq u_{t+1}$. This results in a new approximate regression model with the unknown function g evaluated at the prespecified points u_t, $t = 0, \ldots, M$ as parameters. Because this last regression model suffers from a high degree of multicollinearity due to the interpolation, we use ridge regression to calculate the parameter estimates. We refer to Verbeke, Lesaffre and Brant (1996) for all technical details.

5 Example

As an example, we use repeated measures of prostate specific antigen (PSA) taken on 54 participants of the Baltimore Longitudinal Study of Aging (BLSA). Eighteen of them were identified as prostate cancer cases (4 of them being metastatic cancer cases), 20 participants have benign prostatic hyperplasia (BPH) and there were 16 controls with no clinical sign of prostate disease. The number of repeated measures varies from 4 to 15, while the follow-up period was always between 6.9 and 25.3 years. Pearson et al. (1994) analysed these data with a linear mixed model, assuming that the average evolution of $\ln(1+PSA)$ is a quadratic function of years before diagnosis, within each of the 4 diagnostic groups separately. Further, they corrected for age differences at the time of diagnosis and they included random intercepts and random slopes for the linear as well as quadratic effect of years before diagnosis. All remaining variability was assumed to be measurement error. We now use their model to illustrate the above results.

We first compared the standard errors of the fixed effects obtained from $\widehat{A}_{N,11}^{-1}/N$ with those obtained from the observed Fisher information matrix $\widehat{A}_N^{-1}/N$. The latter ones take account of the extra variability due to the estimation of D and σ^2 and are therefore all larger than the 'naive' standard errors; however, the ratio was never larger than 1.03. Further, we compared the observed Fisher information matrix with our sandwich estimate $\widehat{A}_N^{-1}\widehat{B}_N\widehat{A}_N^{-1}/N$. The ratio of the corrected to the uncorrected standard errors was between 0.52 and 1.72 for all parameters in the marginal model, while the same ratio is between 0.21 and 2.76 for any linear transformation of these parameters. This suggests that the random effects are not quite normally distributed.

In a second step, we fitted several heterogeneity models to the restricted data set of controls and cancer patients only, ignoring our prior diagnostic classification but correcting for age-differences. We found (see Verbeke and Lesaffre 1996a) that a three-component mixture of three-dimensional normals is needed to describe the natural heterogeneity in the random-effects population. These three components correspond to subjects whose PSA-value hardly increases, subjects whose PSA-value increases exponentially fast after a period of very small increase, and subjects whose PSA-value increases exponentially from their enrollment in the study. Posterior classification of the subjects did not coincide with the prior diagnostic classification. This may explain why we found that the random effects are probably not normally distributed.

Finally, based on our extended sample semi-variogram, we found (see Verbeke, Lesaffre and Brant 1996) that measurement error is not sufficient to describe the residual variability. We improved the model of Pearson et al. (1994) considerably by splitting up this remaining variability into an exponential serial correlation component and measurement error, yielding two sources of random variability which are about equally important in the sense that they have similar variances.

6 Conclusions

We have shown how certain distributional assumptions of the linear mixed model can be checked and we have described their impact on the MLE's of all parameters in the marginal model as well as on the EB estimates for the random effects. Further, the normality assumption for these random effects has been relaxed to accomodate clusters in their population.

A different class of model diagnostics are those based on the detection of outliers and influential subjects. Lesaffre and Verbeke (1996) have recently used the local influence approach (see e.g. Cook 1986) to detect influential subjects in the context of the linear mixed model and to describe the influence of each subject to specific characteristics of its covariates and residuals.

7 References

[1] Butler, S.M. and Louis, T.A. (1992), Random effects models with nonparametric priors, *Statistics in Medicine*, **11**, 1981–2000.

[2] Chi, E.M. and Reinsel, G.C. (1989), Models for longitudinal data with random effects and AR(1) errors, *Journal of the American Statistical Association*, **84**, 452–459.

[3] Cook, R.D. (1986), Assessment of local influence, *Journal of the Royal Statistical Society, Series B*, **48**, 133–169.

[4] De Gruttola, V., Lange, N., and Dafni, U. (1991), Modeling the progression of HIV infection, *Journal of the American Statistical Association*, **86**, 569–577.

[5] Diem, J.E. and Liukkonen, J.R. (1988), A comparative study of three methods for analysing longitudinal pulmonary function data, *Statistics in Medicine*, **7**, 19–28.

[6] Diggle, P.J. (1988), An approach to the analysis of repeated measures, *Biometrics*, **44**, 959–971.

[7] Diggle, P.J., Liang, K.Y., and Zeger, S.L. (1994), *Analysis of longitudinal data*, Clarendon Press, Oxford.

[8] Laird, N.M. and Ware, J.H. (1982), Random-effects models for longitudinal data, *Biometrics*, **38**, 963–974.

[9] Lange, N. and Ryan, L. (1989), Assessing normality in random effects models, *The Annals of Statistics*, **17**, 624–642.

[10] Lesaffre, E. and Verbeke, G. (1996), Local influence in linear mixed models, *Submitted for publication.*

[11] Liang, K.Y. and Zeger, S.L. (1986), Longitudinal data analysis using generalized linear models, *Biometrika*, **73**, 13–22.

[12] Mansour, H., Nordheim, E.V., and Rutledge, J.J. (1985), Maximum likelihood estimation of variance components in repeated measures designs assuming autoregressive errors, *Biometrics*, **41**, 287–294.

[13] Núñez-Antón, V. and Woodworth, G.G. (1994), Analysis of longitudinal data with unequally spaced observations and time-dependent correlated errors, *Biometrics*, **50**, 445–456.

[14] Pearson, J.D., Morrell, C.H., Landis, P.K., Carter, H.B., and Brant, L.J. (1994), Mixed-effects regression models for studying the natural history of prostate disease, *Statistics in Medicine*, **13**, 587–601.

[15] SAS Institute Inc., Cary, NC: SAS Institute Inc. (1996), *SAS/STAT Software : Changes and Enhancements through Release 6.11.*

[16] Sharples, K. and Breslow, N.E. (1992), Regression analysis of correlated binary data : some small sample results for the estimating equation approach, *Journal of Statistical Computation and Simulation*, **42**, 1–20.

[17] Strenio, J.F., Weisberg, H.J., and Bryk, A.S. (1983), Empirical bayes estimation of individual growth-curve parameters and their relationship to covariates, *Biometrics*, **39**, 71–86.

[18] Verbeke, G. and Lesaffre, E. (1996a), A linear mixed-effects model with heterogeneity in the random-effects population, *Journal of the American Statistical Association*, **91**, 217–221.

[19] Verbeke, G. and Lesaffre, E. (1996b), The effect of misspecifying the random effects distribution in linear mixed models for longitudinal data, *Computational Statistics and Data Analysis*. To appear.

[20] Verbeke, G., Lesaffre, E., and Brant, L.J. (1996), The detection of residual serial correlation in linear mixed models, *Submitted for publication.*

[21] Waternaux, C., Laird, N.M., and Ware, J.H. (1989), Methods for analysis of longitudinal data : Bloodlead concentrations and cognitive development, *Journal of the American Statistical Association*, **84**, 33–41.

Modeling the Order of Disability Events in Activities of Daily Living Using Discrete Longitudinal Data

Dorothy D. Dunlop[†,‡] and Larry M. Manheim[†,††] *

Northwestern University

United States

ABSTRACT Longitudinal data are used to develop an empirical model for the ordering of a set of events. The empirical ordering is based on the median times to the separate events obtained from estimated survival distributions from a learning dataset. Nonparametric methods are used to validate the empirical order within a person. Also, the probability of developing a specific event is modeled given time-dependent covariates. The approach is used to order the age of initial disability in activities of daily living (ADL) using longitudinal data collected biennially over six years of followup on 5151 elderly people participating in the Longitudinal Study on Aging. Due to the presence of disabilities for some people on study entry and to the periodic nature of data collection, event times are interval censored. The median age to initial disability is estimated for each ADL using survival distribution methods for truncated and interval censored data from a learning dataset. An empirical model, based on the ordered median ages across ADLs, is supported by the test dataset validation. This model differs from orderings proposed in the literature using cross-sectional data. The probability of developing disability in a specific ADL is modeled using a generalized linear model that relates the discrete hazard rate to a time dependent disability profile.

*From the [†]Institute for Health Services Research and Policy Studies, [‡]Department of Preventive Medicine, Northwestern University, Evanston and Chicago IL and [††]Midwest Center for Health Services and Policy Research, VA Hospital, Hines IL. The authors gratefully acknowledge the comments of Ajit Tamhane, Ph.D. and the programming assistance of MaryAnn Chamberlain, M.S. and Karen Ruth, Ph.D. Work for this project was supported in part by Multipurpose Arthritis Center Grant No. AM 30692. The National Center for Health Statistics (NCHS) is the original source of these data from the Longitudinal Study of Aging, 1984-1990. Address correspondence to Dorothy D. Dunlop, Institute for Health Services Research and Policy Studies, 629 Noyes St., Evanston IL 60208

Key words: Repeated Measures, Discrete Time, Ordered Events

1 Introduction

Understanding the order in which older persons acquire disabilities in basic activities of daily living (ADLs) has important public health ramifications in regard to caring for our aging U.S. population. The problem of modeling the order in which older persons acquire disabilities in ADLs has received much attention in recent years [4, 5, 6, 7, 8, 9]. However, these studies have generally used cross-sectional data to infer an order of developing ADL disabilities. In the present paper we address this problem in a novel way by utilizing information from longitudinal data to develop and test a model for the order of incident ADL disabilities within people. In addition, we model the probability of acquiring a specific ADL disability given a person's disability profile. Such a model can be used to identify high risk populations for the purpose of targeting prevention programs. We apply this model to data from the Longitudinal Study on Aging [1], a prospective study of 5151 elderly persons interviewed biennially from 1984 to 1990, to evaluate the order of initial disability occurrence across ADLs.

These longitudinal data collected at discrete time intervals have serious missing data problems. Since the cohort is observed in two year intervals, the exact times of incident ADL disabilities are not observed but are interval censored or right censored. In addition, due to the presence of disability in some people at study entry, those event times are left censored. We use the ordered median ages of initial disability across ADLs, estimated from survival distribution methods for truncated and interval censored data, to develop an empirical ordering. Nonparametric methods are used to validate the empirical order within a person. A discrete hazard rate is used to model the probability of developing an ADL disability utilizing time dependent covariate information.

2 Background of the Study

Data were obtained from the Longitudinal Study of Aging (LSOA) [1]. The LSOA is a prospective study of 5151 community dwelling persons aged 70 years and older who were initially interviewed in the 1984 National Health Interview Survey, Supplement on Aging [2, 3]. Participants were reinterviewed in 1986, 1988 and 1990. The disability status (none versus some) of the ADL functions of walking, bathing, dressing, transferring (getting in or out of bed or chairs), toileting and feeding was measured via self-report at each LSOA interview. Disability for a specific ADL is defined as difficulty in performing that function. The study sample was restricted to 5029 individuals having complete baseline data on all six ADL functions.

3 Statistical Methods

An empirical order of initial disability across the six ADL tasks can be obtained from the ordered median ages to incident difficulty. This ordering is estimated from a learning dataset (50% of the data) and validated using a test dataset. As noted before, the data are interval-censored because interviews are approximately two years apart. A survival distribution using Turnbull's [10] method of estimation for interval censored and truncated data, implemented within the Survival Module of SYSTAT [11], was used to estimate the age distribution of incident disability for each ADL. The ordered estimated median ages of initial disability across the six ADLs are used to determine the empirical order.

While the order of the estimated median ages across ADLs reflects population trends, it may not reflect the order in which events occur within a person. A test of the empirical model based on the within person ordering of incident ADL events is obtained using Hollander's nonparametric test for ordered alternatives [12]. A test dataset is used to test the hypotheses

$$H_0 : \tau_1 = \cdots = \tau_p \text{ versus } H_1 : \tau_1 \leq \cdots \leq \tau_p$$

where τ_i is the median age of incident disability of the ith ordered ADL for ADL functions $i = 1, \cdots, p$. Rejection of the null hypothesis validates the empirical ordering.

One can build on the information from a validated ordering to identify high risk profiles that predict disability in a specific ADL task. One approach is to model discrete time utilizing longitudinal covariate information in which covariates, representing ADL disabilities, are entered into a nested model according to the empirical ordering. Let the discrete time period $T_D = 1, \cdots, K$ be the interval between successive interviews which occur in continuous time at $T = 0, 1, \cdots, K$, as shown in Figure 1. The conditional probability of an event in interval k, given an event-free status in interval $k-1$, is the discrete hazard rate (DHR) associated with T_D given by

$$\theta_k = \Pr\{T_D = k \mid T_D > k-1\} \quad (k = 1, 2, \ldots).$$

The covariate information for the ith individual at interview k is summarized in $x_{ik} = \{x_{ijk}, 1 \leq j \leq J\}, 1 \leq i \leq N$ where J is the number of covariates and N is the number of people. Let θ_{ik} denote the value of θ_k for the ith individual. We fit a generalized linear model with complementary

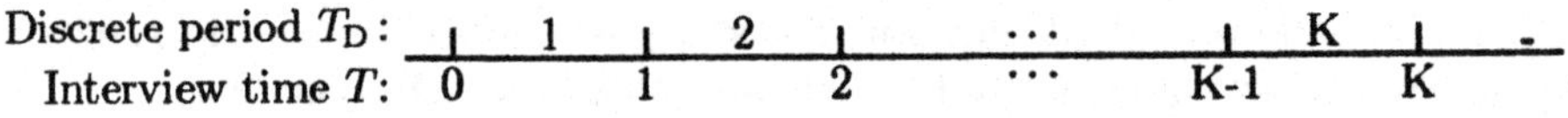

Discrete period T_D : | 1 | 2 | ⋯ | K |
Interview time T: 0 | 1 | 2 | ⋯ | K-1 | K

FIGURE 1. Data Collected at Discrete Time Intervals

log-log (CLL) link to θ_{ik} given by

$$\ln\left[-\ln\left(1-\theta_{ik}\right)\right]=\beta_{0k}+\sum_{j=1}^{J}\beta_{jk}x_{ij;k-1} \tag{1}$$

where the β's are unknown parameters to be estimated. The DHR of 1 is the discrete analogue of the Cox proportional hazard rate [13, 14]. Data on the θ_{ik}'s are available through the indicator variable Y_{ik} where $Y_{ik}=0$ or 1 depending on whether or not the event occurred during the kth period. Thus,

$$\theta_{ik}=\Pr\left(Y_{ik}=1 \mid Y_{i1}=\cdots=Y_{ik-1}=0\right).$$

Assuming independence between individuals, the likelihood function can be written as

$$\mathcal{L}=\prod_{i=1}^{N}\prod_{k=1}^{K_i}\theta_{ik}^{y_{ik}}\left(1-\theta_{ik}\right)^{1-y_{ik}}$$

where y_{ik} is the observed value of Y_{ik}. The GLIM [15] package produces iterative weighted least squares estimates of the β's and their estimated covariance matrix.

4 Results

An empirical order of the occurrence of initial disability across the six ADL functions was determined by estimating the age distribution of initial disability for each ADL from a learning set of 2548 observations using Turnbull's method of estimation of the survival distribution [10]. Figure 2 shows the cumulative proportion of the learning sample with initial disability by age for each ADL. These six curves show good separation in their interquartile ranges, although the dressing and toileting curves are close together. These curves indicate that the ages of ADL disability onset are ordered such that initial disability can be expected to occur first in walking, followed by bathing, transferring, dressing, toileting and finally by feeding.

The ordered median age in years to initial disability is 84 for walking, 87 for bathing, 90 for transferring, 92 for dressing, 93 for toileting and 100 for feeding. For simplicity we represent the empirical ordering as

$$\text{Empirical Model: Walk} \rightarrow \text{Bath} \rightarrow \text{Transfer} \rightarrow \text{Dress} \rightarrow \text{Toilet} \rightarrow \text{Feed} \tag{2}$$

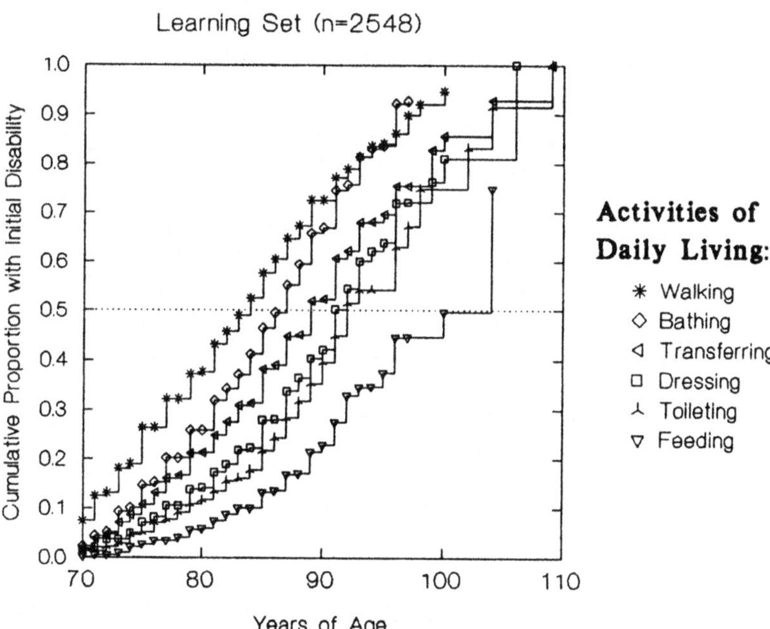

FIGURE 2. Age Distribution of Initial Disability in Activities of Daily Living from LSOA Data.

where the notation A $\rightarrow$ B $\rightarrow$ C is used to indicate that event A occurs first, followed by B, followed by C.

This empirical model 2 differs from other orderings based on cross-sectional data [4, 5, 6, 7, 8, 9]. In particular, it differs from a well-studied conceptual model which postulates that people lose abilities and become disabled based on primary biological and psychosocial function [16]. The conceptual ordering of ADL disability is given by

$$\text{Conceptual Model: Walk} \rightarrow \text{Bath} \rightarrow \text{Dress} \rightarrow \text{Toilet} \rightarrow \text{Transfer} \rightarrow \text{Feed}. \quad (3)$$

While both models indicate that walking and bathing disabilities occur early and feeding disability occurs last, the order of the intermediate disabilities is different. Specifically, the empirical model 2 orders transferring ahead of dressing and toileting disabilities, while the conceptual model 3 orders transferring after dressing and toileting disabilities. There is little debate in the literature regarding the early and late disability events, but different orderings of the intermediate events are investigated elsewhere [5]. Because relatively few people in the LSOA acquired all six ADLs and the outstanding question is in regard to the order of intermediate events, we focus on the order of the intermediate disability events of transferring, dressing and toileting.

A test dataset was used to evaluate the order in which events occur within a person, with respect to the intermediate ADL disability events.

$$\text{Intermediate Empirical Order:} \qquad \text{Transfer} \rightarrow \text{Dress} \rightarrow \text{Toilet} \quad (4)$$

All three intermediate events can be ranked within an individual for 420 persons from the test dataset. The empirical order 4 was tested by the hypotheses $H_0 : \tau_1 = \tau_2 = \tau_3$ versus $H_1 : \tau_1 \leq \tau_2 \leq \tau_3$ where τ_1, τ_2, and τ_3 represent the median initial age of transferring, dressing and toileting disabilities, respectively. The sum of the ranks were 742.5, 849.0 and 937.5 for transferring, dressing and toileting disabilities, respectively. Hollander's ordered alternative statistic [12] based on these rank sums was 5235, which has an asymptotic normalized value of $z = 6.728$ with $p < .001$. This result strongly supports the alternative hypothesis of empirical order among these three events.

An ordering among incident ADL disabilities suggests that a profile of ADL disabilities may be informative to estimate the probability of developing a specific ADL problem. Although a model was developed for each ADL task, we illustrate the development of DHR model for toileting. The problem of toileting dependency is particularly interesting since disability in that function has been associated with poor short term prognoses [17](e.g., institutionalization or death). We model the probability of initial toileting disability in the next two years using a DHR with a CLL link function 1. There were 3804, 2830, 2147 pairs of observations from two-year intervals beginning with 1984, 1986, 1988, respectively, which were used to estimate the DHR of initial toileting disability, controlling for age at an interview and years of education, a proxy for socio-economic status. Age at an interview k was represented using two covariates: age at study entry (centered at 80 years) to evaluate a cohort effect due to age, and elapsed periods k from study entry to evaluate a longitudinal effect of aging. ADLs were entered as indicator variables (0=no disability, 1=disability) in the order indicated by the empirical model 2. Individual covariate terms were assessed by comparing the change in deviances (−log likelihood ratios) corresponding to a particular term with a χ^2 critical value. Due to the multiplicity of tests, a Bonferroni adjustment for a simultaneous .05 level of $\alpha = \frac{.05}{8} = .00625$ was used. This estimated DHR model is:

$$\begin{aligned}\ln[-\ln(1-\theta_{k+1})] &= -2.77 - 0.070k + .085(\text{Entry Age} - 80)\\ &\quad -0.029(\text{Education}) + 0.73(\text{Walk}_k) + 0.64(\text{Bath}_k)\\ &\quad +0.34(\text{Transfer}_k) + 0.73(\text{Dress}_k). \qquad (5)\end{aligned}$$

Standard errors of the estimated parameters are shown in Table 1. The fitted model 5 indicates that the probability of incident toileting disability in the next two years increases with age at study entry, decreases with more years of education, and increases with disability in each ADL which preceded toileting in the empirical model 2. Disability in feeding was not significant, as expected, since it occurs after toileting in the empirical ordering 2. Note from Table 1 that discrete time k is a nonsignificant predictor based on the low magnitude of its associated t-statistic$= \hat{\beta}/\widehat{\text{SE}}(\hat{\beta}) = -.070/.052 = -1.35$. Since time was a strong predictor before the ADL profile was entered, this may indicate that disabilities which often accompany aging, rather than aging itself, increase the risk of losing the ability to independently toilet.

A second model was developed by entering a covariate representing the number of ADLs (NADL) for which a person reported disability (NADL$= 0,\cdots,5$) immediately after the demographic covariates. When the ADL profile was entered after NADL, none of the ADLs were significant. This estimated DHR model is:

$$\begin{aligned}\ln[-\ln(1-\theta_{k+1})] &= -2.60 - 0.070k + .084(\text{Entry Age} - 80)\\ &\quad -0.029(\text{Education}) + 0.59(\text{NADL}_k). \qquad (6)\end{aligned}$$

Standard errors of the estimated parameters are shown in Table 1. Again, discrete time k is a nonsignificant predictor in 6 based on its associated t-statistic$= \hat{\beta}/\widehat{\text{SE}}(\hat{\beta}) = -.070/.051 = -1.37$. The change in deviance associated with NADL in this DHR model 6 was −340 with 1 d.f. In contrast, the change in deviance associated with the four ADLs in the previous model 5 was −346 with 4 d.f. Also, the remaining coefficients (constant, time, entry age and education) are virtually unchanged. It is evident that almost all the model improvement which resulted when the profile of ADLs were

TABLE 1. Complementary Log Log Models for Initial Toileting Disability from LSOA Data

Term	$\hat{\beta}$	$\hat{SE}(\hat{\beta})$	Term	$\hat{\beta}$	$\hat{SE}(\hat{\beta})$
Constant	−2.614	0.118	Constant	−2.601	0.118
Time k	0.070	0.052	Time k	0.070	0.051
Entry Age−80	0.084	0.007	Entry Age−80	0.085	0.007
Education	−0.031	0.010	Education	−0.029	0.010
Walking	0.730	0.101	NADL	0.590	0.030
Bathing	0.652	0.109			
Transfer	0.341	0.109			
Dressing	0.732	0.124			

entered can be attained by entering only NADL in their place. This suggests that it is the number of ADLs, rather than the profile of ADLs, which is predictive of a toileting problem within the next two years. Secondary models which incorporated interactions terms to indicate combinations of ADL problems (e.g., walking×bathing) were also investigated. However, such interactions were not significant when entered after NADL.

Similar models were developed for the other ADL tasks. In all cases, NADL accounted for a large portion of the change in the deviance associated with the profile of ADLs.

5 Discussion

Longitudinal data are used to develop an empirical model for the ordering of a set of ADL disability events based on the median times to the individual events using data from the LSOA. The median times are obtained from survival distributions estimated from a learning dataset. The empirical model is validated on a test dataset using Hollander's test for ordered alternatives which utilizes the ranking of event times within individuals. The empirical ordering, which is strongly supported by the test dataset validation, differs from a well-studied conceptual ordering [4, 5, 6, 7] supported from cross-sectional studies.

The probability of developing initial disability in a specific ADL is modeled using a generalized linear model that relates the DHR to a time dependent profile of disability in other ADLs. The modeling of the DHR is illustrated for the ADL task of toileting. The probability of incident toileting disability in the next two years is modeled as a function of demographics and walking, bathing, transferring and dressing. However, the model improvement due to the entry of these four ADL terms was almost attained by entering a single term in their place, representing the number of ADL difficulties. This result suggests that the number of problems is as informative as the specific nature of the problems for predicting a future toileting disability. Since there appears to be an ordering to the initial occurrence of ADL disabilities, it is counterintuitive that the profile of ADL difficulties contains little information beyond the number of ADL problems. One explanation may be that ADL difficulties can resolve [18, 19]. For example, an elderly person who reports a walking disability may resolve that difficulty through a hip replacement. Thus, the number of disabilities experienced by a person may be as informative as the nature of the problems for predicting a future disability.

6 References

[1] National Center for Health Statistics: Longitudinal Study of Aging, 1984-1990 [database on CDROM]. CD-ROM LSOA, No. 1. SETS Version 1.21. Washington: U.S. Government Printing Office, 1993. 1 compact disc. Accompanied by: 1 manual. System Requirements: IBM PC 286, 396, 486 or full compatible; hard disk with at least 5 MB free space; MS-Dos 3.1 or higher; printer recommended; Microsoft CD-ROM Extensions version 2.0 or higher; CD-ROM reader.

[2] Kovar MG and Pie G (1981), "The design (1973-84) and procedures (1975-83) of the National Health Interview Survey," *Vital Health Statistics* [1];18, Hyattsville. MD: National Center for Health Statistics.

[3] Fitti J and Kovar MG (1987), "The Supplement on Aging to the 1984 National Health Interview Survey," *Vital Health Statistics* [1];21, Hyattsville, MD: National Center for Health Statistics.

[4] Katz S., Akpom Ca. (1976), "A measure of primary sociobiological functions," *International Journal of Health Services* 6:493-507.

[5] Lazaridis EN, Rudgerg MA, Furner SE and Cassel CK (1994), "Do activities of daily living have a hierarchical structure? An analysis using the longitudinal study on aging". *Journal of Gerontology: Medical Sciences* 49:M47-M51.

[6] Siu AL, Reuben DB, Hayes RD (1990), "Hierarchical measures of physical function in ambulatory geriatrics," *Journal of the American Geriatric Society* 38:1113-1119.

[7] Travis SS and McAuley WJ (1990), "Simple counts of the number of basic ADL dependencies for long-term care research and practice," *Health Services Research* 25:349-60.

[8] Kempen GIJM, Suurmeijer TPBM (1990), "The development of a hierarchical polychotomous ADL-IADL scale for noninstitutionalized elders," *Gerontologist* 30:497-502.

[9] Varekamp I, Smit C, Rosendaal FR, Bruckler-Vriends, Briet, van Dijck H and Suurmeijer TPMB (1989),"Employment of individuals with hemophilia inn the Netherlands," *Social Sciences Medicine* 28:261-270.

[10] Turnbull BW (1976), "The empirical distribution function with arbitrarily grouped, censored and truncated data," *Journal of the Royal Statistical Society.B*,38,290-295.

[11] Steinburg D. and Colla P (1988), *SURVIVAL: A supplementary module for SYSTAT*, Evanston, IL: SYSTAT, Inc.

[12] Hollander M (1967), "Rank tests for randomized blocks when the alternatives have an a priori ordering," *Annals of Mathematical Statistics*62:939-949.

[13] Prentice, R.L., and Gloeckler L.A. (1978), "Regression analysis of group survival data with application to breast cancer data" *Biometrics*, 34: 57-67.

[14] Dunlop D.D., Tamhane A.C., Chmiel, J.S. and Phair, J.P (1994), "A model-based approach to estimate the AIDS-free time distribution in homosexual men using longitudinal data," *Journal of Biopharmaceutical Statistics*, 4: 129-146.

[15] GLIM Rel 3.77 (1987), Numerical Algorithm Group Inc., Downers Grove, Il.

[16] Katz S, Ford AB, Moskowitz RW, Jackson BA and Jaffe MW (1963), "Studies of Illness in the aged," *Journal of the American Medical Association*,185:914-919.

[17] Falconer JA, Naughton BJ, Dunlop DD, Elliot JR Srtasser DD and Sinacore JM (1994), "Predicting stroke inpatient rehabilitation outcome using a classification tree approach," *Archives of Physical Medicine and Rehabilitation*,75:619-625.

[18] Manton KG (1988), "A longitudinal study of functional change and mortality in the U.S," *Journal of Gerontological Social Sciences*,43:S153-S161.

[19] Mor, V, Wilcox V, William R, and Jeffrey H (1994), "Functional transitions among the elderly: patterns, predictors and related hospital use," *American Journal of Public Health*84:1274-1280.

Estimation of Subject Means in Fixed and Mixed Models with Application to Longitudinal Data

Edward J. Stanek III *

University of Massachusetts
United States

ABSTRACT The purpose of this paper is to present a clear definition and interpretation of random effects that is consistent with the classical finite population context, and summarize results that identify optimal estimates of random effects. We identify when best linear unbiased predictors should and should not be used for estimating realized random effects. The development is based on traditional frequentist finite population methods, and provides a valuable bridge between frequentist and Bayesian methods. A key aspect of the results is definition of an appropriate sample space for evaluating properties of random effects. We motivate and illustrate these results via a simple example, summarizing more general results.

Key words and phrases: Best linear unbiased predictors, prediction, shrinkage estimator, bias.

1 Introduction

Estimation of linear combinations of fixed and random effects in mixed models is increasingly popular (Littell et al. (1996)). Methods of estimation called best linear unbiased prediction (BLUP) are commonly used for estimating random effects. These methods were developed by Goldberger (1962) and Henderson (1984) and more recently summarized by others (McLean et al. (1991), Robinson (1991), Searle et al. (1992)). Such methods are the basis for computing strategies used in SAS PROC Mixed, as

---

*This work was supported in part by the National Heart Lung and Blood Institute through the Seasons Project, Grant NHLBI-R01-HL4492. Author's address: 404 Arnold House, Department of Biostatistics and Epidemiology, University of Massachusetts, Amherst, MA 01003-0430 U.S.A.

discussed by Wolfinger (1992).

The BLUP estimates of random effects differ from traditional ordinary least squares (OLS) estimates of fixed effects emphasized by Scheffe (1959), Wilk and Kempthorne (1955), Searle (1987, Chapters 1-10), and Hinkelmann and Kempthorne (1994), even though the results of Henderson and others have been discussed by many of these authors (see for example Henderson et al. (1959), and Searle (1987, chapter 11)). Estimation of "random effects" is not discussed in traditional experimental design and linear model texts since their expected value is zero. We motivate comparison of BLUP and OLS estimates of fixed and random effects in a finite population with a simple example.

2 The Dispute

Suppose that a simple random sample of patients is selected from the population of patients in a clinic practice, with the idea of estimating serum cholesterol (SC) levels in the population. For each selected patient, assume that a single independent measure of SC is made. Although primary interest is in the overall average SC level for the population, clinicians would also like to estimate SC levels for each subject selected in the sample. For simplicity, we focus attention on estimating the SC level on one subject, say Harry, who was included in the sample. Although the problem seems simple enough, someone suggests that the clinicians consult a statistician to advise them as to how to best estimate Harry's SC level. Unfortunately, the clinicians make the "mistake" of contacting two statisticians!

One statistician, the "traditional" statistician, proposes using Harry's measure of serum cholesterol to estimate Harry's SC level. This value will be an estimate, not Harry's true SC level, since it is known that SC levels can not be measured without error. The estimate of Harry's SC will differ from Harry's true SC by this measurement error, where past history has shown that σ_e =10 mg/dl. Harry's measure of SC will be an unbiased estimate of his true SC, with variance given by σ_e^2. The estimation approach taken by the first statistician is sensible, and meets with immediate acceptance by the clinicians.

A second statistician, the "modern" statistician, claims that a better estimate of Harry's SC is a weighted average of the overall mean cholesterol in the sample of patients, plus the estimated deviation from that mean of Harry's SC measure. Calling such an estimate a best linear unbiased predictor (BLUP), this statistician claims that the BLUP estimate is closer to the true mean SC for Harry, and hence better. The clinicians have trouble understanding the rational for this approach, asserting that the patients in the sample are unrelated to each other. Why should other patient's SC values affect the estimate of serum cholesterol for Harry? Is there some hidden "biologic" assumption underlying the second estimation approach? The clinicians are suspicious of the second statistician's proposed solution, but resist the temptation to simply disregard the second statistician's advice. Instead they ask the two statisticians to meet and resolve their differences.

This example sets the stage for a heated debate between the two statisticians. The "traditional" statistician rightfully claims that his estimate is unbiased, and for the given subject, has well known optimal properties (BLUE) that clearly demonstrate that the "traditional" estimate is best. Since the "traditional" estimate is unbiased, the "modern" estimate must be biased, so there is obviously something wrong with the "modern" statisticians claim that it is a "best linear unbiased predictor".

The "modern" statistician is sympathetic, but then cites a long list of complicated theoretical papers to support the claim that the "traditional" estimate is inferior. Besides, the BLUP estimates have a Bayesian interpretation which makes them much more general than the traditional estimates. At this point, the conversation breaks down, with the traditional statistician yelling "Subjective!" and the modern statistician shaking her head. Finally, the traditional statistician challenges the modern statistician to "show me" that she is right. The two agree to construct a particularly simple example, evaluate proposed estimators, and see which one is really best.

3 An Example

We consider a simple example corresponding to a study of SC where a simple random sample (without replacement) of $m = 2$ patients is selected from a clinic population of $M = 3$ patients (Sam, Beth and Harry), with $n = 1$ measure made on each selected patient. In the hypothetical example, we assume that the true serum cholesterol levels for the patients are given by 184.9, 192.4, and 222.7 mg/dl, respectively. The true SC values are not observed for patients in the sample since there is measurement error. The measurement error is independent and identically distributed, and limited to take on only two values (-10 or +10) with equal probability. The two statisticians agree that with a population of size 3, there are 3 distinct simple random samples of subjects that can be selected of size 2 and for each sample, 2^2=4 possible patterns of measurement error, or a total of 12 possible sample responses. The results for the 12 samples are given in Table 1. The "traditional" statistician takes as his estimator of Harry's SC the simple measure of SC on Harry, given by $p_1 = Y_{Harry}$. The "modern" statistician takes as her estimator the quantity $p_2 = \overline{Y} + K(Y_{Harry} - \overline{Y})$, where $\overline{Y}$ is the average of the cholesterol levels in the sample, and $K = n\sigma_M^2/(\sigma_e^2+n\sigma_M^2)$, with σ_M^2 representing the variance between true SC levels of patients in the population, where σ_M=20, and σ_e^2 represents the response variance, with σ_e =10.

TABLE 1. Observed Serum Cholesterol Responses for 12 Simple Random Samples

Sample number	Sam (184.9 mg/dl)	Beth (192.4 mg/dl)	Harry (222.7 mg/dl)
1	174.9	182.4	.
2	194.9	182.4	.
3	174.9	202.4	.
4	194.9	202.4	.
5	174.9	.	212.7
6	194.9	.	212.7
7	174.9	.	232.7
8	194.9	.	232.7
9	.	182.4	212.7
10	.	202.4	212.7
11	.	182.4	232.7
12	.	202.4	232.7

The two statisticians focus on the eight sample estimates of SC for Harry (sample numbers 5-12 in Table 1). Upon review of the observed response and BLUP estimates that are summarized in Table 2, the "traditional" statistician exclaims "Ah Ha! Your estimates are biased!". The "modern" statistician, somewhat chagrined, counters, "They may be biased, but they are closer to Harry's true SC." The two agree to compute the variance and mean square error comparing the estimators (Table 3). The mean square error for the traditional estimate of Harry's SC is given by 100, and is larger than the MSE for the BLUP estimates (given by 93.7). Similar results hold for the other patients.

Although the "modern" statistician rests her case, the "traditional" statistician still is bothered by the results in Table 3. After some time, he returns with a second example, this time with $M = 4$ patients in the population (Ira, Xiong, Mark, and Pam), where simple random samples of $m = 3$ patients are selected. True SC values for the patients are 116.7, 116.7, 116.7, and 450.0 mg/dl, respectively, resulting in σ_M=166.7. Measurement error is set identical to the first example. Table 4 summarizes the results of the 32 possible samples for the estimators p_1 and p_2. Once again, the observed response (p_1) is an unbiased estimate of the true SC for a patient, while the BLUP estimate (p_2) is biased. However, when comparing the MSE of the two estimators, the BLUP estimate has smaller MSE only for Ira, Xiong, and Mark, whereas for Pam, the MSE of the simple observed response (p_1) is smaller. "You see," said the traditional statistician, "not only is the BLUP estimate biased, but it also has larger MSE! For Pam the OLS estimate given by her observed response is the best estimate of

TABLE 2. Observed Response and BLUP estimates for Harry from Simple Random Sample with $m = 2$, where Harry's True Serum Cholesterol=222.7 mg/dl

Observed Response	BLUP Estimate	Obs.-True Serum C.	BLUP-True Serum C.
212.7	208.9	-10.0	-13.8
212.7	209.7	-10.0	-13.0
212.7	210.9	-10.0	-11.8
212.7	211.7	-10.0	-11.0
232.7	226.9	10.0	4.2
232.7	227.7	10.0	5.0
232.7	228.9	10.0	6.2
232.7	229.7	10.0	7.0
		Sum: 0.0	-27.2

her SC." We summarize and discuss more general results that lead to these examples next.

4 Populations, Parameters, Sampling and Models

We define the population and parameters, and describe the sampling, models and estimation that lead to the results illustrated in the simple examples in Section 3. Consider a population of $s = 1, ..., M$ subjects, where the kth measure on subject s differs from the expected response, μ_s, by response error, such that $Y_{sk} = \mu_s + e^*_{sk}$. We assume that $E_R[e^*_{sk}] = 0$ for all s and k, and that $E_R[e^*_{sk}, e^*_{sk*}] = \sigma^2_e$ when $k = k*$ for all $s = 1, ..., M$, and zero otherwise. We use the subscript R to denote expectation over response error. These assumptions imply that response error has the same first and second moment for all subjects, and is uncorrelated. The expected responses, μ_s for $s = 1, ..., M$, are fixed parameters in the finite population of M subjects. We define population parameters for the mean and variance in terms of these parameters as $\mu = \sum_{s=1}^{M} \frac{\mu_s}{M}$ and $\sigma^2_M = \sum_{s=1}^{M} \frac{(\mu_s - \mu)^2}{M-1}$.

The population model is often expressed using a different parameterization. We define the subject s effect, β_s, as the difference between the population mean μ, and the expected response for subject s, μ_s, such that $\beta_s = \mu_s - \mu$, noting that by definition, the sum over $s = 1, .., M$ of β_s is zero. Using this parameterization, a model for subject s is given as $Y_{sk} = \mu + \beta_s + e^*_{sk}$. Let $j = 1, ..., m$ index the subject selections in a simple random without replacement sample of size m, and define the indicator random variable $S_j(s)$ to equal one if subject s is the jth subject selected from the population, and zero otherwise. With these definitions, we express a model for the jth selected subject as

TABLE 3. Expected Value, Bias, Variance and MSE for Observed Response (p_1) and BLUP (p_2) estimates of Serum Cholesterol (mg/dl) for $M = 3$ Patients from all possible Simple Random Samples with $m = 2$, where Response Var=100, Pop Var=400

	Sam	Beth	Harry
True SC mg/d	184.9	192.4	222.7
Average $E(p_1)$	184.9	192.4	222.7
Ave BLUP $E(p_2)$	187.1	193.6	219.3
Bias (p_1)	0.0	0.0	0.0
Bias (p_2)	2.3	1.1	-3.4
Var (p_1)	100.0	100.0	100.0
Var (p_2)	84.3	85.6	82.1
MSE (p_1)	100.0	100.0	100.0
MSE (p_2)	89.4	86.9	93.7

$$\sum_{s=1}^{M} S_j(s)Y_{sk} = \sum_{s=1}^{M} S_j(s)\mu_s + \sum_{s=1}^{M} S_j(s)e^*_{sk}$$

or $y_{jk} = \mu + B_j + e_{jk}$ where $B_j = \sum_{s=1}^{M} S_j(s)\beta_s$ and $e_{jk} = \sum_{s=1}^{M} S_j(s)e^*_{sk}$ and where $S_j(s)$ and e^*_{sk} are assumed independent such that $var_R(e^*_{sk}) = var_R(e_{jk})$. We use upper case Y for a particular subject (say subject s), and lower case y for a randomly selected subject (say the jth selected subject), to help maintain the distinction between the two settings. The subject effect B_j is random due to the fact that we don't know in advance which subject will be selected on the jth selection. Note that

$$E_S[B_j] = \sum_{s=1}^{M} E_S[S_j(s)]\beta_s = 0$$

since $E_S[S_j(s)] = \frac{1}{M}$, where we use the subscript S to denote expectation with respect to sampling without replacement. The random variables B_j are commonly called random effects. Using standard finite population sampling results (Cochran, 1977),

$$E_S[S_j(s)S_{j^*}(s^*)] = \begin{cases} \frac{1}{M} & \text{if } s = s^* \text{ and } j = j^* \\ \frac{1}{M(M-1)} & \text{if } s \neq s^* \text{ and } j \neq j^* \\ 0 & \text{otherwise,} \end{cases}$$

implying that

$$var_S(B_j, B_{j^*}) = \begin{cases} \frac{M-1}{M}\sigma_M^2 = \sigma_M^{*2} & \text{if } j = j^* \\ -\frac{1}{M}\sigma_M^2 & \text{if } j \neq j^*. \end{cases}$$

TABLE 4. Expected Value, Bias, Variance and MSE for Observed Response (p_1) and BLUP (p_2) estimates of Serum Cholesterol (mg/dl) for $M = 4$ Patients from all possible Simple Random Samples with $m = 3$, where Response Var=100, Pop Var=27,778 (values rounded)

	Ira	Xiong	Mark	Pam
True SC mg/d	116.7	116.7	116.7	450.0
Average $E(p_1)$	116.7	116.7	116.7	450.0
Ave BLUP $E(p_2)$	116.9	116.9	116.9	449.2
Bias (p_1)	0.0	0.0	0.0	0.0
Bias (p_2)	0.3	0.3	0.3	-0.8
Var (p_1)	100.0	100.0	100.0	100.0
Var (p_2)	99.6	99.6	99.6	99.5
MSE (p_1)	100.0	100.0	100.0	100.0
MSE (p_2)	99.6	99.6	99.6	100.2

Although $E_S[B_j] = 0$ for random effects, $E_S[\beta_s] = \beta_s$ for the fixed effects. With these assumptions and notation, we can summarize a model for n independent measures on each of a simple random sample of m subjects as

$$\mathbf{y} = \mathbf{X}\mu + \mathbf{Z}\mathbf{U} + \mathbf{e}$$

where $\mathbf{y} = (\mathbf{y}_1' \, \mathbf{y}_2' \cdots \mathbf{y}_m')$; $\mathbf{y}_j' = (y_{j1} \, y_{j2} \cdots y_{jn})$; $\mathbf{X} = \mathbf{1_m} \otimes \mathbf{1_n}$; $\mathbf{Z} = \mathbf{I_m} \otimes \mathbf{1_n}$; $\mathbf{U}' = (\mathbf{B}_1 \, \mathbf{B}_2 \ldots \mathbf{B}_m)$; and $\mathbf{e}' = (\mathbf{e}_1' \, \mathbf{e}_2' \ldots \mathbf{e}_m')$; $\mathbf{e}_j' = (e_{j1} \, e_{j2} \ldots e_{jn})$; and var_{SR} $(\mathbf{y}) = \mathbf{\Omega} = \mathbf{Z}\mathbf{G}\mathbf{Z}' + \mathbf{R}$ with $\mathbf{G} = \sigma^2_{\mathbf{M}}[\mathbf{I_m} - \frac{\mathbf{J_m}}{\mathbf{M}}]$ and $\mathbf{R} = \sigma^2_{\mathbf{e}}\mathbf{I_m} \otimes \mathbf{I_n}$.

This is the standard mixed model defined by McLean et al. (1991) and others in a finite population context. If the population of subjects is very large such that $M \to \infty$, the only change in the model is that $\mathbf{G} = \sigma^2_{\mathbf{M}}\mathbf{I_m}$.

5 Estimating Realized Random Effects

In a mixed model, although both B_j and e_{jk} are random variables, we use the term "random effects" to refer only to B_j. The distinction between the random variables is that B_j is random solely due to sampling. Conditional on the selected sample, B_j is no longer a random variable, whereas e_{jk} still is random. This distinction has a long history, and underlies the difference between fixed, mixed, and random effects models in the experimental design literature. A realized random effect corresponds to a selected subject. The part of the model that is realized is the set of indicator random variables that identify the particular subject. For the jth selection, we denote the selected subject by $s_j = \sum_{s=1}^{M} S_j(s)s$ to indicate that $S_j(s) = 1$ when $s = s_j$, and hence that subject s_j was selected. We identify the set of m realized subjects in a sample by $s = \left\{s_j = \sum_{s=1}^{M} S_j(s)s;\ j = 1, \ldots, m\right\}$.

We use a similar notation to represent the realized random effects in the mixed model. For the jth realized subject, we represent the model as $Y_{s_jk} = \mu_{s_j} + e^*_{s_jk}$ denoting the jth realized subject mean as $\mu_{s_j} = \mu_j \mid s = \mu + \beta_{s_j}$. The examples in Section 3 were focused on estimating realized subject means.

There are some simple, but important distinctions that need to be made when discussing and evaluating estimates of realized subject means, as opposed to fixed effects (like μ). First of all, although we can discuss a "realized random effect" generically (for example, as the deviation for a subject that resulted from the jth selection), to interpret an estimate of this effect, we need to focus on the specific realized subject. Thus, our attention for a realized random effect is focused on μ_{s_j} or β_{s_j}, not B_j. In the context of the first example in Section 3, when Harry is a realized subject, we are interested in estimating SC for Harry, and not for the jth selected subject in a sample.

Traditional experimental design literature has not focused on estimating random effects, since the random effects were defined generically (as B_j) and hence have expected value (over S) of zero. In contrast, more recent presentations of mixed models (Searle et al. (1992), Littell et al. (1996)) have extensive discussion of realized random effects, which (while poorly defined), correspond in concept to β_{s_j}.

There are consequences of this distinction. The most obvious consequence is that there is little interest in estimating a "realized random effect" for a subject that is not "realized". The implication is that we will form estimates for a realized subject, s_j, only in samples that include the subject. If we denote the set of samples that include a particular realized subject as S^*, then estimates of the realized random effect will only be made for the $\begin{pmatrix} M-1 \\ m-1 \end{pmatrix}$ samples (S^*) as opposed to the $\begin{pmatrix} M \\ m \end{pmatrix}$ samples (S) formed by all possible selections of subjects. This difference in sample spaces has implication for the definition of estimates of realized random effects, and their evaluation. For example, "unbiased" is a common criteria that is used when developing estimators. The estimator p_1 is derived under the unbiased assumption $E_{S^*R}[p_1] = \mu_{s_j}$, while the BLUP estimator is derived under the unbiased assumption $E_{SR}[p_2] = \mu$, which we refer to as "unconditional unbiased" since unbiased is evaluated over all samples, including samples that do not include the realized random subject (see Stanek and O'Hearn (1996)). It is this difference that leads to the paradox resulting from UNBIASED in the acronym "best linear unbiased predictor (BLUP)" in contrast to "BIAS" when evaluated in Tables 3 and 4. Specifically, conditional on the realized random effect, $E_{S^*R}[p_2] \neq \mu_{s_j}$ as illustrated in the examples.

The difference in sample spaces also has implication for evaluating estimators. Each of the estimators of the realized random effects can be derived as the linear estimator that minimizes the MSE, subject to the unbiased constraints. However, for p_1, the MSE is evaluated with respect to S^* and R, while for p_2 the MSE is evaluated with respect to S and R. The consequence is that each estimator is "best" in the context in which it is derived. These contexts differ due to the difference between the sample space S^* and S. Any comparison of the estimators must be based on the same sample space, and one that is relevant to the goal of the analysis– estimating the parameter for a realized subject. The natural set of samples for comparison is S^*, the set of samples that include the realized random subject. A summary of the properties of the estimators when evaluated over this sample space (as well as others) is given in Table 5, where

$$C_1 = (1-K^2)\left(\frac{m-1}{m}\right)\frac{\sigma_e^2}{n} - (1-K)^2\left(\frac{m-1}{m}\right)\frac{1}{m}\left[\frac{M-m}{M-2}\right]\sigma_M^2$$

and

$$C_2 = -(1-K)^2\left(\frac{m-1}{m}\right)\frac{1}{m}\left(\frac{M}{M-2}\right)\left[m-\left(\frac{M}{M-1}\right)\right].$$

The results indicate that the BLUP estimator is biased, while the OLS estimator is unbiased. Neither estimator has uniformly smaller MSE.

Since the BLUP estimate is biased, we use the MSE evaluated with respect to S^* and R to determine which estimator is best. This difference is given by

$$\Delta(\beta_{s_j}) = MSE_{S^*R}(p_1) - MSE_{S^*R}(p_2) = C_1 + C_2\beta_{s_j}^2.$$

The first term in this expression may be positive, while the second term is negative, indicating that neither estimator has uniformly smaller MSE. Setting the difference to zero, we can evaluate ranges of β_s where the BLUP will have smaller MSE than the OLS estimate . When both M and m are large (ie. $\frac{M}{M-2} \cong 1$, $\frac{m-1}{m} \cong 1$, and $\frac{m}{M-2} \cong 0$), we can ignore the functional dependence of σ_M^2 on β_s and conclude that the BLUP estimate will have smaller MSE whenever $\mid \beta_{s_j} \mid < \sqrt{\frac{\sigma_e^2}{n} + 2\sigma_M^2}$. Similar results when evaluated for finite M and m accounting for the dependence of σ_m^2 on β_s lead to the lack of uniformly smaller MSE for BLUP estimates illustrated in Table 4.

6 Application to the Worcester Seasonal Cholesterol Study

We relate the example to a longitudinal study (the Season study) of $m = 600$ adults in Worchester, MA, with SC measured once each season($n = 4$) on each subject, focusing on winter–summer differences in SC for a realized subject. For simplicity, we assume that $M >> m$, where the true population

TABLE 5. Expected Value, Bias, Variance and MSE of OLS (p_1) and BLUP (p_2) of a Realized Subject over Response error (R), All Samples (S) and Samples containing the Realized Subject (S*). Note: $\phi = (1 - K^2)\left(\frac{m-1}{m}\right)$.

Property	$p_1 = \bar{y}_{s_j}$	$p_2 = \bar{y} + K(\bar{y}_{s_j} - \bar{y})$
E_R	μ_{s_j}	$\mu_{s_j} + (K-1)(\beta_{s_j} - \beta_s)$
var_R	σ_e^2/n	$(\sigma_e^2/n)\,[1-\phi]$
MSE_R	σ_e^2/n	$(\sigma_e^2/n)\,[1-\phi] + (K-1)^2(\beta_{s_j} - \bar{\beta}_s)^2$
E_{SR}	μ	μ
var_{SR}	$\sigma_e^2/n + (\frac{M-1}{M})\sigma_M^2$	$[1-\phi]\,(\sigma_e^2/n) + [\frac{M-1}{M} - \phi]\sigma_M^2$
MSE_{SR}	$var_{SR} + \beta_{s_j}^2$	$[1-\phi]\,(\sigma_e^2/n) + [\frac{M-1}{M} - \phi]\sigma_M^2 + \beta_{s_j}^2$
E_{S*R}	μ_{s_j}	$\mu_{s_j} + (K-1)(\frac{(m-1)M}{(M-1)m})\beta_{s_j}$
var_{S*R}	σ_e^2/n	$\sigma_e^2/n - C_1 + C_2\left(\frac{M-m}{m(M-1)-M}\right)\left(\frac{\beta_{s_j}^2}{M-1}\right)$
MSE_{S*R}	σ_e^2/n	$\sigma_e^2/n - C_1 - C_2\beta_{s_j}^2$

mean SC is 205 mg/dl, with $\sigma_M = 43$, and $\sigma_e = 20$. BLUP estimates of SC based on the four measures will be biased 5% towards the population mean, since $K = 0.95$, but will have smaller MSE than OLS estimates whenever the true SC of the realized subject is within 63 mg/dl of the population mean.

An important goal of the Season study is estimation of the seasonal effect (winter-summer difference in SC) for realized subjects in the study. Conditional on a realized subject, the summer and winter measures of SC can be assumed independent, such that the difference will have within subject variance equal to $2\sigma_e^2 = 800(mg/dl)^2$. At present, although the average seasonal difference (winter-summer) is thought to be 20 mg/dl, little is known about the variance of the latent distribution of seasonal differences. We evaluate the shrinkage factors for these estimators (K) for several possible latent distribution variances (σ_M^2=4, 25, 100, and 400), and the range where BLUP estimates of seasonal difference have smaller MSE. Shrinkage factors for the BLUP estimates with different latent distribution variance are given as 0.005, 0.03, 0.1, and 0.3, respectively. The shrinkage factors are all small, indicating that the study design will have little ability to distinguish individual subject seasonal effects unless they are very large. Next, we evaluate the range of realized random effects (values of β_s) where the BLUP estimates will have smaller MSE. The ranges are given by ±28, ±29, ±31, and ±40 mg/dl, respectively for the various possible latent distribution variances. These ranges correspond to 14, 6, 3, and 2 standard deviations of the corresponding latent distributions. The results indicate that BLUP estimates will have smaller MSE than OLS estimates for virtually all subjects if σ_M^2=5 , 25, or 100, and for the vast majority of subjects (approximately 95 % of subjects if the latent distribution of seasonal differences is normally distributed) when σ_M^2=400.

7 Discussion

The dispute and examples all relate to a very simple problem, but one that identifies core issues in estimating a realized subject's mean response in longitudinal studies, and interpreting the results. A key aspect of results is choice of the sample space for evaluating estimates of realized random effects. As illustrated in Table 1, a given subject (say Harry) will be realized in only a subset of possible samples. We argue that estimates of the realized subject should be evaluated over the set of samples where the subject is realized. This simple notion, which we consider to be self-evident, leads to the conclusion that BLUP estimates have smaller MSE for subjects whose parameters do not differ dramatically from the population mean, but have larger MSE than OLS estimates for subjects whose parameters are far away from the population mean. Thus, when evaluated over the set of samples that contain a realized subject, BLUP estimates are not uniformly best. The results in Table 5 provide a detailed summary of these conclusions, and identify the extent of the differences.

There are many implications from these results. We focus on one important implication, referring broader discussion to Stanek and O'Hearn (1996). The implication is that the traditional understanding of fixed and random effects requires modification. Traditionally, when $m = M$, subject effects have been called "fixed", whereas when $M > m$, subject effects have been called "random". Expressions in Table 5 describe properties of OLS and BLUP estimates for samples of size m from populations of size M. There is no requirement in these expressions that $M > m$, and in fact all expressions can be evaluated when $M = m > 2$. Since the interpretation of a realized random effect is not altered by the finite population size, this implies that the traditional distinction between fixed and random effects is artificial. We can view a vector of M responses as an exchangeable vector of random variables even when $M = m$. Hence, the results imply that BLUP estimates of what have been traditionally referred to as "fixed" effects are better (ie. have smaller MSE) for certain true effects. We consider these results to have far reaching implications for practice.

8 References

[1] Cochran, W. (1977). *Sampling Techniques.* John Wiley and Sons, New York.

[2] Goldberger, A.S. (1962). Best linear unbiased prediction in the generalized linear regression model, *Journal of the American Statistical Association* 57:369-375.

[3] Henderson, C. (1984). *Applications of Linear Models in Animal Breeding*, Guelph, Canada: University of Guelph.

[4] Henderson, C.R., Kempthorne, O., Searle, S.R., and Von Krosigk, C.M. (1959). Estimation of environmental and genetic trends from records subject to culling, *Biometrics*, 15:192-218.

[5] Hinkelmann, K. and Kempthorne, O. (1994). *Design and Analysis of Experiments, Volume I. Introduction to experimental design.* John Wiley and Sons, New York.

[6] Littell, R.C.; Milliken, G.A.; Stroup, W.W.; and Wolfinger, R.D. (1996). *The SAS System for Mixed Models*, SAS Institute, Cary, NC

[7] McLean, R.A., Sanders, W.L. and Stroup, W.W. (1991). A unified approach to mixed linear models, *The American Statistician* 45:54-63.

[8] Robinson, G.K. (1991). That BLUP is a good thing: the estimation of random effects, *Statistical Science* 6:15-51.

[9] Scheffe, H. (1959). *The Analysis of Variance.* John Wiley and Sons, New York.

[10] Searle, S.R. (1987). *Linear Models for Unbalanced Data*, John Wiley and Sons, New York.

[11] Searle, S.R., Casella, G., and McCulloch, C.E. (1992). *Variance Components*, John Wiley, New York.

[12] Stanek, E.J.III and O'Hearn, J.R. (1996). Estimating realized random effects, submitted to *Communications in Statistics.*

[13] Wilk, M.B. and Kempthorne, O. (1955). Fixed, mixed, and random models, *Journal of the American Statistical Association*, 50:1144-1167.

[14] Wolfinger, R. (1992). *A Tutorial on Mixed Models*, SAS Institute, Cary, N.C.

Modeling Toxicological Multivariate Mortality Data: a Bayesian Perspective

Debajyoti Sinha*

University of New Hampshire
United States

Dipak K. Dey and Hui-May Chu

University of Connecticut
United States

ABSTRACT We propose a Bayesian method for the modeling and analysis of toxicological mortality data from large families observed over discrete time periods. The discrete mortality rate for a family of subjects at a given time depends on the time and the common toxic level experienced by the family and the observed value of any other relevant covariate present at that time. Markov Chain Monte Carlo technique is used to find posterior estimates of the model parameters and mortality rates and other several quantities of interest. Further, Bayesian methods are used for several plausible model comparisons. An illustrative example involving the mortality data for several families of fishes in presence of water hardening and added toxic NaScN at different concentration levels is analyzed using our proposed Bayesian methodologies.

Key words and phrases. Gaussian martingale process, linear models, mortality rate, random effects.

---

*Send correspondence to: D. Sinha, Dept. of Mathematics, Univ. of New Hampshire, Durham, NH 03824, USA. E-mail: sinha@purabi.unh.edu . Dr.Sinha's research was supported by the NCI grant R29-CA69222-02.

1 Introduction.

In many toxicological studies, each family of related subjects exposed to a particular level of a toxic material are observed at discrete time points to monitor the effect of the toxin on the mortality rate of the family. In animal toxicological experiment in O'Hara Hines and Lawless (1993), (this will be referred to as OHL), for each of the six levels of toxic NaSCN there were 6 tanks each containing 95 trout fish eggs. The indicator variable of the water hardening was the other available covariate beside the level of NaSCN associated with each of the $n = 36$ tanks. In this experiment, mortality counts for each tank were taken at $t_1 = 1$, $t_2 = 6$, $t_3 = 13$, $t_4 = 20$ and $t_5 = 27$ days after the application of the toxin. In other examples the times of observation of the mortality counts may differ from one family to another.

The dependence within family members makes this problem different from the grouped survival data problem considered by Prentice and Gloeckler (1978), Lawless (1982), Sinha et al. (1993), and etc. The fishes within a tank are related by birth and also through the same shared environment. So, it is unwise to assume that the mortality rates of the fishes within the same family are conditionally independent given the water hardening condition and the level of the toxin the family is exposed to.

Typical multivariate survival models such frailty models (Oakes, 1989) are also neither useful nor computationally feasible in this situation, because the family sizes (95 for fish data) are typically very large compared to the number of families (36 for fish data). We introduce a time-dependent random effects model which allow the familial random effects on the mortality rates to vary over time. Let us define the random mortality rate for the the fishes at risk in I_j at the k-th tank as

$h_{kj} = P\Big(\text{dying in the interval } I_j \text{ at tank k} \mid \text{alive till } t_{j-1}\Big),$

for $k = 1, \cdots, 36$, $j = 1, \cdots, 5$ and $I_j = (t_{j-1}, t_j]$. The number of fishes dying in I_j at the k-th tank out the fishes at risk there is Binomial with random success probability h_{kj}. For an increasing link function η,

$$\eta(h_{kj}) \;=\; \alpha_o + \beta X_k + g_\gamma(t_j) + e_{kj}\ , \tag{1}$$

where g_γ is a known function of time with unknown parameters γ (possibly vector valued), $\beta = (\beta_1, \beta_2)$ are the regression parameters to the covariates X_{1k} (level of toxin in the tank) and X_{2k} (the indicator of water hardening condition of the tank). Here α_0 is the overall mean in (1). Given the e_{kj}'s (the random effects to the mortality rates associated with the fishes at the k-th tank in different time intervals), the fishes within a tank are indendent with each other.

We impose a martingale structure to this time-dependent familial random effects to incorporate the correlation of the mortality rates of a family over time. The discrete gaussian martingale structure of the random effects within a tank is given by

$$e_{k,j+1}|e_{kj},\cdots,e_{k1} \sim N(e_{kj},\sigma_2^2) \tag{2}$$

for $k = 1,\cdots,36$ and $e_{k1} \sim N(0,\sigma_1^2)$. Other suitable distributions besides normal (e.g. scale mixture of normals) can be considered in (2) to relax the gaussian assumption of the martingale. Unlike OHL, we avoid imposing any completely restrictive functional form on the mortality rates of different families.

Higher values of σ_1 imply the existence of higher magnitude of initial heterogeneity among different families. Again, higher values of σ_2^2 signify greater possibility for a big change in the familial effect of the k-th tank in the j-th interval from the familial effect of the the same tank in the previous (j-1)st time interval.

Depending on two different functional forms of $g_\gamma(t)$, we entertain two different models based on the logit link for analyzing this fish tank data. These models are as follows: $\mathcal{M}_1$: logit link with $g_\gamma(t) = \gamma_1 log(t)$;
$\mathcal{M}_2$: logit link with $g_\gamma(t) = \gamma_1 log(t) + \gamma_2(log(t))^2$;

Note that, $\mathcal{M}_1$ and $\mathcal{M}_2$ are random-effects versions of the logistic-hazard model proposed by Efron (1988) for univariate survival data. One may consider other links such as complementary log-log link as alternative models. In the next section, we talk about the likelihood and priors associated with these models. Section 3 deals with Bayesian computation for this problem using MCMC algorithm. Section 4 gives a Bayesian analysis of the OHL's fish tank data. Section 5 deals with the Bayesian model selection methods for this problem.

2 The Likelihood and The Hierarchical Model

Let us denote $\eta(h_{kj})$ by y_{kj}, $(\alpha_0 + \beta\mathbf{X_k} + g_\gamma(t_j))$ by μ_{kj} and the observed data by $\mathbf{D} = \{(d_{kj}, r_{kj}) : k = 1,\cdots,36; j = 1,\cdots,5\}$. Where, d_{kj} is the number of deaths and r_{kj} is the number of subjects at risk in the j-th interval at the k-th tank. The likelihood of the parameters $\mathbf{Y} = \{y_{kj}$: for all k's and j's$\}$ based on the data $\mathbf{D}$ is given by

$$L_1(\mathbf{Y}|\mathbf{D}) \propto \prod_{k=1}^{K}\prod_{j=1}^{m_k}(h_{kj})^{d_{kj}}(1-h_{kj})^{r_{kj}-d_{kj}} . \tag{3}$$

The joint distribution of the random effects, $\mathcal{E} = \{e_{kj} : k = 1,\cdots,36; j = 1,\cdots,5\}$, is derived from (2) as

$$\pi(\mathcal{E}|\sigma_1,\sigma_2) \propto \left[\prod_{k=1}^{K}\phi(e_{k1}|0,\sigma_1^2)\right] \times \left[\prod_{k=1}^{K}\prod_{j=2}^{m_k}\phi(e_{kj}|\ e_{k,j-1},\sigma_2^2)\right] , \tag{4}$$

where $\phi(x|a, b^2)$ is the normal density with mean a and standard deviation b evaluated at x. The likelihood of the parameter vector $\Theta = (\alpha_0, \beta, \gamma, \sigma_1, \sigma_2)$ given the data **D** can be evaluated by multiplying L_1 in (3) with π in (4) and then integrating the vector of random effects. The likelihood is obviously very complicated to evaluate for any of our models. The prior distributions of the other parameters are as follows:

$$\pi(\alpha_0) \sim N(\theta_0, \sigma_0^2); \text{ and } \pi(\beta_i) \sim N(0, \sigma_{\beta i}^2) \text{ for } i = 1,2;$$

$$\pi(\sigma_i^2) \sim IG(a_i, b_i) \text{ for } i = 1,2, \qquad (5)$$

where, $IG(a_i, b_i)$ means $\frac{1}{\sigma_i^2}$ has gamma distribution with mean $\frac{a_i}{b_i}$ and variance $\frac{a_i}{b_i^2}$. All the hyperparameters associated with the above priors are assumed to be known. Though the forms of these prior distributions are chosen primarily to facilitate an easier computational tool, these prior distributions are also found to be often adequate for all practical purposes.

3 Bayesian Computation.

The Gibbs sampling algorithm (Gelfand and Smith 1990; Geyer, 1992; Tanner 1993) is used for this problem to compute the approximate posterior estimates of the mortality rates and the marginal posteriors of the parameters of interest. The Gibbs sampling algorithm is an iterative Markov chain Monte Carlo algorithm to sample from the joint distribution of a vector of random variables, when only the conditional distributions are available to sample from.

For using the Gibbs sampling algorithm, we need the conditional posteriors for each of the parameters and random effects given the rest. We are going to use the notation [parameter|*rest*] to denote the conditional posterior of the particular quantity given the rest of the parameters and random effects and the observed data **D**. For the linear marginal time effect model $\mathcal{M}_1$: $[\alpha_0|rest] \sim N(\mu_\alpha, v_\alpha^2)$, where,

$$\mu_\alpha = \frac{\theta_0\sigma_1^2 + \sum_{k=1}^{36} \sigma_0^2\{y_{k1} - \beta_1 x_{1k} - \beta_2 x_{2k} - \gamma log(t_1)\}}{36\sigma_0^2 + \sigma_1^2}$$

and $v_\alpha^2 = \frac{\sigma_1^2\sigma_0^2}{36\sigma_0^2+\sigma_1^2}$, and $[\beta_i|rest] \sim N(\mu_i, v_i^2)$ for $i = 1,2$, where

$$\mu_i = \frac{\sum_{k=1}^{36} \sigma_{\beta_i}^2\{y_{k1} - \alpha_0 - \beta_j x_{jk} - \gamma log(t_1)\}}{\sigma_1^2 + \sigma_{\beta_i}^2 \sum_{k=1}^{36} x_{ik}^2}$$

and

$$v_i^2 = \frac{\sigma_1^2\sigma_{\beta_i}^2}{\sigma_1^2 + \sigma_{\beta_i}^2 \sum_{k=1}^{36} x_{ik}^2},$$

where j=2 when i=1 and j=1 when i=2. Finally, $[\gamma|rest]$ is also normal with mean

$$\mu_\gamma = \frac{\sigma_\gamma^2 \sum_{k=1}^{36} [t'_1\sigma_2^2(y_{k1} - \mu_k^{(\gamma)}) + \sigma_1^2\{t'_1(y_{k1} - y_{k2}) + t'_5(y_{k5} - y_{k4}) + \sum_{j=2}^4 t'_j y_{kj}^*\}]}{\sigma_\gamma^2\sigma_2^2 t_1'^2 + 36\sigma_\gamma^2\sigma_1^2[\sum_{j=1}^4\{t'_j - t'_{j+1})\}] + \sigma_1^2\sigma_2^2}$$

(where $t' = log(t)$) and variance

$$v_\gamma^2 = \frac{\sigma_1^2\sigma_2^2\sigma_\gamma^2}{36\{t'_1\}^2\sigma_2^2\sigma_\gamma^2 + 36\sigma_1^2\sigma_\gamma^2[\sum_{j=1}^4\{t'_j - t'_{j+1}\}] + \sigma_1^2\sigma_2^2}.$$

Here, $\mu_k^{(\gamma)}$ denotes $(\alpha_0 + \beta_1 x_{1k} + \beta_2 x_{2k})$ and y_{kj}^* denotes $(2y_{kj} - y_{k,j-1} - y_{k,j+1})$ for $j = 2, 3, 4$. The conditional posterior of γ_2 in $\mathcal{M}_2$ and can be evaluated as normal with certain mean and variances with similar expressions.

The conditional posterior of y_{kj} depends on the link function η. For a logit link function and linear time effect in $\mathcal{M}_1$, $[y_{kj}|rest]$ has density proportional to

$$exp\left[-\frac{1}{2\sigma_2^2}\left\{2y_{kj}^2 - 2y_{kj}(\gamma t_j^* + y_{k,j-1} + y_{k,j+1} + \sigma_2^2 d_{kj})\right\}\right] \times (1 + e^{y_{kj}})^{-r_{kj}},$$

where $t_j^* = \{2log(t_j) - log(t_{j-1}) - log(t_{j+1})\}$.

For both models, $[\sigma_1^2|rest]$ is $IG(a_1 + 18\ ,\ b_1 + \frac{1}{2}\sum_{k=1}^{36} e_{k1}^2)$ and $[\sigma_2^2|rest]$ is $IG(a_2 + 18 \times 4,\ b_2 + \frac{1}{2}sum_{k=1}^{36}\sum_{j=1}^4(e_{k,j+1} - e_{kj})^2)$.

4 Results for Fish Tank Data

As an illustration of our Bayesian models and methodologies for multivariate mortality data, we present the results of the re-analysis of the fish tank data of OHL. For this example, as we do not have any substantial prior information about the parameters, we use independent $N(0, 10)$ priors for the parameters $\alpha_0, \beta_1, \beta_2$ and γ, and independent $IG(3, 1000)$ for σ_1 and σ_2. The first two moments of each of these priors exist but the distribution is very flat. In practice, the statistician who will be directly associated with the study from the beginning will be likely to have more precise prior information about the parameters, and hence the statistician will probably choose more informative priors. Here our particular choices of the priors are driven by the objective to make inference solely from the data information.

TABLE 1. Bayes Posterior Estimates For $\mathcal{M}_1$

Parameter	Mean	St. dev.	Median	95% C.I.
α	-3.633	0.600	-3.652	(-4.889,-2.483)
β_1	0.245	0.225	0.258	(-0.197,0.701)
β_2	-0.030	0.093	-0.029	(-0.210,0.163)
γ_1	0.175	0.170	0.169	(-0.176,0.514)
σ_1^2	0.456	0.111	0.438	(0.288,0.717)
σ_2^2	4.468	0.521	4.426	(3.552,5.608)

TABLE 2. Bayes Posterior Estimates For $\mathcal{M}_2$

Parameter	Mean	St. dev.	Median	95% C.I.
α	-4.143	0.584	-4.140	(-5.339,-2.879)
β_1	0.252	0.222	0.253	(-0.198,0.693)
β_2	-0.018	0.089	-0.019	(-0.211,0.164)
γ_1	0.170	0.168	0.169	(-0.155,0.496)
γ_2	0.552	0.110	0.553	(0.332,0.772)
σ_1^2	0.456	0.104	0.436	(0.287,0.717)
σ_2^2	3.971	0.487	3.930	(3.136,5.037)

The approximate means, and medians of the marginal posteriors of different parameters of $\mathcal{M}_1$ are given in Table 1 along with the approximate standard deviations of the marginal posteriors and the 95% credible intervals. These posteriors estimates are obtained from the samples from 5 independent chains of the Gibbs algorithm after 2,000 iterations of each chain. Though, each chain seems to have converged long before 2,000 iterations. The marginal posterior means and standard deviations indicate only moderate evidence of the linear log-time effect on the mortality rates of the groups. The effects of the covariates on the mortality rates are also found to be insignificant, at least from the marginal posteriors of the regression parameters. Definitely the marginal posteriors of σ_1 and σ_2 indicates strong evidence of dispersion among families and variability of these familial effects over time.

Table 2 indicates that under the logit link, inclusion of the new term in $g_\gamma(t)$ does not have much effect on the marginal posteriors of the covariate effects and the linear term in time. The marginal credible region for each of those parameters still contains 0. The marginal posterior of σ_1 is also nearly unchanged from the marginal posterior of the σ_1 under $\mathcal{M}_1$. But, both the posterior mean and the standard deviations of σ_2 are lower under this new model compared to $\mathcal{M}_1$. This suggests that under the new model the group effects in adjacent intervals are less fluctuating compared to those under $\mathcal{M}_1$. Also, the marginal posterior estimate of the quadratic term suggests a significant quadratic log-time effect on the mortality rate.

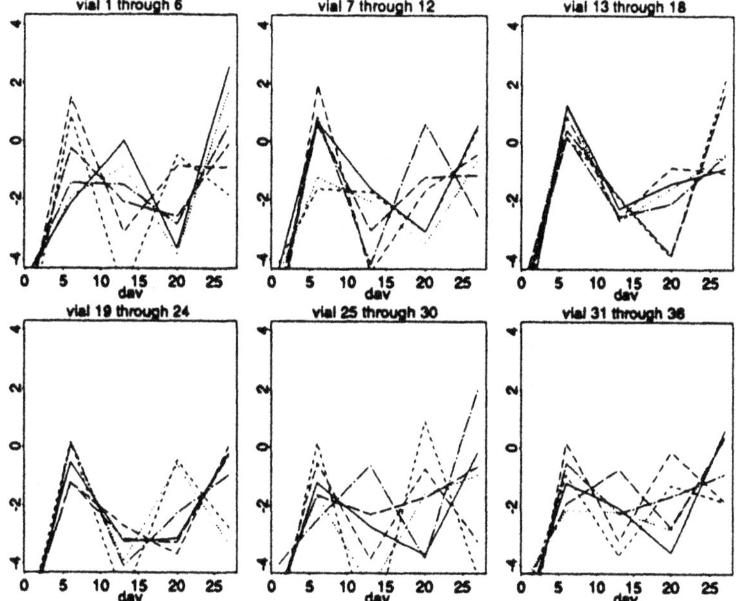

FIGURE 1. Bayesian Residual Plots for 36 families under $\mathcal{M}_1$

Figure 1, the residual plot associated with $\mathcal{M}_1$, shows high negative residuals at initial time points and the magnitudes of the residuals are found to be decreasing and leveling of over time. This pattern of residuals indicate a possible time quadratic model. Figure 2 shows that after including the quadratic component of time in the model the residuals are now smaller in magnitude and the fit is particularly better at early time points. In practice, there may be huge number of choices for possible model of the time trend (e.g. polynomials of different orders and even splines of different orders). These plots may at least suggest, from this extremely large class of possible models, which models we

should compare with each other using formal Bayesian procedures. For this problem, more formal methods of Bayesian model determination are developed in the next section.

5 Bayesian Model Selection.

A good Bayesian analysis should include at least some method to compare different competing models. Here, we propose a model selection method using criterion based on Bayes factor (Kass and Raftery, 1995).

Suppose that there m models $M_1, M_2, \ldots, M_m$ in our consideration. De-

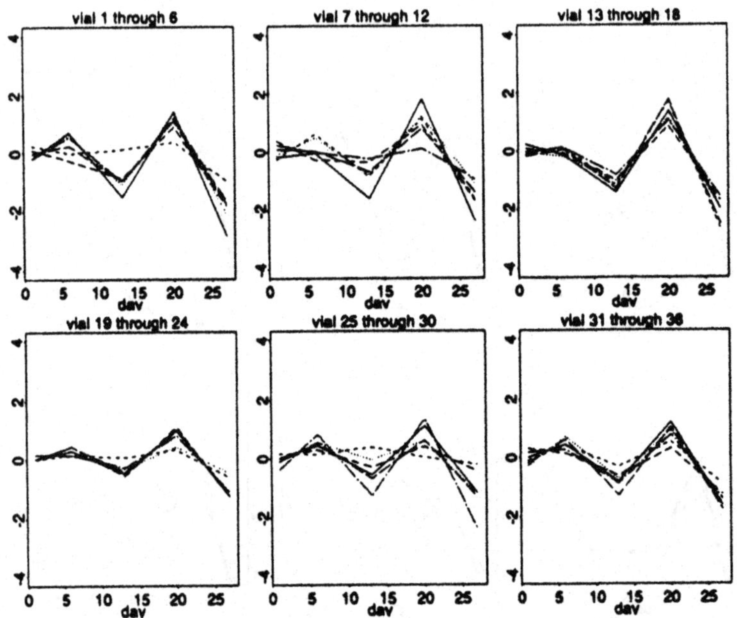

FIGURE 2. Bayesian Residual Plots for 36 families under $\mathcal{M}_2$

note $f(\Theta|y_{obs}, M_i)$ to be the posterior distribution for model M_i. Here, for the sake of simplicity we use the same notation, i.e., Θ, to denote all parameters for each model. However, in our application, the dimension of Θ vary from model to model. Also denote $f(y_{obs}|M_i)$ to be the marginal likelihood for model M_i, that is,

$$f(y_{obs}|M_i) = \int f(\Theta|y_{obs}, M_i)d\Theta \tag{6}$$

then, a Bayes factor for comparing models i and i^* is defined as

$$B_{ii^*} = \frac{f(y_{obs}|M_i)}{f(y_{obs}|M_{i^*})}. \tag{7}$$

The posterior model probability of model M_i can be calculated as

$$P(M_i|y_{obs}) = \frac{f(y_{obs}|M_i)P(M_i)}{\Sigma_{i^*=1}^{m} f(y_{obs}|M_{i^*})P(M_{i^*})} \tag{8}$$

where $P(M_i)$ denotes the prior probability of model M_i. When the prior information for model M_i is not available, $P(M_i)$ is typically chosen to be $1/m$. Therefore, model M_i is preferred over M_{i^*} when $B_{ii^*} > 1$; see Kass and Raftery (1995) for detailed discussion. In the context of model comparison, we choose the model which yields the largest posterior probability $P(M_i|y_{obs})$.

Recently, many effective simulation based Monte Carlo methods for computing a Bayes factor or model posterior probabilities have been developed, which include bridge sampling, path sampling, a data-augmentation-based method to estimate the marginal density, ratio importance sampling, and computing Bayes factor with different dimensions of model parameter spaces.

In this article, the calculation of Bayes factor is done by adopting the data-augmentation-based approach of Chib (1995), which exploits the fact that marginal density can be expressed as the prior times the likelihood function over the posterior density. An estimate of the posterior density can be obtained, since all complete conditional densities used in the Gibbs sampler have closed-form expressions and the posterior density is also estimated at a high density point to improve accuracy.

We write the posterior density at the selected point as

$$\pi(\Theta^*|Y) \;=\; \pi(\Theta_1^*|Y) \times \pi(\Theta_2^*|Y, \Theta_1^*) \times \ldots \times \pi(\Theta_B^*|Y, \Theta_1^*, \ldots, \Theta_{B-1}^*) \ ,$$

where B is the number of parameter in the model, then the log of the marginal likelihood is

$$\ln\hat{m}(Y) \;=\; \ln f(Y|\Theta^*) + \ln\pi(\Theta^*) - \sum_{r=1}^{B} \ln\hat{\pi}(\Theta_r^*|Y, \Theta_{s(s<r)}^*) \ .$$

To compute the Bayes factor for the two models, that is, $m(Y|M_1)/m(Y|M_2)$, the following estimate is used :

$$\hat{B}_{12} \;=\; \exp\{\ln\hat{m}(Y|M_1) - \ln\hat{m}(Y|M_2)\} \ .$$

We found that the $\mathcal{M}_2$ with quadratic effect in time is the more preferable model among the two.

6 Concluding Remarks.

There are already some models available for overdispersed multinomial data. Some of the more appropriate ones among these models are mentioned by OHL. First, one of these models is the Dirichlet-multinomial model (McCullagh and Nelder, 1989). The main advantages of our present model over the Dirichlet-multinomial model are in two aspects. Unlike our model, Dirichlet-multinomial model can not be used to model the mortality-rate h_{kj}. Secondly, the plots of estimated π_{kj}'s for different groups from Dirichlet-multinomial model tend to cross each other too frequently. For an individual from the k-th group, π_{kj} is defined as the probability of dying in the time interval I_j.

After recognizing the limitations of the Dirichlet-multinomial model, OHL proposed at least three more models for the fish data. The main idea behind these models is to build overdispersion with the basic model,

$$\eta(\pi_{kj}) = \mu_o + \beta X_k + \tau_{\nu_k}(t_j) , \tag{9}$$

where $\tau(\cdot)$ is known function of time with unknown parameter vector ν_k. OHL developed three models using a constant, linear and quadratic function of time as τ. In their models, the ν_k's are different for each group. A random effect version of this kind of model can be expressed as $\nu_k = \nu_0 + e_k$, where e_k's are i.i.d. univariate (if τ is a constant function) or multivariate random variables (if τ is either linear or quadratic). The estimates of the π_{kj}'s for different groups in OHL's models do not cross with each other frequently. But, this model allows the response times of a family to have only a constant shift. Say, when τ is linear, this model will allow only the scale and location shifts of the response time for each family. Our new model will allow the flexibility to have any kind of change in the response time of each family, but it will also allow the change to be somewhat smooth over time and avoid too jaggered changes in the response time for each family.

Another disadvantage of OHL's model and analysis are that they use the Taylor's series expansion of the model to get an approximate expression of the covariance structure which is then used for inference. But, when the τ is more complicated as splines, the approximate expressions for the covariance matrices are difficult to obtain. In many practical situations, especially when m_k's (number of observation times) are moderately large, data may suggest a spline model for the response time. Even in our analysis with quadratic model for the mortality rate, the Figure 2 shows that most of the e_{kj}'s are positive for observation time 13 and many of the e_{kj}'s are negative for observation times 20 and 27. This may suggest that even the quadratic model may not be too satisfactory. If this data would have even a couple of observations between 20 and 27 then a spline model would have been warrantied.

Our model in (1), is very appropriate when each family has relatively large number of subjects compared to the number of time points of observation and the total number of families under study. For such data sets, we have lot of informations about the variability among families at every time point as the data from each family contribute substantial information on the mortality rate for that family at each of these few time points. The model in (1) also permits the marginal mortality rate of each family to vary over time from other families without forcing the marginal mortality rates to cross each other too many times.

7 REFERENCES

[1] Chib, S. (1995). Marginal likelihood from the Gibbs output. *J. Amer. Statist. Assoc.*, **90**, 1313-1321.

[2] Efron, B. (1988). Logistic regression, survival analysis, and the Kaplan-Meier curve. *J. Amer. Statist. Assoc.*, **83**, 414-424.

[3] Gelfand, A. E. and Smith, A. F. M. (1990). Sampling based approaches to calculating marginal densities. *J. Amer. Statist. Assoc.*, **85**, 398-409.

[4] Geyer, C. J. (1992). Practical Markov chain Monte Carlo. *Statist. Sc.* **7**, 473-483.

[5] Kass, R. E. and Raftery, A. E. (1995). Bayes factors. *J. Amer. Statist. Assoc.*, **90**, 773-795.

[6] Lawless, J. F. (1982) *Statistical Models and Methods for Lifetime Data.* Wiley: New York.

[7] Oakes, D. (1989). Bivariate survival models induced by frailties. *J. Amer. Statist. Assoc.*, **84**, 487-493.

[8] O'Hara Hines, R. J. and Lawless, J. F. (1993), Modelling overdispersion in toxicological mortality data grouped over time. *Biometrics*, **49**, 107-122.

[9] Prentice, R. L. and Gloeckler, L. A. (1978), Regression analysis of grouped survival data with application to breast cancer data. *Biometrics*, **34**, 57-67.

[10] Sinha, D., Tanner, M. A. and Hall, W. J. (1993), Maximization of the marginal likelihood of grouped survival data. *Biometrika*, **81**, 53-60.

[11] Tanner, M. A. (1993). Tools for Statistical Inference: Observed Data and Data Augmentation Methods. *Lecture Notes in Statistics*, Springer-Verlag.

Comparison of Methods for General Nonlinear Mixed-Effects Models

Thérèse A. Stukel* and Eugene Demidenko

Dartmouth Medical School
United States

ABSTRACT We extend the usual nonlinear mixed-effects model (Lindstrom and Bates, 1990) to analyze either a subset of the individual regression parameters or a characteristic of the curve, when the characteristic is expressed as a nonlinear function of the individual regression curve parameters. We also compare methods of estimation for these models proposed by Lindstrom and Bates (1990), Vonesh and Carter (1992), and a two-stage estimator proposed by Pocock et al. (1981) and Berkey and Laird (1986). Based on simulations, when the model is correctly specified, the Lindstrom-Bates estimators have the smallest bias and MSE, and when the model is misspecified, the two-stage estimators are optimal. Unless the random effects enter linearly and the variances are small, the Vonesh-Carter method produces biased estimates and standard errors. In addition, the two-stage method can easily analyze characteristics of the regression curve without resorting to reparametrization. We apply these results to a study of factors affecting small cell carcinoma of the lung (SCCL) tumor growth in mice.

Key words and phrases: Longitudinal data, random effects, tumor growth.

1 Introduction

Longitudinal analyses have been used in both human and animal studies in a variety of biomedical applications such as tumor biology, pharmacokinetics and dose-response analyses. Techniques for the analysis of linear mixed-effects models with normal errors are well established (Laird and Ware, 1982). Estimation for nonlinear mixed-effects models is considerably more

---

*The authors are grateful to Nan Laird, Ed Vonesh, Bob Glynn and Mark Segal for useful suggestions and O. Pettengill for use of her data. This work was supported by National Cancer Institute grant CA52192. Corresponding author address: Thérèse Stukel, Dartmouth Medical School, 7927 Strasenburgh, Hanover, NH 03755-3861

complex. A major problem is that the marginal likelihood consists of functions containing integrals that do not often have a closed form expression. To circumvent this problem, several authors have proposed approximate estimation methods. Their statistical properties have been investigated by Vonesh and Carter (1992) and Demidenko (1997).

In this paper, we extend the usual nonlinear mixed-effects model to analyze either a subset of the individual regression parameters, or a characteristic of the curve that can be expressed as a function of the original regression parameters. We explore the practical implications of the asymptotic conditions for consistency and efficiency by comparing three methods of estimation under a variety of conditions.

2 General Nonlinear Mixed-Effects Model

We denote the repeated observations for subject i as $(y_{ij}, \mathbf{x}_{ij})$, $j = 1, ..., n_i$, $i = 1, \ldots, N$. The y_{ij} are serial measurements and $\mathbf{x}_{ij}$ is an $m \times 1$ vector of within-subject covariates. The within-subjects regression curve is written as

$$\mathbf{y}_i = \mathbf{f}_i(\mathbf{X}_i; \mathbf{a}_i) + \boldsymbol{\epsilon}_i, \quad i = 1, \ldots, N, \tag{1}$$

where $\mathbf{y}_i = (y_{i1}, \ldots, y_{in_i})'$, $\mathbf{X}_i = (\mathbf{x}_{i1}, \ldots, \mathbf{x}_{in_i})'$ is a matrix of within-subject covariates, $\mathbf{f}_i$ is a known nonlinear vector function and $\mathbf{a}_i = (a_{i1}, \ldots, a_{im})'$ is an $m \times 1$ vector of random parameters with unknown marginal means $\boldsymbol{\alpha}_i$ and covariance matrix $\boldsymbol{\Omega}$. The $\boldsymbol{\epsilon}_i$ are independent normal errors with zero means and covariance matrix $\sigma^2\mathbf{I}$. In the usual nonlinear mixed-effects model, the effect of population covariates on the individual regression parameters $\mathbf{a}_i$ is expressed through the second-stage model,

$$\mathbf{a}_i = \mathbf{Z}_i\boldsymbol{\beta} + \mathbf{b}_i, \tag{2}$$

where $\mathbf{Z}_i$ is an $m \times r$ between-subjects design matrix of population covariates such that $\sum_i \mathbf{Z}_i'\mathbf{Z}_i$ is nonsingular, $\boldsymbol{\beta}$ is an $r \times 1$ vector of population parameters and $\mathbf{b}_i$ are independent, normal errors with zero means and covariance matrix $\boldsymbol{\Omega}$ (Lindstrom and Bates, 1990). A model is specified for all parameters in the second stage, whether or not these are meaningful.

In the general nonlinear mixed-effects model that we propose, the parameters of interest are denoted as the $k \times 1$ subvector $\mathbf{a}_{i1}$, where $\mathbf{a}_i' = (\mathbf{a}_{i1}', \mathbf{a}_{i2}')$, $k \leq m$. The second stage model is written as

$$\mathbf{a}_{i1} = \mathbf{Z}_{i1}\boldsymbol{\beta}_1 + \mathbf{b}_{i1}, \tag{3}$$

where $\mathbf{Z}_{i1}$ is the $k \times p$ submatrix of $\mathbf{Z}_i$ corresponding to the $\mathbf{a}_{i1}$ with $\sum_i \mathbf{Z}_{i1}'\mathbf{Z}_{i1}$ nonsingular, $\boldsymbol{\beta}_1$ is a $p \times 1$ vector of population parameters and the $\mathbf{b}_{i1}$ are independent, normal errors with zero means and covariance matrix $\boldsymbol{\Omega}_{11}$, where $\boldsymbol{\Omega}_{11}$ is the submatrix of $\boldsymbol{\Omega}$ corresponding to the $\mathbf{a}_{i1}$.

The model for the remaining regression parameters $\mathbf{a}_{i2}$ is left unspecified. The general nonlinear mixed-effects model (1, 3) is identical to the usual model (1, 2) when $k = m$ and $p = r$. It is also possible to collapse (3) to (2) by specifying the marginal mean of the $\mathbf{a}_{i2}$; however, the general model is more flexible because it does not require making such assumptions. Model (1, 3) is similar in form to the general linear growth curve model proposed by Stukel and Demidenko (1997).

3 Estimation Methods

The likelihood function for the mixed-effects models can be written in terms of the marginal density of $\mathbf{y}$, $p(\mathbf{y}) = \int p(\mathbf{y}|\mathbf{b})p(\mathbf{b})d\mathbf{b}$. Since the marginal expectation of $\mathbf{y}$ is a nonlinear function of $\mathbf{b}$, there is no closed form expression for this density, leading to computational problems during estimation (Pinheiro and Bates, 1995). To circumvent this problem, alternative methods, described below, have been proposed.

3.1 Lindstrom-Bates Method

Lindstrom and Bates (1990) proposed an estimation procedure for model (1, 2) that produces maximum likelihood estimators for a linear mixed-effects model when the expectation function is linear, and the usual nonlinear least squares estimator when there are no random effects. It assumes model (1, 2) and requires specification of a model for all regression parameters $\mathbf{a}_i$. Estimation consists of a penalized nonlinear least squares step to estimate $\boldsymbol{\beta}$ and $\mathbf{b}_i$, conditional on σ^2 and $\boldsymbol{\Omega}$, and a linear mixed-effects step to estimate σ^2 and $\boldsymbol{\Omega}$, based on a first-order Taylor expansion of the model about the current estimates of $\boldsymbol{\beta}$ and $\mathbf{b}$. These steps are iterated until convergence. Details concerning implementation of the algorithm are given by Pinheiro and Bates (1995).

3.2 Vonesh-Carter Method

Due to the computational problems inherent in $\mathbf{f}_i$ being a nonlinear function of $\mathbf{b}_i$, Vonesh and Carter (1992) considered a nonlinear mixed-effects model that is linear in the random effects,

$$\mathbf{y}_i = \mathbf{f}_i(\mathbf{X}_i, \mathbf{Z}_i, \boldsymbol{\beta}) + \mathbf{A}_i\mathbf{b}_i + \boldsymbol{\epsilon}_i. \tag{4}$$

When $\mathbf{A}_i = \partial\mathbf{f}_i/\partial\mathbf{b}_i|_{\mathbf{b}_i=\mathbf{0}}$, (4) is a first-order approximation to model (1, 2). For model (4), Vonesh and Carter developed a noniterative estimation procedure that consists of a generalized weighted nonlinear least squares estimator for $\boldsymbol{\beta}$ and moment estimators for the variance parameters. They have shown that the resulting estimator $\widehat{\boldsymbol{\beta}}$ is consistent, asymptotically efficient, and normally distributed for model (4) when $N \to \infty$ and $n_i \to \infty$. Demidenko (1997), however, has shown that $\widehat{\boldsymbol{\beta}}$ is inconsistent for a model where the random effects enter the model nonlinearly, as in (1, 2).

3.3 Two-Stage Estimation Procedure

Several authors have proposed a two-stage method of estimation based on the two-stage model used to describe the response (Pocock, Cook and Beresford, 1981; Steimer et al., 1984; Berkey and Laird, 1986). The method is computationally simple and has intuitive appeal. The estimation procedure is implemented in two stages. First, one estimates the individual regression parameters $\hat{\mathbf{a}}_i^o$ from model (1) using nonlinear least squares (Bates and Watts, 1988). In the second step, one regresses the $\widehat{\mathbf{a}}_i^o$ on the $\mathbf{Z}_i$ in (2), weighting by the inverse marginal variance of $\widehat{\mathbf{a}}_i^o$, denoted $\mathbf{M}_i^{-1}$. These steps lead to the two-stage estimator of $\boldsymbol{\beta}$,

$$\widehat{\boldsymbol{\beta}}= \left(\sum\nolimits_i \mathbf{Z}_i'\mathbf{M}_i^{-1}\mathbf{Z}_i\right)^{-1} \left(\sum\nolimits_i \mathbf{Z}_i'\mathbf{M}_i^{-1}\widehat{\mathbf{a}}_i^o\right), \tag{5}$$

where $\mathbf{M}_i = E(var(\widehat{\mathbf{a}}_i^o \mid \mathbf{a}_i))+var(E(\widehat{\mathbf{a}}_i^o \mid \mathbf{a}_i)) = \mathbf{V}_i+\boldsymbol{\Omega}$. $\widehat{\mathbf{V}}_i \approx \widehat{\sigma}^2(\mathbf{G}_i'\mathbf{G}_i)^{-1}$ is the approximate variance of $\widehat{\mathbf{a}}_i^o$ from model (1), $\widehat{\sigma}^2$ is the pooled within-subjects mean square error from model (1) and $\mathbf{G}_i = \partial\mathbf{f}_i/\partial\mathbf{a}_i \,|_{\hat{\mathbf{a}}_i^o}$ (Bates and Watts, 1988).

An estimator for the random effects variance $\boldsymbol{\Omega}$ based on maximum likelihood was proposed by Pocock et al. (1981) and later generalized to the multivariate situation by Berkey and Laird (1986). For one parameter, $\mathbf{a}_i = a_i$, the following recurrence formula for ω was suggested.

$$\omega_{k+1} = \omega_k \frac{\sum_i(\widehat{a}_i^o - \mathbf{z}_i'\widehat{\boldsymbol{\beta}})^2(\widehat{v}_i + \omega_k)^{-2}}{\sum_i(\widehat{v}_i + \omega_k)^{-1}}, \quad k = 0, 1, \ldots \tag{6}$$

where $\omega_0 = N^{-1}\sum_i[(\widehat{a}_i^o - \mathbf{z}_i'\widehat{\boldsymbol{\beta}}^o)^2 - \widehat{\sigma}^2]$ is an initial estimate of ω and $\widehat{\boldsymbol{\beta}}^o = (\sum_i \mathbf{z}_i\mathbf{z}_i')^{-1}(\sum_i \mathbf{z}_i\widehat{a}_i^o)$ is the ordinary least squares estimator of $\boldsymbol{\beta}$. To obtain the two-stage estimator of $\boldsymbol{\beta}$, one first computes $\widehat{a}_i^o$, $\widehat{\sigma}^2$, ω_0 and $\widehat{\boldsymbol{\beta}}^o$ and then iterates between (6) and (5) until convergence.

4 Comparison of Methods via Simulation

To compare the performance of the three methods, we simulated growth curve data under various conditions, and assessed the effects of second stage model misspecification. We investigated two different growth curves, the Gompertz,

$$y_{it} = a_0 \exp(-\exp(-a_1(t - a_2))) + e_{it}, \quad t = 1, \ldots, n_i, \; i = 1, \ldots, 100,$$

and the modified exponential,

$$y_{it} = a_0 - \exp(-a_1(t - a_2)) + e_{it}, \quad t = 1, \ldots, n_i, \quad i = 1, \ldots, 100.$$

Two different second stage models were simulated for each growth curve. In the first, only a_{i1}, which was related to rate of growth, was affected by treatment ($z_i = 0$ or 1):

$$E\begin{pmatrix} a_{i0} \\ a_{i1} \\ a_{i2} \end{pmatrix} = \begin{pmatrix} 1 & 0 & 0 & 0 \\ 0 & 1 & z_i & 0 \\ 0 & 0 & 0 & 1 \end{pmatrix} \begin{pmatrix} \beta_1 \\ \beta_2 \\ \beta_3 \\ \beta_4 \end{pmatrix}. \tag{7}$$

In the second, a_{i0} was also affected by age:

$$E\begin{pmatrix} a_{i0} \\ a_{i1} \\ a_{i2} \end{pmatrix} = \begin{pmatrix} 1 & age_i & 0 & 0 & 0 \\ 0 & 0 & 1 & z_i & 0 \\ 0 & 0 & 0 & 0 & 1 \end{pmatrix} \begin{pmatrix} \beta_0 \\ \beta_1 \\ \beta_2 \\ \beta_3 \\ \beta_4 \end{pmatrix}. \tag{8}$$

Age was continuous (range, 20 to 70 years) and uncorrelated with treatment for the Gompertz models; it was binary (<45, 45+ years) and correlated with treatment for the modified exponential models.

We used the three different methods to analyze the treatment effect for both types of growth curves and for models (7) and (8). We ignored the effect of age on α_{i0} and assumed only that treatment affected the rate of growth a_{i1}. All three methods correctly specified the dependence of a_{i1} on treatment. Differences among methods occurred in the models for the secondary parameters that were not of interest in the analysis, a_{i0} and a_{i2}. The usual mixed-effects model (1, 2) proposed by Lindstrom and Bates included a population mean for a_{i0} and a_{i2}. The general model (1, 3) ignored a_{i0} and a_{i2} and assumed only that $E(a_{i1}) = \beta_2 + \beta_3 z_i$. The Vonesh-Carter method requires a special form of design matrix $\mathbf{Z}_i$ whereby the model for each growth curve parameter is identical, even though the effects of treatment on a_{i0} and a_{i2} were not significant. The detailed models are given in Stukel and Demidenko (1997).

We generated data with a small number of observations per individual, 12 (Gompertz curve) or 17 (modified exponential curve). In the unbalanced case, length of followup varied randomly between times 6 and 11 (Gompertz) or 8 and 16 (modified exponential). The individual regression parameters were either marginally correlated ($r = .8$) or uncorrelated. For each set of conditions, we generated 100 data sets, each consisting of $N = 100$ growth curves. Tables 1 and 2 report the percent relative bias in the treatment effect $\widehat{\beta}_3$, the empirical and model-based standard errors of $\widehat{\beta}_3$, and the ratio of the MSE of each estimate with respect to the usual nonlinear mixed-effects model (Lindstrom-Bates) estimate.

TABLE 1. Results of the Simulation Study to Compare Estimates of Treatment Effect β_3 using the Gompertz Growth Curve From Three Nonlinear Mixed-Effects Models Under Different Conditions. The true $\beta_3 = 1.2$.

Data	Method*	% Rel. Bias	Empir. $SE(\widehat{\beta}_3)$	Model-Based $SE(\widehat{\beta}_3)$	MSE/ MSE(LB)
		True Model (7)			
Balan./ $r = .8$	2-S	-24.4	.106	.093	9.2
	VC	-84.6	.089	.090	98.1
	LB	1.7	.101	.092	1.0
Unbal./ $r = .8$	2-S	-32.2	.129	.120	5.0
	VC	-83.5	.208	.123	31.2
	LB	5.4	.171	.133	1.0
		True Model (8)			
Balan./ $r = .8$	2-S	-2.7	.036	.034	0.6
	VC	-51.4	.085	.077	99.6
	LB	0.6	.062	.029	1.0
Unbal./ $r = .8$	2-S	-2.8	.046	.047	0.1
	VC	-46.6	.238	.094	16.1
	LB	12.3	.034	.040	1.0

*2-S refers to the Two-Stage, VC to the Vonesh-Carter, LB to the Lindstrom-Bates Estimation Methods

When the true model is (7), the usual nonlinear mixed-effects model (1, 2), and thus the LB model, is correct. Accordingly, the LB method produces nearly unbiased estimates and the smallest MSE. The two-stage and VC estimates are biased. When the true model is (8), both the LB and the VC methods misspecify the model for a_{i0}. The two-stage method, which ignores the model for a_{i0}, is nearly unbiased and has smallest MSE. The effect on bias of ignoring age can be pronounced for the VC estimates.

In both situations, the LB and two-stage methods produced comparable and valid standard errors. Standard errors from the VC method were usually larger than those from the other two methods, and were underestimates of the true standard errors. Adjusting the estimate of Ω for the LB method when it became non positive-definite did not materially change these results. Lack of correlation of the growth curve parameters (results not shown) and lack of balance had no effect on these results.

TABLE 2. Results of the Simulation Study to Compare Estimates of Treatment Effect β_3 using the Modified Exponential Growth Curve From Three Nonlinear Mixed-Effects Models Under Different Conditions. The true $\beta_3 = 0.03$.

Data	Method*	% Rel. Bias	Empir. SE($\widehat{\beta}_3$)	Model-Based SE($\widehat{\beta}_3$)	MSE/ MSE(LB)
			True Model (7)		
Balan./	2-S	-27	.007	.007	1.9
$r = .8$	VC	5.5	.031	.016	17
	LB	3.1	.008	.006	1.0
Unbal./	2-S	-35	.008	.007	3.2
$r = .8$	VC	-3.4	.027	.013	14
	LB	2.5	.007	.012	1.0
			True Model (8)		
Balan./	2-S	-.08	.003	.004	0.5
$r = .8$	VC	2.1	.008	.006	3.0
	LB	6.0	.004	.003	1.0
Unbal./	2-S	-2.0	.004	.004	0.5
$r = .8$	VC	-8.9	.011	.006	3.9
	LB	7.9	.005	.004	1.0

*2-S refers to the Two-Stage, VC to the Vonesh-Carter, LB to the Lindstrom-Bates Estimation Methods

5 Model for Characteristics of Nonlinear Regession Curves

Model (1, 3) can be further generalized to analyze a characteristic of the curve, defined as a nonlinear function of the individual regression parameters, $c_i = c(\mathbf{a}_i)$, where c is a nonlinear function. The effects of population covariates on this characteristic can be written,

$$c_i = \mathbf{z}_i'\beta + b_i, \tag{9}$$

similarly to model (3). This model lends itself naturally to the two-stage method of estimation described previously. The two-stage estimator is written (5) as before, replacing $\widehat{a}_i^o$ by $\widehat{c}_i^o$ and $\widehat{v}_i$ by $\widehat{u}_i$, where $\widehat{u}_i = E(var(\widehat{c}_i^o|c_i)) \approx \widehat{\sigma}^2\mathbf{d}_i'(\mathbf{G}_i'\mathbf{G}_i)^{-1}\mathbf{d}_i$, and $\mathbf{d}_i = \partial c/\partial \mathbf{a}_i \mid_{\widehat{\mathbf{a}}_i^o}$, using a first-order Taylor expansion of $\mathbf{f}_i$ about $\widehat{c}_i^o$ (Bates and Watts, 1988). Because the LB and VC methods consider only models for the $\mathbf{a}_i$, model (1, 9) cannot easily be analyzed using these methods without resorting to a reparametrization of the original nonlinear regression curve (1).

TABLE 3. **Analysis of the Effects of Cell Line on the "Growth Rate" a_1 of SCCL Tumors in Mice Using Three Estimation Methods.**

Cell Line	$\widehat{\beta} \pm SE(\widehat{\beta})$		
	LB*	2-S*	VC*
DMS79	.041±.004	.031±.003	.028±.004
DMS114	.050±.004	.049±.004	.048±.013
DMS92	.045±.006	.050±.008	.040±.011
DMS153	.042±.004	.045±.003	.035±.005

***2-S refers to the Two-Stage, VC to the Vonesh-Carter, LB to the Lindstrom-Bates Estimation Methods**

6 Factors affecting SCCL tumor growth in mice

Experimental studies of tumor growth in an animal model system can elucidate the pathobiology of human tumor cell types. Pettengill et al. (1980) inoculated nude, athymic mice with four established cell lines of small cell carcinoma of the lung (SCCL). Mice were treated with intraperitoneal injections of antilymphocyte serum (ALS), antithymocyte serum (ATS) or not at all (controls), to assess the effect of increased immunosuppression on tumor growth of the naturally immunodeficient mice. After the appearance of the tumors, volume was measured weekly in three dimensions with calipers.

The resulting growth curves are plotted in Figure 1 by sex and cell line. We fitted the following modified exponential growth curve to the serial tumor volumes from each mouse,

$$y_{it} = a_0(\exp(a_1 t) - 1) + e_{it}, \quad t = 1, \ldots, n_i, \; i = 1, \ldots, 161,$$

and assessed the effects of cell line on the "growth rate" a_1. The regression parameters and standard errors from the three estimation methods were similar (Table 3).

Using the two-stage estimator, we also studied the effects of sex, treatment and cell line on second quadrupling time, or time for the tumor to grow from 0.4 to 1.6 cm^3, a nonlinear characteristic of the curve defined as $a_1^{-1} \log((1.6 + a_0)/(0.4 + a_0))$. Our results show that quadrupling time was longer for males than for females and was shortest for the DMS114 cell line, but was not affected by immunosuppression treatment (Table 4).

Although the results of the analysis of the "growth rate" made biological sense, this parameter was not of interest to the tumor biologists. Doubling and quadrupling times are common measures of tumor growth delay used by tumor biologists but they are not easily analyzed except with the two-stage method, being nonlinear characteristics of the curve.

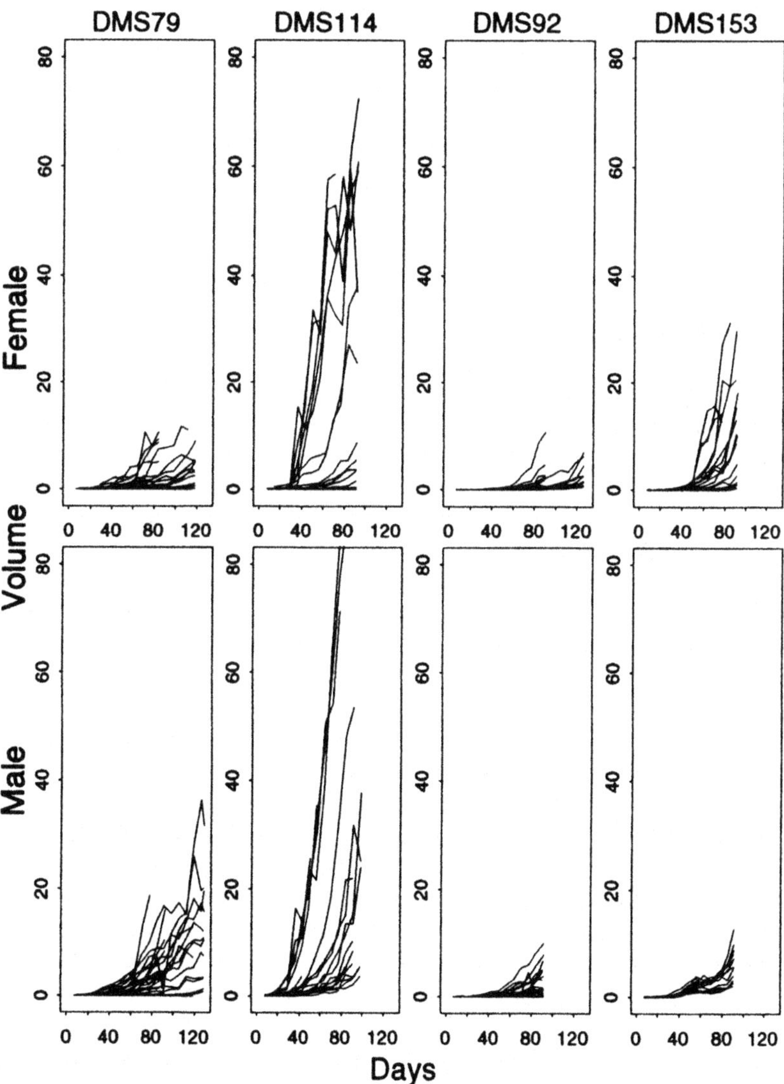

FIGURE 1. SCCL Tumor Growth in Mice According to Sex and Cell Line.

TABLE 4. Analysis of Factors Affecting the Second Quadrupling Time of Tumors Using the Two-Stage Estimation Procedure.

Factor	$\widehat{\beta} \pm SE(\widehat{\beta})$
Male	4.29±1.37
ATS	.35±1.65
ALS	-.66±1.62
DMS79	13.5±1.7
DMS153	10.1±1.7
DMS92	10.3±2.7
Intercept	10.9±1.6

7 Discussion

In this paper, we generalize the usual nonlinear mixed-effects model (1, 2) to study the effects of population covariates on a subset of the regression parameters, or on a characteristic of the regression curve defined as a nonlinear function of the individual regression parameters. When interest focuses on the entire set of growth curve parameters, the model reverts to (1, 2). While it is possible to analyze a subset of the individual regression parameters using all three methods described in the paper, it is not possible to analyze a characteristic of the curve easily using anything but the two-stage method, unless a complex reparametrization of the original nonlinear regression curve formula (1) is undertaken to make one of the new parameters correspond to the characteristic of interest.

To apply the two-stage method, the number of observations per individual must be large enough for the individual regression parameters in (1) to be estimable for all i. Dropping individuals from the study could lead to selection bias and invalid estimates. On the other hand, the LB method involves complex nonlinear optimization and can encounter problems with convergence. Most such problems we encountered were a result of lack of positive-definiteness of $\boldsymbol{\Omega}$, which could be corrected. The VC method also failed occasionally for reasons of extreme lack of fit of the model. Failure to converge for these models can result in loss of information from an entire data set.

The simulation study demonstrated that when the true model is known, the LB estimator has the least bias and smallest standard errors. This is likely due to the fact that it is an approximation to maximum likelihood, which is asymptotically optimal in terms of bias and efficiency. If the model for a secondary parameter is misspecified, the two-stage method was nearly unbiased and had lowest MSE. Because it makes assumptions only about parameters that are of interest in the analysis, the two-stage method may be robust to model misspecification of the remaining parameters. Finally, unless the random effects are known to enter the expectation function linearly, the VC method will not produce valid estimates or standard errors. However, when the random effects are linear, the variances, σ^2 and $\mathbf{\Omega}$, are small, and the model for the mean is correct, the VC method can perform quite well (Vonesh et al., 1996). These results are similar to our previous findings for general linear mixed-effects models (Stukel and Demidenko, 1997) and are consistent with the asymptotic properties of these nonlinear mixed-effects models (Demidenko, 1997).

8 REFERENCES

[1] Bates DM and Watts DG, (1988), Nonlinear Regression Analysis and Its Applications. New York: Wiley and Sons.

[2] Berkey, C.S. and Laird, N.M. (1986), "Nonlinear Growth Curve Analysis: Estimating the Population Parameters," *Annals of Human Biology,* **13**, 111-128.

[3] Demidenko, E. (1997), "Asymptotic Properties of Nonlinear Mixed-Effects Models," Modelling Longitudinal and Spatially Correlated Data: Methods, Applications, and Future Directions. Springer Lecture Notes in Statistics. New York: Springer-Verlag.

[4] Laird, N.M. and Ware, J.H. (1982), "Random-Effects Models for Longitudinal Data," *Biometrics*, **38**, 963-974.

[5] Lindstrom, M.J. and Bates, D.M. (1990), "Nonlinear Mixed Effects Models for Repeated Measures Data," *Biometrics*, **46**, 673-687.

[6] Pettengill, O.S., Curphey, T.J., Cate, C.C., Flint, C.F., Maurer, L.H. and Sorenson, G.D. (1980), "Animal Model for Small Cell Carcinoma of the Lung," *Experimental Cell Biology,* **48**, 279-297.

[7] Pinheiro, J.C. and Bates, D.M. (1995), "Approximations to the Log-Likelihood Function in the Nonlinear Mixed-Effects Model," *Journal of Computational and Graphical Statistics*, **4**, 12-35.

[8] Pocock, S.J., Cook, D.G. and Beresford, S.A.A. (1981), "Regression of Area Mortality Rates on Explanatory Variables: What Weighting is Appropriate?" *Applied Statistics,* **30**, 286-295.

[9] Steimer, J.L., Mallet, A., Golmard, J.L. and Boisvieux, J.F. (1984) "Alternative Approaches to Estimation of Population Pharmacokinetic Parameters: Comparison with the Nonlinear Mixed-Effect Model," *Drug Meta-bolism Reviews,* **15**, 265-292.

[10] Stukel, T.A. and Demidenko, E. (1997) "Two-Stage Method of Estimation for General Linear Growth Curve Models," *Biometrics,* **53**, 340-348.

[11] Vonesh, E.F. and Carter, R.L. (1992), "Mixed-Effects Nonlinear Regression for Unbalanced Repeated Measures," *Biometrics*, **48**, 1-17.

[12] Vonesh, E.F. (1992), "Non-Linear Models for the Analysis of Longitudinal Data," *Statistics in Medicine*, **11**, 1929-1954.

[13] Vonesh, E.F., Chinchilli, V.M. and Pu, K. (1996), "Goodness-of-Fit in Generalized Nonlinear Mixed-Effects Models," *Biometrics*, **52**, 572-587.

Repeated Measures Analysis Using Mixed Models: Some Simulation Results

S. Paul Wright
University of Tennessee
United States

Russell D. Wolfinger
SAS Institute Inc.
United States

ABSTRACT Currently available software (e.g., the MIXED procedure in SAS) makes it easy to analyze repeated measures data having such "non-standard" features as incomplete observations and structured covariance matrices. Unfortunately, in small samples, the hypothesis tests based on the asymptotically valid Wald chi-square statistics and related F statistics can be grossly inaccurate. Previously reported simulations showed that accurate results could be obtained from adjusted F statistics using both univariate (Greenhouse-Geisser and Huynh-Feldt) and multivariate (Lawley-Hotelling trace) approaches to adjustment. Both approaches worked well when using the potentially time-consuming REML estimates of covariances, but not with the faster, non-iterative MIVQUE0 estimates. The present paper reports encouraging results from new simulations comparing REML with alternative non-iterative SSCP estimates based on sums-of-squares-and-cross-products of residuals — in effect, using 2-stage least squares.

Key words and phrases: Geisser-Greenhouse adjustment, Huynh-Feldt adjustment, Lawley-Hotelling trace, REML, MIVQUE0.

1 Introduction and Summary

With the availability of software such as the MIXED procedure in SAS/STAT, it is now easy to fit a variety of linear models for repeated measures data. In particular, models with structured covariance matrices for data sets with possibly incomplete observations are easily handled. The software provides the user with many options both for model specification (e.g., fixed and random effects, various covariance structures), parameter estimation (e.g., ML, REML, MIVQUE0, SSCP) and hypothesis testing (e.g., Wald chi-square tests, F tests, Lawley-Hotelling type test statistics). Unfortunately, in small samples, the hypothesis tests based on the asymptotically valid Wald chi-square statistics and related F statistics can be grossly inaccurate. This paper reports results from simulations to investigate the accuracy of modified F statistics based on (1) the widely used univariate adjustments of Greenhouse-Geisser and Huynh-Feldt and (2) the multivariate approach using the Lawley-Hotelling trace.

Both the adjusted univariate and the multivariate approaches worked well when the covariance matrix was estimated by REML or by SSCP but not when MIVQUE0 was used. Unfortunately, the non-iterative SSCP method, which is much faster than the iterative REML method, often produced a singular matrix. Some ways of handing the singular matrix problem are discussed.

Only the highlights of the simulation results are reported here. Complete tables of simulation results, as well as additional details about the computations, are available on request from the first author.

2 The Study Design

The design studied here was a two-way repeated measures ANOVA with one between-subjects factor (GROUP) having three levels and one within-subjects factor (TIME) having four levels. There were five subjects per group. (A few simulations were done with 20 subjects per group.) The design is shown in Table 1. This setup was simulated with various patterns of covariances among the four times and with various methods for testing the hypotheses of no main effects or interaction. Each simulation "run" consisted of 1000 simulated datasets. In some of the runs there were three missing values. An "X" in Table 1 identifies the location of a missing value in those runs. The methods for hypothesis testing are discussed in subsequent sections. The covariance matrices used in the simulations are described below. In every case except the RC structure, the variances were set to 100.

(1) CS (compound symmetry) with an intraclass correlation of .50. Box's (1954) epsilon for this matrix is 1.00.

(2) AR1 (1st order autocorrelation) with an autocorrelation of .92. Epsilon = 0.6734.

(3) Toeplitz with correlations on successive off-diagonals of .90, .75, .50. Epsilon = 0.4580.

(4) UN (unstructured) with off-diagonal correlations (in lower triangle) of .75, .25 .50, .01 .04 .09. Epsilon = 0.7554.

(5) RC (random coefficients) with elements in lower triangle of 17, 25 42, 34 57 81, 43 73 103 134. Epsilon = 0.3708. This matrix was based

Table 1. A Two-Way Repeated Measures ANOVA Layout

Group	Subject	Time1	Time2	Time3	Time4
	1	.	.	.	.
	2	X	.	.	.
1	3	.	.	.	.
	4	.	.	.	.
	5	.	.	.	.
	6	.	.	.	.
	7	.	X	.	.
2	8	.	.	.	.
	9	.	.	.	.
	10	.	.	.	.
	11	.	.	.	.
	12	.	.	X	.
3	13	.	.	.	.
	14	.	.	.	.
	15	.	.	.	.

on two random coefficients (an intercept and a slope) with variances of 5 and 7 and covariance equal to 2, and an error covariance matrix equal to an identity matrix. The TIME values used were 1, 2, 3 ,4.

3 Background

When there are no missing data, the analysis of a repeated measures design such as that in Table 1 typically uses one (or both) of two approaches. The univariate mixed-model approach produces exact F tests for all effects (both between- and within-subjects) when the covariance matrix of the repeated measurements has Type-H structure (Huynh & Feldt, 1970). See Aitkin (1981) and Yates (1982) for an interesting discussion of many issues pertaining to the univariate approach. When the Type-H assumption is tenuous, two adjustments are popular for tests of within-subjects factors: the Greenhouse-Geisser (G-G) adjusted F test (Greenhouse & Geisser, 1959) and the Huynh-Feldt (H-F) adjusted F test (Huynh & Feldt, 1976). Lecoutre (1991) has given a correction to the H-F adjustment.

A second common approach to analyzing repeated measures is the multivariate approach (see Morrison, 1990). This method makes no assumptions about the structure of the covariance matrix for all measurements on the same subject. Indeed, the usual unstructured estimate of the covariance matrix, based on ordinary least squares residuals, is *required* in the calculation of the various multivariate statistics that are commonly used used for testing within-subjects factors (Wilks' lambda, Lawley-Hotelling trace, Pillai trace, Roy's largest root).

A third approach which is implemented, for example, in the MIXED procedure in SAS/STAT (and is therefore called the MIXED approach in this paper) is a generalization of the above univariate mixed-model approach. It includes both the above approaches as special cases. This approach uses a univariate representation of the multivariate data, i.e., the multiple responses for all individuals are stacked into a single vector, but observations on the same individual are allowed to covary. Type-H structure and "unstructured" are just two of many available covariance structures that can be fitted.

The penalty that is paid for the additional generality of this approach is that, in general, only asymptotic results are available for tests of hypotheses, even when there is no missing data. In the MIXED procedure, Wald-type test statistics are used. (Likelihood ratio tests can be constructed from the log-likelihood information included in the output by running the procedure more than once and subtracting the values obtained.) The asymptotic chi-square approximation is available, but the default is to use an F approximation. This F reduces to the traditional univariate mixed-model F when a CS (compound symmetry) structure is fitted. When an unstructured matrix is fitted, the resulting F is related to the multivariate Lawley-Hotelling trace statistic (see Kleinbaum 1973); but it is *not* one of the F approximations that multivariate programs usually report. In general, this F approximation can be quite inaccurate in small samples (and the chi-square approximation is even less accurate). An obvious remedy is to apply the traditional "adjustments" (G-G, H-F, and multivariate tests) in this more general MIXED approach. The purpose of the current study was to see how well these adjustments, which are intended for the case of no missing data and (in the multivariate approach) an unstuctured covariance matrix, perform when there is missing data and structured covariance matrices are fitted. Related simulation studies have been done by Schwertman *et al.* (1985), Schlucter & Elashoff (1990), and Wright (1995).

4 What is the Problem?

Table 2 displays the empirical type 1 error rate for the TIME effect at significance levels of .01, .05 and .10. (Results for the GROUP-by-TIME interaction are similar and are not reported here.) The covariance structure used to generate the data was compound symmetry (CS), and there were no missing values. The three methods used to analyze the data were: (1) Method U: the traditional unadjusted univariate mixed model approach; (2) Method M:

Table 2. Empirical Type 1 Error Rate for the TIME Effect. True Structure: CS; Fitted Structure: UN. 15 Subjects; No Missing Values.

	Alpha		
Method	.010	.050	.100
U	.011	.055	.112
M	.013	.050	.106
X	.051 ++	.148 ++	.215 ++

++ = more than 3 standard errors above nominal alpha.

the multivariate approach using McKeon's (1974) F approximation for the Lawley-Hotelling trace statistic; (3) Method X: the large-sample F statistic from SAS's MIXED procedure fitting an unstructured covariance matrix (SAS Institute Inc., 1996, Chapter 18).

Method X clearly has a problem. Methods U and M both gave accurate results in this case, as they should when the covariance matrix has the CS structure. But method X, which is asymptotically equivalent to Method M, had a grossly inflated type 1 error rate in this small sample. So why not simply use method U or M instead of X? One problem with method M is that, as usually implemented, it uses only complete records; observations with missing data are omitted. Method X uses all the data, including observations with missing values. (The MIXED procedure does implement method M with missing data; see section 6 below.) A second problem with method M is that it applies only when the estimated covariance matrix is unstructured. Consequently method M may lose power in cases where the true covariance structure has only a few parameters. Method X applies with structured as well as unstructured covariance matrices.

Table 3 presents results from another simulation run that illustrates a problem with method U. This method is valid only in the case of a Type-H covariance structure of which compound symmetry is a special case. The results in Table 3 are for data sets generated from the Toeplitz covariance matrix. In this case (and all the other cases except the CS structure), method U produces excessive type 1 errors. (Methods G and L in Table 3 are Greenhouse-Geisser and Lecoutre (Huynh-Feldt) adjustments, respectively. They are discussed below.)

5 Adjusting the Univariate Results

Standard approaches to testing within-subjects effects in the absence of compound symmetry (or of Type-H structure) are (1) to use the multivariate approach (e.g., Method M) or (2) to apply adjustments to the univariate results. Two commonly used adjustment methods are the Greenhouse-

Table 3. Empirical Type 1 Error Rate for the TIME Effect. True Structure: Toeplitz; Fitted Structure: UN. 15 Subjects; No Missing Values.

	Alpha		
Method	.010	.050	.100
U	.044 ++	.097 ++	.142 ++
M	.011	.046	.105
X	.046 ++	.142 ++	.216 ++
G	.014	.060	.096
L	.016	.066 +	.102

+ = more than 2 standard errors above nominal alpha.
++ = more than 3 standard errors above nominal alpha.

Geisser (1959) method and the Huynh-Feldt (1976) method. Lecoutre's (1991) corrected version of the Huynh-Feldt adjustment was used in this study. Methods G and L in Table 3 show the results with the Greenhouse-Geisser and Lecoutre (Huynh-Feldt) adjustments, respectively. Both methods generally produced accurate error rates, though method L was slightly liberal at alpha=.05.

6 Handling Incomplete Records

Results given above are for data sets with no missing values. One of the attractive features of the MIXED approach is its ability to estimate covariance matrices and conduct hypothesis tests in the presence of incomplete observations. Table 4 shows results when there were three missing values (see Table 1) and the true covariance structure was AR1. Three different methods were used to estimate the covariance matrix (all three methods give the same result when there is no missing data): (1) REML (restricted or residual maximum likelihood), (2) SSCP (sums of squares and cross products of ordinary least squares residuals), and (3) MIVQUE0 (minimum variance quadratic unbiased with a zero initial value). The important lesson in Table 4 is that the adjusted univariate (methods G and L) and the multivariate (method M) tests produced excessive type 1 errors when MIVQUE0 was used. The REML and SSCP methods produced accurate or only slightly liberal results. (The unadjusted methods U and X generally produced excessive type 1 errors, as expected.)

What is not shown in Table 4 is a potentially serious problem with the SSCP method. It frequently produced a singular estimated covariance matrix. Table 5 shows how frequently this occurred in the simulations. Thus in Table 4, the SSCP results using methods M and X are based on only

Table 4. Empirical Type 1 Error Rate for the TIME Effect. True Structure: AR1; Fitted Structure: UN. 15 Subjects; 3 Missing Values.

Method	Covariance	Alpha		
		.010	.050	.100
U	REML	.030++	.070+	.121+
U	SSCP	.029++	.066+	.101
U	MIVQUE0	.062++	.120++	.173++
M	REML	.012	.066+	.124+
M	SSCP	.012	.053	.094
M	MIVQUE0	.040++	.089++	.128+
X	REML	.073++	.160++	.234++
X	SSCP	.056++	.135++	.203++
X	MIVQUE0	.097++	.150++	.193++
G	REML	.009	.050	.088
G	SSCP	.007	.051	.079−
G	MIVQUE0	.045++	.090++	.146++
L	REML	.017+	.058	.099
L	SSCP	.018+	.056	.086
L	MIVQUE0	.054++	.104++	.158++

+ = more than 2 standard errors above nominal alpha.
++ = more than 3 standard errors above nominal alpha.
− = more than 2 standard errors below nominal alpha.

978 "successful" runs rather than 1000. It is worth noting that a singular matrix is a problem only for the multivariate approach. The univariate adjustments can be computed even on a singular matrix.

7 Using Structured Covariance Matrices

Another attractive feature of the MIXED approach to repeated measures is that the estimated covariance matix need not be unstructured. This allows a more parsimonious model to be used. For example, the unstructured 4-by-4 covariance matrix in the simulation contains ten parameters while the CS and AR1 matrices have only two parameters and the Toeplitz and RC matrices have only four.

Table 6 shows the results when an AR1 matrix was fitted to data that was in fact generated from an AR1 covariance structure. As before, the MIVQUE0 method produced inaccurate results. With REML and SSCP, the adjusted univariate results were accurate, but the multivariate results were

Table 5. The Number of Singular Estimated Covariance Matrices in 1000 trials using the SSCP Method.

True Structure	Estimated Structure	Sample Size	Missing Values	Number Singular
CS	UN	15	3	5
AR1	UN	15	3	22
Toeplitz	UN	15	3	198
Toeplitz	UN	60	3	0
RC	UN	15	3	43
UN	UN	15	3	26
Toeplitz	Toeplitz	15	0	271
Toeplitz	Toeplitz	60	0	43
Toeplitz	Toeplitz	15	3	308
Toeplitz	Toeplitz	60	3	64

too conservative. Heuristically, this can be attributed to "overadjustment" since the multivariate approach assumes that an unstructured covariance matrix is used; it does not take into account that only 2, not 10, covariance parameters were estimated.

Also note that (with REML and SSCP), the results from the MIXED approach (method X) were accurate in this case. This is in sharp contrast to the previously reported examples. Again this is due to the fact that only two covariance parameters were estimated. MIXED's inaccuracy in the other examples is a consequence of failure to account for additional variability caused by estimating covariance parameters. In effect, MIXED treats the covariances as known. The fewer covariance parameters there are, the less impact their estimation has on the results.

Table 5 shows that using the SSCP method to estimate *structured* covariance matrices can also produce singular covariance matrices, at least with certain covariance structures. The SSCP method for obtaining CS and AR1 matrices ensures their non-singularity, but this is not the case for Toeplitz and unstructured. Note especially that fitting a Toeplitz structure by SSCP can produce a singular matrix even when there are no missing data!

8 Conclusions, Discussion, Unanswered Questions

Based on these simulation results, some general recommendations can be made for testing within-subjects effects in repeated measures analysis with missing data. (Error rates for tests of between-subjects effects were near their nominal levels for all cases in our simulations.)

Table 6. Empirical Type 1 Error Rate for the TIME Effect. True Structure: AR1; Fitted Structure: AR1. 15 Subjects; 3 Missing Values.

Method	Covariance	Alpha .010	.050	.100
U	REML	.030++	.070+	.121+
U	SSCP	.029++	.066+	.101
U	MIVQUE0	.062++	.120++	.173++
M	REML	.001−	.007−−	.035−−
M	SSCP	.001−	.009−−	.026−−
M	MIVQUE0	.037++	.075++	.105
X	REML	.011	.057	.118
X	SSCP	.009	.045	.083
X	MIVQUE0	.078++	.130++	.173++
G	REML	.014	.056	.092
G	SSCP	.011	.051	.079−
G	MIVQUE0	.044++	.091++	.145++
L	REML	.020++	.061	.105
L	SSCP	.017+	.058	.091
L	MIVQUE0	.057++	.107++	.163++

+ = more than 2 standard errors above nominal alpha.
++ = more than 3 standard errors above nominal alpha.
− = more than 2 standard errors below nominal alpha.
−− = more than 3 standard errors below nominal alpha.

(1) Use REML to estimate covariances if possible. Use SSCP when REML is impractical (i.e., when the sample size is large and/or there are many covariance parameters to be estimated). Avoid MIVQUE0. (See below for some hints on dealing with singular SSCP matrices.)

(2) Be wary when using Wald chi-square and F tests with small samples. Use the adjusted univariate or the multivariate tests instead. Or, perhaps better, select a more parsimonious covariance structure, if appropriate, before testing.

(3) Use a structured covariance matrix, when appropriate, to reduce the number of covariance parameters to be estimated. This is especially helpful when using REML. (SSCP actually requires *more* computation to obtain a structured matrix than an unstructured one in most cases, so there is little reason to do so.)

(4) The adjusted univariate tests, i.e. Greenhouse-Geisser method G and Lecoutre (Huynh-Feldt) method L, performed well in all cases studied. For the simulations as a whole (including cases not reported here), method L was somewhat liberal in a small number of cases; method G was somewhat conservative in a small number of cases.

(5) The multivariate tests can be used when the estimated covariance matrix is unstructured, but not when a structured covariance is used.

Regarding recommendation (1), there are (at least) two ways to deal with the singular matrices produced by SSCP. One easy solution is to use only complete observations to estimate the unstructured covariance matrix; i.e., to use "listwise deletion." The method used in this study was "pairwise deletion." Listwise deletion is practical only when the amount of missing data is small. Additional work is needed to determine how much missing data is too much to permit effective use of listwise deletion. A second solution is to modify the MIXED methodology to permit a singular covariance matrix. See Schwertman & Allen (1979).

Regarding (3), a question needing more investigation is: What are the consequences of using an inappropriately structured covariance matrix? For example, how would the results change if the true structure were Toeplitz but an AR1 structure was fitted?

The above recommendations raise the question: Which approach to repeated measures analysis is "best," the adjusted univariate, the multivariate, or the general mixed model approach with structured covariance matrices? Regarding univariate versus multivariate tests, the answer from simulation studies having no missing data seems to be, "It depends." See, for example, Rogan, Keselman & Mendoza (1979) and Maxwell & Arvey (1982). For data sets with missing values, additional simulations are needed to study the power characteristics of the various alternatives.

9 References

[1] Aitkin, M. (1981). Response to "Regression Models for Repeated Measurements." *Biometrics* **37,** 831-832.

[2] Box, G. E. P. (1954). Some Theorems on Quadratic Forms Applied in the Study of Analysis of Variance Problems, II. Effects of Inequality of Variance and of Correlation Between Errors in the Two-Way Classification. *Annals of Mathematical Statistics* **25,** 484-498.

[3] Greenhouse, S. W. & Geisser, S. (1959). On Methods in the Analysis of Profile Data. *Psychometrika* **24,** 95-112.

[4] Huynh, H. & Feldt, L. S. (1970). Conditions Under Which Mean Square Ratios in Repeated Measurements Designs Have Exact F-

Distributions. *Journal of the American Statistical Association* **65,** 1582-1589.

[5] Huynh, H. & Feldt, L. S. (1976). Estimation of the Box Correction for Degrees of Freedom from Sample Data in Randomized Block and Split-Plot Designs. *Journal of Educational Statistics* **1,** 69-82.

[6] Kleinbaum, D. G. (1973). Testing Linear Hypotheses in Generalized Multivariate Linear Models. *Communications in Statistics* **1,** 433-457.

[7] Lecoutre, B. (1991). A Correction for the $\tilde{\epsilon}$ Approximate Test in Repeated Measures Designs With Two or More Independent Groups. *Journal of Educational Statistics* **16,** 371-372.

[8] Maxwell, S. E. & Arvey, R. D. (1982). Small Sample Profile Analysis With Many Variables. *Psychological Bulletin* **92,** 778-785.

[9] McKeon, J. J. (1974). *F* Approximations to the Distribution of Hotelling's T_0^2. *Biometrika* **61,** 381-383.

[10] Morrison, D. F. (1990). *Multivariate Statistical Methods,* 3rd Edition. New York: McGraw-Hill.

[11] Rogan, J. C., Keselman, H. J. & Mendoza, J. L. (1979). Analysis of Repeated Measurements. *British Journal of Mathematical and Statistical Psychology* **32,** 269-286.

[12] SAS Institute Inc. (1996). *SAS/STAT Software: Changes and Enhancements through Release 6.11.* Cary, NC: SAS Institute Inc.

[13] Schwertman, N. C. & Allen, D. M. (1979). Smoothing an Indefinite Variance-Covariance Matrix. *Journal of Statistical Computation and Simulation* **9,** 183-194.

[14] Schwertman, N. C., Flynn, W., Stein, S. & Schenk, K. L. (1985). A Monte Carlo Study of Alternative Procedures for Testing the Hypothesis of Parallelism for Complete and Incomplete Growth Curve Data. *Journal of Statistical Computation and Simulation* **21,** 1-37.

[15] Schlucter, M. D. & Elashoff, J. D. (1990). Small-Sample Adjustments to Tests with Unbalanced Repeated Measures Assuming Several Covariance Structures. *Journal of Statistical Computation and Simulation* **37,** 69-87.

[16] Wright, S. P. (1995). Adjusted *F* Tests for Repeated Measures with the MIXED Procedure. In SAS Institute Inc., *Proceedings of the Twentieth Annual SAS Users Group International Conference.* Cary, NC: SAS Institute Inc. 1154-1159.

[17] Yates, F. (1982). Response to Aitkin (1981). *Biometrics* **38,** 850-853.

Object Identification Using Markov Random Field Segmentation Models at Multiple Resolutions of a Rectangular Lattice

Jeffrey D. Helterbrand and Noel Cressie*

Iowa State University

United States

ABSTRACT One of the most powerful uses for Markov random fields is in the area of image analysis, where the (noisy) image is observed on a rectangular lattice. In Bayesian approaches, Markov chain Monte Carlo (McMC) algorithms are usually suggested as a means to obtain a maximum *a posteriori* (MAP) prediction. The particular problem we consider here is that of contextual image segmentation. In practice, approximations to theoretically optimal McMC algorithms are necessary but these algorithms tend to restrict movement through the space of potential segmentations. In this paper, efficient multi-resolution techniques are used to obtain a good initial labeling and to allow more movement through the label configuration space. Examples of both natural images and synthetic images are presented.

Key words and phrases: Image analysis, Bayesian methods, Markov chain Monte Carlo.

1 Introduction

This research is concerned with digital image analysis, where an image Y consists of the observed intensities on an $n \times m$ rectangular lattice of pixel

---

*Contact address: Noel Cressie, Department of Statistics, Iowa State University, Ames, IA 50011–1210, USA. Jeffrey D. Helterbrand is currently with Lilly Research Laboratories, Eli Lilly and Company, Indianapolis, IN 46285. The research was supported by the Office of Naval Research (N00014–93–1–001) and an Iowa State University Research Grant (Carver Grant). The authors are grateful to Michail A. Esterman for providing the glomerulus image.

locations. Image restoration corresponds to the prediction of the true image θ from the (noisy image) data Y. By contrast, image segmentation is a very broad term describing procedures that break the image up into regions having different properties, as desired by the user. Due to frequency-band attenuations, motion, recording instrument characteristics, and digitization, the observed image is often distorted from the true scene.

Schalkoff (1989, pp. 262) separates segmentation algorithms into two classes. In *noncontextual* segmentation, spatial relations among pixels or regions are ignored; though often computationally efficient, the performance of these techniques is adversely affected by noise in the image-recording process. In *contextual* segmentation, the segmentation process employs neighboring relations among pixels and regions. Contextual classification is often more successful because the local image information typically reinforces a classification decision. For a review of statistical approaches to both image restoration and image segmentation, see Cressie and Davidson (1997).

In statistical image analysis, many authors have considered (contextual) *Bayesian* segmentation algorithms, where an intensity model is defined and a MRF prior model is placed on a label process to promote desired characteristics in the final label estimate (segmentation); see, for example, Elliot et al. (1986), Derin and Elliot (1987), Devijver (1988), Pitas (1988), Short (1993), and Johnson (1994). Grenander and Miller (1994) define an elegant probability model on a space of deformable templates, variable in number and with textured interiors, to identify objects in medical images. Their strategy requires a parameterization of the basis templates prior to implementation; this can be extremely difficult to do in many situations. A template-based approach was considered also by Cooper et al. (1993) for recognizing objects in 3-D space. Markov chain Monte Carlo (McMC) algorithms with single-site updating are typically suggested as a means to obtain a maximum *a posteriori* (MAP) segmentation based on the specified model; see Besag and Green (1993) for a good description. Unfortunately, to use these techniques in practice, approximations to the statistically optimal segmentation are necessary. These approximation algorithms, such as Iterated Conditional Modes (ICM) (Besag, 1986), tend to be too local; movement through the label-configuration space is hindered by the single-site updating. One approach, to allow more movement through the label-configuration space, is to consider a Markov-chain algorithm with multiple-site updating (Amit and Grenander, 1991); this adds computational complexity to the optimization algorithm. The localness of the approximation algorithms also places additional pressure on the user to obtain a good initial label estimate. Efficient procedures to obtain good initial segmentations are lacking. In addition, the number of objects in a scene is often unknown. These problems are addressed and resolved in this paper.

Our goal is to give a Bayesian segmentation methodology that is practical for scientists and engineers, and we do it through a multi-resolution approach. Our algorithm has three features: 1) it allows more movement through the label-configuration space; 2) it obtains a good initial labeling in an efficient manner; and 3) the number of segments does not have to be prespecified. Specifically, we use the hybrid median filter (Russ, 1992, p. 68) and a modification of the multi-resolution, pyramid-based, image-segmentation algorithm of Hong and Rosenfeld (1984) to allow efficient spatial clustering at a coarse resolution. Second, a MRF segmentation algorithm is used at multiple resolutions to consider more global movements through the label-configuration space yet still refine the segmentation at the finest resolution of interest. This methodology can be applied to general clustering problems where the (possibly multivariate) data can be expressed on a (spatial or nonspatial) lattice.

In Section 2, the problem to be considered is specified and the Bayesian formulation and solution to the image-segmentation problem is summarized. In Section 3, a class of statistical segmentation models is presented. A multi-resolution algorithm is proposed in Section 4. In Section 5, application of the multi-resolution algorithm on a real image is presented and the performance of the algorithm is assessed using an artificial image. Extensions of the multi-resolution techniques described here are discussed in Section 6.

2 Problem Specification

Let $\mathbf{D}$ denote the $n \times m$ lattice array of pixel locations. Let $Y(\mathbf{s})$ denote the observed intensity at pixel locations $\mathbf{s} = (s^1, s^2) \in \mathbf{D}$. Arbitrarily, the pixel location (1,1) is selected to be the upper left pixel in the lattice; then $\mathbf{s} \equiv (s^1, s^2)$ denotes the center of a pixel with the first index indicating the center of the column s^1 and the second index indicating the center of row s^2, where $s^1 \in \{1, 2, \ldots, n\}$ and $s^2 \in \{1, 2, \ldots, m\}$.

Define $W(\mathbf{s})$ to be the value of the label process at location $\mathbf{s} \in \mathbf{D}$, and assume that there are P distinct objects present in the image. Then $W(\mathbf{s}) \in \{1, \ldots, P\}$; $\mathbf{s} \in \mathbf{D}$. The value of P may be unknown *a priori*.

Let Ω_W denote the set of all possible *label configurations*. The goal of contextual segmentation is to identify objects via the optimal (in a statistical sense) labeling $\omega^* \in \Omega_\mathrm{W}$ of the pixel sites, given the available information in the form of observed pixel intensities and prior knowledge regarding the scene of interest.

For $\omega \in \Omega_\mathrm{W}$ and $\mathbf{y} \equiv \{y(\mathbf{s}) : \mathbf{s} \in \mathbf{D}\}$, define $\Pr(\mathbf{y}|\omega) \equiv \Pr(Y(\mathbf{s}) = y(\mathbf{s}) : \mathbf{s} \in \mathbf{D}|\omega)$ to be the *probability mass function* (pmf) of pixel intensities, where $\Pr(A|B)$ denotes the probability of A given B. Also, for $\omega \in \Omega_\mathrm{W}$, denote the *prior pmf* of the label process by $\Pr(\omega)$. The distribution of interest is $\Pr(\omega|Y(\mathbf{s}) : \mathbf{s} \in \mathbf{D})$; $\omega \in \Omega_\mathrm{W}$, which is referred to as the *posterior pmf* of the label process. By Bayes' Theorem, $\Pr(\omega|\mathbf{y}) \propto \Pr(\mathbf{y}|\omega) \cdot \Pr(\omega)$; $\omega \in \Omega_\mathrm{W}$.

Our goal is to obtain a label configuration $\omega^* \in \Omega_W$ that maximizes the posterior label process pmf, that is, find the maximum *a posteriori* (MAP) estimator. Such a choice is equivalent to a Bayes decision procedure when considering a 0–1 loss function (e.g., Cressie, 1993, p. 511).

For most imaging problems, a direct search for the optimal labeling ω^* is infeasible. Using an McMC algorithm, an irreducible Markov chain with state space Ω_W and limiting pmf equal to the posterior pmf is constructed (Geman and Geman, 1984). Let $\omega^{(t)} \in \Omega_W$ denote the state (labeling) of the Markov chain at time t. By running the chain sufficiently long, one can obtain a configuration $\omega^{(\nu)} \in \Omega_W$ (ν large) that can be considered a sample from $\Pr(\omega|Y(\mathbf{s}) : \mathbf{s} \in \mathbf{D})$ on Ω_W. To reduce complexity, single-site updating is typically used; that is, the labeling $\omega^{(t-1)}$ is updated to labeling $\omega^{(t)}$ by changing the value of $\{W(\mathbf{s}) : \mathbf{s} \in \mathbf{D}\}$ at no more than one site in $\mathbf{D}$. To obtain the MAP estimator, one can use *simulated annealing* (Geman and Geman, 1984), although convergence can be slow.

In an attempt to approximate the MAP estimator for image reconstruction, Besag (1986) introduced the ICM algorithm, which is iterative. However, use of the approximation algorithm comes with its own difficulties. At a fine resolution, movement through the space of label configurations is restricted. Our approach is to apply statistical labeling algorithms at multiple-resolution representations of the image domain along with a good initial labeling; see Section 4.

3 Statistical Segmentation Models

Pixel Intensity Models: In an uncorrupted image, one may identify objects as regions where the intensity value $X(\mathbf{s})$ is approximately constant. It is assumed that $\{X(\mathbf{s}) : \mathbf{s} \in \mathbf{D}\}$ is a random field with realizations *constant within connected regions* of $\mathbf{D}$ (Cristi, 1990).

For a label configuration $\omega \in \Omega_W$, define

$$R_i(\omega) \equiv \{\mathbf{s} \in \mathbf{D} : W(\mathbf{s}, \omega) = i\} \; ; \quad i = 1, 2, \ldots, P \; ,$$

where the argument ω in $W(\mathbf{s}, \omega)$ is included here to indicate clearly the dependence on the label configuration being considered. We assume $X(\mathbf{s}) = \mu_i$ if $\mathbf{s} \in R_i$, where μ_i denotes the constant intensity corresponding to the region of homogeneity $R_i(\omega)$.

Now denote the *observed* intensities as $\{Y(\mathbf{s}) : \mathbf{s} \in \mathbf{D}\}$. For $\omega \in \Omega_W$ given, we assume that

$$\Pr(Y(\mathbf{s}) : \mathbf{s} \in \mathbf{D}|\omega) = \prod_{i=1}^{P} \Pr(Y(\mathbf{s}) : \mathbf{s} \in R_i(\omega)|\omega) \; ,$$

where $Y(\mathbf{s}) \sim \mathrm{NID}(\mu_i, \sigma^2)$; $\mathbf{s} \in R_i(\omega)$ and 'NID' means 'normal and independently distributed'. Upon letting $n_i(\omega)$ denote the number of distinct sites $\mathbf{s}_{ij} \in R_i(\omega) \subseteq \mathbf{D}$, we obtain

$$\Pr(Y(\mathbf{s}) : \mathbf{s} \in \mathbf{D}|\omega) = \prod_{i=1}^{P} \prod_{j=1}^{n_i(\omega)} (2\pi\sigma^2)^{-1/2} \exp\{-(Y(\mathbf{s}_{ij}) - \mu_i)^2/2\sigma^2\} ,$$

where $\{\mu_i : i = 1, \ldots, P\}$, $\sigma^2 > 0$, and P are parameters. Specification or estimation of the parameters is necessary.

MRF Prior Label Models: A class of simple but flexible MRF prior label models that advocate desirable characteristics in the final segmentation is sought. Define a *Gibbs distribution* (e.g., Kindermann and Snell, 1980) relative to a spatial domain $\mathbf{D}$ and a neighborhood system N as a probability measure $\Pr(\omega)$ on $\Omega_{\mathbf{W}}$ with the following representation:

$$\Pr(\omega) = \frac{1}{Z_0} \exp(-U_0(\omega)) \; ; \quad \omega \in \Omega_{\mathbf{W}} ,$$

where

$$U_0(\omega) \equiv \sum_{C \in \mathcal{C}} V_C(\omega)$$

is the *energy function*, made up of a sum of *potential functions* $\{V_C : C \in \mathcal{C}\}$, $\mathcal{C}$ denotes the set of cliques for the neighborhood system N, and Z_0 is the *normalizing constant* that ensures $Pr(\cdot)$ is a pmf. Any Gibbs distribution relative to $\{\mathbf{D}, N\}$ determines a MRF with neighborhood system N; and a clique is any subset of $\mathbf{D}$ such that any pair of its elements are neighbors or the subset is a singleton. This relationship provides a simple, practical way of specifying MRFs by specifying the values of potential functions.

The selection of a good prior label-process model should be based on any information regarding the scene of interest or on intuition regarding the genesis or behavior of the objects that appear in the image. For example, to discourage excessive boundaries (transitions) and the effects of noise in a label estimate, prior penalties are placed on configurations $\omega \in \Omega_{\mathbf{W}}$ that include many label transitions and many small connected regions. (A set of pixels is considered connected if it is possible to move from any pixel in the set to any other pixel in the set without leaving the set.) These penalties are specified through nonzero potential functions V_C in the Gibbs prior distribution.

For example, letting $\mathbf{s_h} \equiv \mathbf{s} + (1, 0)$ and $\mathbf{s_v} \equiv \mathbf{s} + (0, 1)$, Short (1993) penalizes excessive transitions via,

$$\beta \cdot \sum_{\mathbf{s} \in \mathbf{D}} \chi(W(\mathbf{s_h}) \neq W(\mathbf{s})) + \chi(W(\mathbf{s_v}) \neq W(\mathbf{s})) ,$$

where β is a real-valued parameter and χ denotes the indicator function.

Boundary roughness can be penalized via,

$$\gamma \cdot \sum_{s \in \mathbf{D}} \sum_{i=1}^{4} V_{C_{ri}(s)}(\omega) \, ,$$

where γ is a real-valued parameter and the clique $C_{r1}(s)$ is made up of pixels $\{s,\ s+(-1,-1),\ s+(1,-1),\ s+(-1,0),\ s+(0,1),\ s+(1,0)\}$. If the first three pixels have the same label and all other pixels in the clique have a different label, then potential function $V_{C_{r1}(s)} = 1$; otherwise it is zero. The other three potential functions are similarly defined, in terms of the three cliques that are obtained from $C_{r1}(s)$ by rotating it by 90°, 180°, and 270°, respectively.

Other potential functions can be considered to penalize undesirable segmentations, such as each occurrence of a disjoint region of area equal to two pixel units. Define the clique $C_{21}(s) = \{s,\ s+(1,0),\ s+(2,0),\ s+(1,1),\ s+(0,1),\ s+(-1,0),\ s+(0,-1),\ s+(1,-1)\}$. If the first two pixels have the same label and all other pixels in the clique have a different label, then potential function $V_{C_{21}}(s) = 1$; otherwise it is zero. The potential function $V_{C_{22}}(s)$ is similarly defined, in terms of the clique $C_{22}(s)$ that is obtained by rotating $C_{21}(s)$ by 90°. Then

$$\alpha \sum_{s \in \mathbf{D}} \{V_{C_{21}(s)} + V_{C_{22}(s)}\}$$

penalizes the number of times disjoint regions of area equal to two pixel units occur in ω.

These three potential functions, penalizing excessive transitions, roughness, and small regions, could be added together to yield $U_0(\omega)$, which defines a simple but effective class of MRF prior models. Proceeding in this fashion, other functions to penalize segmentations with many small regions can be defined for $\omega \in \Omega_{\mathbf{W}}$ and used to augment the prior model. The complexity of the image-segmentation algorithm will increase as the number of nonzero potential functions increases.

How the model parameters are specified or estimated is up to the user and depends on the intended application. In a classical Bayesian approach, the distribution of the prior parameters are specified based on the intuition of the user; see Sections 4 and 5 for further consideration of parameter specification.

4 Multiple Resolution Methods

As explained in Section 2, the use of approximation algorithms causes difficulties; movement through the space of label configurations is inhibited and a good initial labeling is necessary. In this section, multi-resolution techniques are proposed to remedy both difficulties.

The algorithm to obtain a good *initial* labeling (starting value) combines the hybrid median filter and the contextual image segmentation algorithm of Hong and Rosenfeld (1984), at a coarse resolution, to permit efficient spatial clustering. The algorithm thus provides an initial labeling of the image domain, an initial estimate of the maximum number of labels to use, and an initial estimate of label-class parameters. Additional movement through the label-configuration space is obtained by applying the statistical model-based segmentation algorithm at multiple resolutions.

The hybrid median filter is an edge-preserving, noise-eliminating, three-step ranking operation. In the 5×5 pixel locations about $\mathbf{s}$, $\mathbf{N}_2(\mathbf{s}) \cup \{\mathbf{s}\}$, pixels are ranked in two different groups, as shown in Figure 4.1. The median values of the "$\times$" and "$+$" shaped groups (both of which include $\mathbf{s}$) are grouped with the central pixel value (at $\mathbf{s}$). The median value of this set of three numbers is then saved as the new pixel value at $\mathbf{s}$. This procedure is computationally efficient, preserves lines and corners that are erased or rounded off by the conventional median filter, and reduces the tendency of intensity noise to propagate at coarser resolutions of the multi-resolution segmentation algorithm; see, for example, Kay (1994).

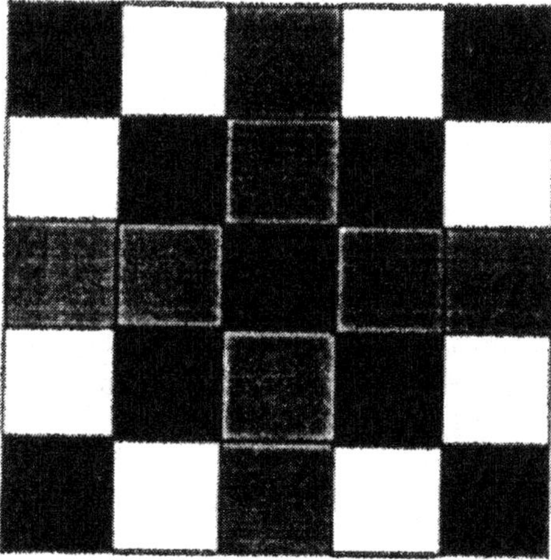

Figure 4.1. For the hybrid median filter, the median values of the "$\times$" and "$+$" shaped groups are grouped with the central pixel value, and the median of these three values is then taken.

The algorithm of Hong and Rosenfeld (1984) uses a multi-resolution ("pyramid") image representation to extract compact regions of homogeneity. In this research, we use Helterbrand's (1996) modification of it, resulting in an initial (contextual) segmentation of $\mathbf{D}$. Importantly, the number of regions, P, to be found in the image need not be specified in advance.

The modified Hong-Rosenfeld algorithm can be used as a pixel-clustering routine at any resolution; however, the computational time required grows quickly with the size of the image. Therefore, in practice, great time savings can be made by implementing the algorithm at a coarse resolution.

Let $\mathbf{D}_1 \equiv \mathbf{D}$. Let $\mathbf{D}_2$ denote the lattice of pixel locations at the next coarsest resolution; $\mathbf{D}_2$ is $(n/2) \times (m/2)$, where it is assumed that n and m are multiples of 2. The pixel location $\mathbf{s} \equiv (s^1, s^2) \in \mathbf{D}_2$ is used to summarize the information contained in pixel locations $(2s^1, 2s^2)$, $(2s^1 - 1, 2s^2)$, $(2s^1, 2s^2 - 1)$, $(2s^1 - 1, 2s^2 - 1) \in \mathbf{D}_1$. Additionally, for $\mathbf{s} \in \mathbf{D}_2$, define its corresponding intensity vector as

$$\mathbf{Y}_2(\mathbf{s}) \equiv [Y(2s^1, 2s^2),\ Y(2s^1 - 1, 2s^2),\ Y(2s^1, 2s^2 - 1),\ Y(2s^1 - 1, 2s^2 - 1)]^T$$

and postulate that the true underlying pixel intensities for $\mathbf{s} \in \mathbf{D}_2$ are constant vectors within compact homogeneous regions. In general, let $\mathbf{D}_z$ denote the lattice of pixel locations at the z-th coarsest resolution, $z = 2, 3, \ldots$; thus, $\mathbf{D}_z$ is $(n/2^{z-1}) \times (m/2^{z-1})$. Each pixel location $\mathbf{s} \equiv (s^1, s^2) \in \mathbf{D}_z$ is then used to summarize the information contained in pixel locations $(2s^1, 2s^2)$, $(2s^1 - 1, 2s^2)$, $(2s^1, 2s^2 - 1)$, $(2s^1 - 1, 2s^2 - 1) \in \mathbf{D}_{z-1}$, and has a corresponding $2^{2(z-1)} \times 1$ intensity vector.

The multiple-resolution Bayesian segmentation algorithm we propose can be specified as follows:

1. For $h = 1$ to $z - 1$:

   (a) Perform the hybrid median filter at the h-th coarsest resolution on $\mathbf{D}_h$;

   (b) Move to the $(h+1)$-th coarsest resolution by defining the value at $\mathbf{s} \in \mathbf{D}_{h+1}$ as the median intensity of the hybrid median filter values at locations $(2s^1, 2s^2)$, $(2s^1 - 1, 2s^2)$, $(2s^1, 2s^2 - 1)$, $(2s^1 - 1, 2s^2 - 1) \in \mathbf{D}_{h+1}$.

2. At resolution z, perform the Hong-Rosenfeld algorithm on the hybrid median filter values to cluster the pixels in $\mathbf{D}_z$; this procedure gives an initial labeling $\{W_z(\mathbf{s}) : \mathbf{s} \in \mathbf{D}_z\}$ at the coarse resolution $\mathbf{D}_z$.

3. For $h = z$ to 1:

   (a) Perform the ICM algorithm with intensity vectors $\{\mathbf{Y}_h(\mathbf{s}) : \mathbf{s} \in \mathbf{D}_h\}$ and starting values $\{W_h(\mathbf{s}) : \mathbf{s} \in \mathbf{D}_h\}$ to obtain an (approximately) optimal labeling $\{W_h^*(\mathbf{s}) : \mathbf{s} \in \mathbf{D}_h\}$;

   (b) Obtain starting value $\{W_{(h-1)}(\mathbf{s}) : \mathbf{s} \in \mathbf{D}_{h-1}\}$ for the next iteration to be given by $W_{h-1}(2s^1, 2s^2) = W_{h-1}(2s^1 - 1, 2s^2) = W_{h-1}(2s^1, 2s^2 - 1) = W_{h-1}(2s^1 - 1, 2s^2 - 1) = W_h^*(s^1, s^2)$; $(s^1, s^2) \in \mathbf{D}_h$.

We recommend choosing σ^2 and the prior penalties based on the finest resolution $\mathbf{D}_1 \equiv \mathbf{D}$ and we have used those same penalities at each resolution. This tends to promote larger, smoother objects at the coarser resolutions. And, importantly, the final segmentation is carried out on $\mathbf{D}_1$, using the result of all previous segmentations to produce an excellent starting value for the final ICM algorithm.

To summarize, the hybrid median filter reduces noise artifacts as one moves to coarse image representations. At a coarse resolution, the Hong-Rosenfeld algorithm is an efficient way to obtain an initial segmentation. Finally, a model-based McMC algorithm is applied at multiple resolutions to allow more movement through the label configuration space yet refine the segmentation at fine resolutions.

5 Examples

Two images are presented in this section. The first image, a 128×128 image of cells in the glomerulus of the kidney of a mouse, is used to illustrate all steps of the multi-resolution segmentation algorithm. The hybrid median filter prevents noise propagation at coarse resolutions and the modified Hong-Rosenfeld algorithm is applied at a 32×32 image resolution to obtain an initial segmentation efficiently. The ICM algorithm is implemented at the 32×32, 64×64, and 128×128 image representations to obtain the final segmentation. The second image, an artificial 128×128 image with four gray levels, will be used to assess the performance of the algorithm at several signal-to-noise ratios.

Glomerulus Image: The observed 128×128 glomerulus image is presented in Figure 5.1(a). The intended application to this scientific problem is to extract automatically the stained regions (white cells) from the observed image. Further processing is then required to characterize properties of the extracted cells. The image is used here to outline the steps of the multi-resolution ICM algorithm.

The multi-resolution segmentation algorithm of Section 4 was applied using $z = 3$ resolutions. The image resulting from the hybrid median filter applied at the fine 128×128 image is displayed in Figure 5.1(b). The hybrid median filter applied at the 64×64 and 32×32 image representations are displayed in Figures 5.1(c) and 5.1(d), respectively. Then, in Figure 5.1(e), the initial labeling obtained using the Hong-Rosenfeld algorithm at the coarse (32×32) resolution is displayed. The ICM algorithm was applied at each resolution with $\sigma^2 = 81$, $\beta = 4$, $\gamma = -0.1$, and small penalties of $\alpha_1 = 2$, $\alpha_2 = 1$, and $\alpha_3 = 1$ for isolated regions of one, two, and three pixel units in area, respectively. Since the parameter β was set large enough to prohibit, severely, transitions in horizontal and vertical directions, the parameter γ was set equal to a small negative value to advocate "roundish" objects. The resulting 32×32, 64×64, and 128×128 segmentations are presented in Figures 5.1(f), 5.1(g), and 5.1(h), respectively. Convergence was achieved after a small number (< 5) of passes for each resolution.

The desirable features of our approach are worth reiterating. It can be seen that the hybrid median filter smoothes the original image, is edge-preserving, and does not allow isolated regions of pixel intensities to propagate to coarse resolutions. The coarse-resolution Hong-Rosenfeld algorithm segments the image domain and identifies several labelings. The multi-resolution ICM algorithm smoothes and refines the segmentation.

Application of this methodology in the medical sciences shows considerable promise. For example, the algorithm has automated glomerulus cells extraction, the counting of overlapping virus plaques in a tissue culture cell sheet, and bone segmentation at Eli Lilly. Moreover, for medical problems, there are often training images avalable, from which the variance estimates and prior specifications can be obtained.

Artificial Image: A 128×128 artificially generated image with true pixel intensities displayed in Figure 5.2 will be used to assess the performance of the multi-resolution segmentation algorithm. The image contains irregularly-shaped regions and regions within regions to test the sensitivity of the multi-resolution algorithm to these features. Here, $z = 3$ resolutions were used.

Define the *signal-to-noise ratio* of an image as

$$\text{SNR} \equiv \frac{\text{minimum intensity difference of adjacent regions in image}}{\text{standard deviation of noise component in image}}.$$

In this experiment, each pixel is corrupted by Gaussian noise with mean zero and variance equal to 2, 4, 8, or 16. Thus, for this experiment, the SNRs we will consider are 2.83, 2, 1.41, and 1, respectively. For each level of noise, the corrupted image, the final segmentation, and the differenced image of the estimated segmentation compared to the *true* segmentation are displayed in Figure 5.3. The differenced image is defined as $D(\mathbf{s}) \equiv |\hat{X}(\mathbf{s}) - X(\mathbf{s})|$; $\mathbf{s} \in \mathbf{D}$, where $D(\mathbf{s})$ is the value of the differenced image at $\mathbf{s}$, $X(\mathbf{s})$ is the true pixel intensity, and $\hat{X}(\mathbf{s})$ is the estimated true pixel intensity, estimated by the sample mean of the pixels in the region to which our algorithm has assigned $\mathbf{s}$. The ICM algorithm was applied at each resolution with σ^2 equal to the variance of the Gaussian error, $\beta = 4$, $\gamma = 0.2$, and small penalties of $\alpha_1 = 2$, $\alpha_2 = 1.5$, and $\alpha_3 = 1$ for isolated regions of one, two, and three pixel units in area, respectively. The large value of β guaranteed that the segmentation would be resilient to independent Gaussian noise for all resolutions. For each SNR and each resolution, two to four passes of the image domain were required for convergence of the ICM algorithm. In this experiment, 99.9% of the pixels were assigned to the appropriate region with SNR = 2.83; further, 99.5%, 98.6%, and 94.4% of the pixels were correctly assigned for the images with SNR $=$ 2, 1.41,

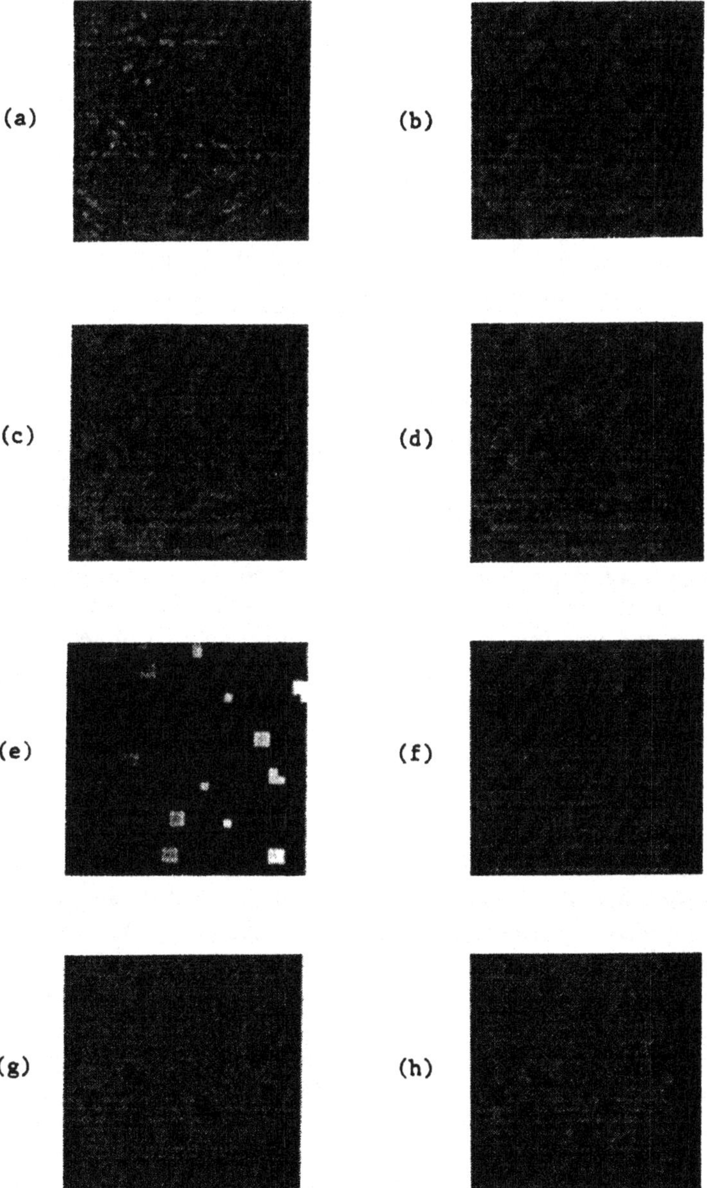

Figure 5.1. (a) The observed glomeruli image; (b)-(d) the hybrid median filter applied to (a) at the 128 × 128, 64 × 64, and 32 × 32 resolutions, respectively; (e) an initial labeling from the Hong-Rosenfeld algorithm; (f)-(h) the ICM labelings at 32 × 32, 64 × 64, and 128 × 128 resolutions, respectively.

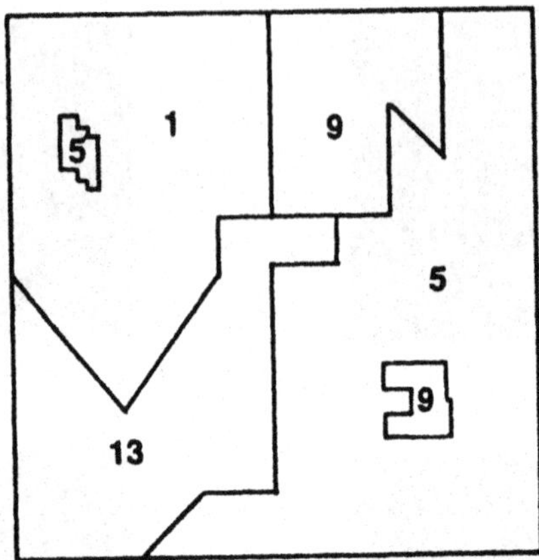

Figure 5.2. True pixel intensities of the artificial image presented.

and 1, respectively. The spatial pattern of the misclassified pixel locations is also informative. As expected, we observe that at low signal-to-noise ratios, the misclassified pixels are generally clustered in regions where the true pixel intensity differences are nonzero but small, and where jagged edges occur in the true image. Thus, even with severely corrupted images, the multi-resolution algorithm based on a simple prior model does an excellent job of clustering pixels into appropriate groups.

6 Discussion

The multi-resolution method described in this paper combines nonstatistical smoothing and clustering algorithms with a statistically based image-segmentation algorithm to construct a methodology that can be implemented in practical applications. The result is a segmentation with desired characteristics obtained in a more efficient manner than single-resolution methods.

It has been our experience that potential functions that penalize the existence of small objects of area two, three, or more pixels are troublesome when combined with the ICM algorithm; the ICM algorithm is a steepest-ascent algorithm and thus often does not allow slightly larger objects to disappear with single-site updating. Coarse-resolution updating can correct this weakness and we have featured this aspect in our method.

There are ways to extend our method to obtain greater movement through the label-configuration space. After a pass through the image domain using single-site updating, the user will have a current segmentation of the image domain. For a small ($<$ 12 pixels, say) regular or irregular region defined by the segmentation, one could consider changing the label of all pixels in

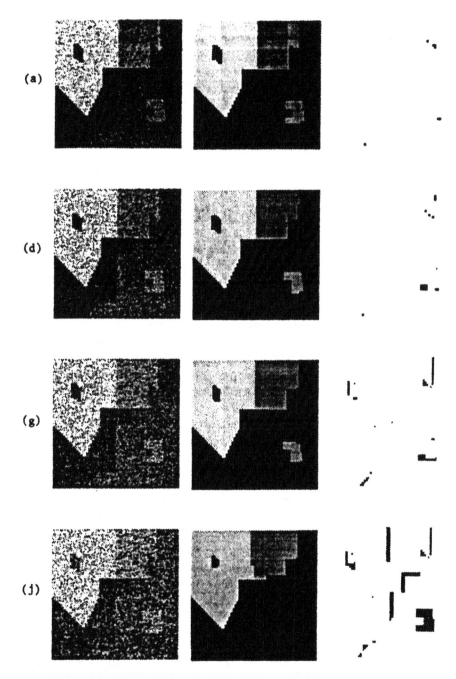

Figure 5.3. (a)-(c), (d)-(f), (g)-(i), (j)-(l) The corrupted image, the final segmentation, and the difference image of the estimated segmentation compared to the true segmentation for SNRs = 2.83, 2, 1.41, and 1, respectively.

the small region with the labeling of an adjacent region, effectively removing the region from the segmentation. By calculating the posterior energy with respect to the old segmentation and the proposed new segmentation, the algorithm can choose the segmentation that achieves the larger of the two. A similar algorithmic adjustment can be made to introduce new regions into the image domain. The resulting algorithm would essentially intersperse a pixel-by-pixel updating scheme with a region-by-region updating scheme. The pixel-by-pixel algorithm would then refine the segmentation of the region-by-region update.

7 References

Y. Amit and U. Grenander (1991). Comparing sweep strategies for stochastic relaxation. *Journal of Multivariate Analysis*, 37:197–222.

J. Besag (1986). On the statistical analysis of dirty pictures. *Journal of the Royal Statistical Society, Series B*, 48:259–279.

J. Besag and P. Green (1993). Spatial statistics and Bayesian computation. *Journal of the Royal Statistical Society, Series B*, 55:25–37.

J. Banfield and A. Raftery (1992). Ice floe identification in satellite images using mathematical morphology and clustering about principle curves. *Journal of the American Statistical Association*, 87:7–16.

N. Cressie (1993). *Statistics for Spatial Data, revised edition*. Wiley, New York.

N. Cressie and J. Davidson (1997). Image processing, entry in *Encyclopedia of Statistical Sciences (Update)*, eds S. Kotz, C.B. Read, and D.L. Banks. Wiley, New York, forthcoming.

R. Cristi (1990). Markov and recursive least squares methods for the estimation of data with discontinuities. *IEEE Transactions on Acoustics, Speech, and Signal Processing*, 38:1972–1980.

D. Cooper, J. Subrahmonia, Y. Hung, and B. Cernuschi-Frias (1993). The use of Markov random fields in estimating and recognizing objects in 3D space, in *Markov Random Fields: Theory and Applications*, eds R. Chellappa and A. Jain. Academic Press, New York, 335–367.

H. Derin and H. Elliot (1987). Modeling and segmentation of noisy and textured images using Gibbs random fields. *IEEE Transactions on Pattern Analysis and Machine Intelligence*, 9:39–55.

P.A. Devijver (1988). Image segmentation using causal Markov random fields models. *Pattern Recognition*, 301:131–143.

H. Elliot, H. Derin, R. Cristi, and D. Geman (1986). Application of the Gibbs distribution to image segmentation, in *Statistical Image Processing and Graphics*, eds E.J. Wegman and D.J. DePriest. Marcel Dekker, New York, 3–24.

S. Geman and D. Geman (1984). Stochastic relaxation, Gibbs distributions, and the Bayesian restoration of images. *IEEE Transactions on Pattern Analysis and Machine Intelligence*, 6:721–741.

D. Geman, S. Geman, C. Graffigne, and P. Dong (1990). Boundary detection by constrained optimization. *IEEE Transactions on Pattern Analysis and Machine Intelligence*, 12:609–628.

U. Grenander and M. Miller (1994). Representations of knowledge in complex systems. *Journal of the Royal Statistical Society, Series B*, 56:549–581.

J. Helterbrand (1996). One-pixel-wide closed boundary identification. *IEEE Transactions on Image Processing*, 5:780–783.

T. Hong and A. Rosenfeld (1984). Compact region extraction using weighted pixel linking in a pyramid. *IEEE Transactions on Pattern Analysis and Machine Intelligence*, 6:222–229.

V. Johnson (1994). A model for segmentation and analysis of noisy images. *Journal of the American Statistical Association*, 89:230–241.

J. Kay (1994). Statistical models for PET and SPECT data. *Statistical Methods in Medical Research*, 3:5–21.

R. Kindermann and J. Snell (1980). *Markov Random Fields and Their Applications*, volume 1. American Mathematical Society, Providence, RI.

I. Pitas (1988). Markovian image models for image labeling and edge detection. *Signal Processing*, 15:365–374.

J. Russ (1992). *The Image Processing Handbook*. CRC Press, Inc., Boca Raton, FL.

R. Schallkoff (1989). *Digital Image Processing and Computer Vision*. Wiley, New York.

T. Short (1993). An algorithm for the detection and measurement of rail surface defects. *Journal of the American Statistical Association*, 88:436–440.

Comparison of Some Sampling Designs for Spatially Clustered Populations

Mary C. Christman*

American University
United States

ABSTRACT Adaptive cluster sampling (Thompson, 1990 *Journal of the American Statistical Association*) is a sampling design in which an initial sample is selected according to some probability scheme and additional units are added to the sample if the originally selected units meet some predefined condition. We compare adaptive cluster sampling in which the initial units are selected according to simple random sampling (*ASRS*) to some other sampling designs, including simple random sampling of equivalent sample size (*SRS*) and balanced sampling excluding contiguous units (*BSEC*) (Hedayat, Rao and Stufken, 1988 *Journal of Statistical Planning and Inference*). Another design we consider is a variation on *ASRS* in which, if a selected unit does not meet the condition for adaptively sampling of its neighbors, then the neighbors are excluded from being included in the final sample (*AESRS*).

Key words and phrases: adaptive sampling, balanced sampling excluding contiguous units, rare populations, sampling efficiency, quadrat sampling.

1 Introduction

Recent years have seen an increasing interest in sampling strategies for estimating the parameters of rare, highly clustered populations. Some examples include multiplicity or network designs (Thompson, 1992), snowball designs (Biernacki and Waldorf, 1981), balanced sampling excluding con-

*Part of this work was supported by a grant from the University Research Support Awards Program at American University and from the National Science Foundation, grant number DMS-9631318. Author address: Department of Mathematics and Statistics, 4400 Massachusetts Avenue NW, Wahington, DC 20016-8050 U.S.A.

tiguous units (Hedayat, Rao, and Stufken, 1988), and designs that use initial screening methods to identify the rare subpopulations (Sudman, 1985). In many cases, the clustering is with respect to geographically aggregated units but it can, of course, refer to clustering on other variables for which the units of interest are of a kind. For example, in studies of the U.S. population, individuals may be clustered by familial or genetic relationships.

For geographic clustering an intuitively appealing design is adaptive cluster sampling (*ACS*), recently described by Thompson (1990, 1992, 1994, 1996) and implemented or modified by several authors, including Roesch (1993), Smith, Conroy, and Brakhage (1995), and Pontius (1996). In *ACS*, an initial sample is taken first according to some probability scheme. If one of the selected units has the rare trait, its "neighbors" are sampled and if any of those units also meet the condition of having the rare trait, then their neighbors are sampled. This continues until no more adaptively sampled neighboring units have the rare trait. Given a definition for a unit's neighborhood, the population is partitioned into distinct networks, each one of which consists only of units who would be sampled as a consequence of a neighbor or itself being selected during sampling (*cf* Thompson, 1990). Hence, a network consists either of a single unit, which does not have the rare trait, or of many units all of which have the rare trait and which would be sampled if any one of them were selected in the initial sample.

Several issues are still unresolved for *ACS*. There has been some effort to determine the conditions under which the design is better, i.e. yields more accurate estimates, than other designs (Thompson, 1994; Thompson and Seber, 1996; Smith *et al.*, 1995; Christman, 1996a). Thompson (1990; 1994), for example, showed that a Hansen-Hurwitz-type estimator (T_{HH}) is unbiased for the population average per quadrat. In addition, he showed analytically that T_{HH} has lower variance than the sample mean $\bar{Y}_{SRS}$ based on simple random sampling (*SRS*) when the within-network variability is a high proportion of the overall variability of the population and when the final sample size is close to the initial sample size. Hence, the more heterogeneous the networks are with respect to the variable being observed and the fewer the networks containing units with the rare trait, the more efficient *ASRS* is relative to *SRS*.

In a study of the efficiency of the *ASRS* design, Christman (1996a) showed that the Hansen-Hurwitz estimator T_{HH} was more efficient than the SRS sample mean only when the trait was very rare and very highly clustered. On the other hand, an alternative estimator based on the Horvitz-Thompson estimator T_{HT}, also developed by Thompson (1990), was more accurate than $\bar{Y}_{SRS}$ for a larger variety of populations. Christman explored the behavior of the two estimators for a wide variety of initial samples sizes, different types of neighborhoods, and for several kinds of populations and showed that (*ASRS*; T_{HT}) outperforms both (*ASRS*; T_{HH}) and (*SRS*; $\bar{Y}_{SRS}$) for more types of populations but that it often does so at the cost of very large final sample sizes.

In their studies of the efficiency of the Horvitz-Thompson estimator under *ASRS*, Smith *et al.* (1995) and Christman (1996a) considered a geographic region which was subdivided into equal sized quadrats. A population consisted of the set of counts per quadrat, $\{Y_1, Y_2, ..., Y_N\}$, and those values of Y that meet some predefined condition C are considered to be rare. The adaptive conditions studied were of the form $C = \{Y \geq k\}$ where k is a given constant. Both Smith *et al.* and Christman considered a neighborhood to be the four adjacent quadrats (the "rook" neighborhood). Both studies showed that, for the populations considered, the efficiency of the Horvitz-Thompson estimator increased as the initial sample size increased but that it generally decreased as the adaptive condition C became more restrictive. This decrease is likely due to the fact that, although the population is essentially redefined by the more restrictive condition to be more rare and tightly-clustered (since less units meet the condition they are more rare), the networks are more homogeneous than under less restrictive conditions.

In this paper, we explore the behavior of the adaptive sampling strategy ($ASRS$; T_{HT}) as compared to (SRS; $\bar{Y}_{SRS}$) for a wider variety of populations and compare ($ASRS$; T_{HT}) to some other sampling strategies. Section 2 describes the simulated populations and Section 3, the sampling designs. The results are given in Section 4.

2 Study Populations

Populations were generated from a variation of a Neyman-Scott process as follows. A random number of parents were generated from a Poisson process with intensity λ_P and randomly distributed over a square spatial region. For each parent, a random number of children from a Poisson process with a mean of 50 were generated and the children were located around the parent according to a bivariate symmetric normal distribution with standard deviation τ (see Christman 1996a for details). Any children randomly located outside of the square were reflected back into the square near the parent rather than using the more common approach of toroidal mapping.

Once the points from the process were located over the region, the population was obtained by subdividing the region into $N = 100$ quadrats of equal size. The population thus consists of the counts of points in each quadrat, i.e. Y_i is the number of points in the ith unit. In this approach, the quadrats with non-zero values tend to cluster contiguously.

For the comparisons of the different sampling strategies, one realization was generated for each of several values of λ_P and τ; see Tables 1 to 3 for a listing of the specific combinations. Note that larger values of either λ_P or τ generally lead to less clustering and more homogeneous networks.

3 Sampling Strategies

3.1 Adaptive Cluster Sampling

We consider adaptive cluster sampling in which an initial sample of size $n_1 = 10$ is randomly selected without replacement from the population and the neighborhood around the quadrat is adaptively sampled if the selected unit satisfies the condition $C = \{Y \geq 1\}$.

Three neighborhoods are studied. The first is the rook neighborhood described in the introduction. The second is based on relabelling the population from doubly-indexed, (i, j), to singly indexed starting in the top left corner and going down the columns consecutively, i.e. as $10 * (j - 1) + i$. The neighborhood of unit i is now defined as units $(i - 1)$ and $(i + 1)$. This is a slight modification of a two-dimensional neighborhood composed of north-south units in that, in our case, if a unit falls at the edge of the study region and its neighborhood is to be sampled, a unit at the opposite side of the square will be included. The reason for this and the next approach to a neighborhood is to allow comparison of the efficiency of the estimator to that of the BSEC estimators described below.

The third neighborhhood is also based on renumbering the units and adaptively sampling the two adjacent units $(i - 1)$ and $(i + 1)$. The renumbering scheme is similar to the one above except that the relabelling is done in a serpentine fashion as follows. Unit (i, j) is reindexed as $10 * (j - 1) + i$ if j is odd and as $10 * (j - 1) + (10 - i + 1)$ if j is even. The neighborhood of unit i again is defined as units $(i - 1)$ and $(i + 1)$. This renumbering scheme and choice of neighborhood has the effect that, for half of the units along the top and bottom edges at least, any unit whose neighbors are sampled will have its neighbors be physically contiguous.

For each neighborhood and population we calculated the expected final sample size $E[\nu]$ and variance of the Thompson-Horvitz estimator using the equations given in Thompson (1990). In addition, the proportion (σ_W/σ) of the total variance of the population that is the variance within networks was calculated. Also calculated was the number of black-white joins $(\#BW)$, defined as the number of adjoining sides of quadrats where one quadrat satisfies the condition but the other does not. Let $X_i = I[Y_i \in C]$ indicate where $I[\cdot]$ is the usual indicator function and let $W_{i,j}$ be the indicator variable for whether units i and j have a side in common. Then the number of black-white joins is given by

$$\#BW = \frac{1}{2} \sum_i \sum_j W_{i,j} [X_i - X_j]^2$$

(*cf.* Upton and Fingleton, 1985). High values indicate possible negative spatial autocorrelation while low values imply positive spatial autocorrelation. The relative efficiency of the unbiased estimator T_{HT} is calculated as $R[T_{HT}] = var[\bar{Y}_{SRS}]/var[T_{HT}]$ where $var[\bar{Y}_{SRS}]$ is the variance of

$(SRS; \bar{Y}_{SRS})$ calculated for without replacement sampling with a sample of size equivalent to the expected size for ASRS.

3.2 Balanced Sampling Excluding Contiguous Units

Balanced sampling designs excluding contiguous units were described by Hedayat, Rao, and Stufken (1988, 1995) as designs in which the probability that units k and $(k+1)$ are both included in a sample is zero. The design is similar to systematic sampling in that sampled units are spread out among the population but the sampled units need not be "equidistant" (e.g. every k^{th} unit as in systematic sampling). In addition, the design is balanced in that second-order inclusion probabilities are either 0 or a constant and the first order inclusion probabilities are constant for every unit in the population. Hence, the Horvitz-Thompson estimator of the population mean and its variance are easily obtained.

BSEC sampling has been demonstrated to exist for singly-indexed populations but has not been shown yet to exist for two-dimensional, i.e. doubly-indexed, populations (Stufken, personal communication). In order to compare BSEC to ASRS, we reindexed all populations to single indices in one of two ways as described in Section 3.1. The serpentine renumbering scheme is subsequently referred to as BSEC-1; the other as BSEC-2.

BSEC sampling requires that the sample size, which is fixed, be smaller than one-third of the population size. For those populations in which the expected sample size under ACS was sufficiently small, the variances of the BSEC estimators were calculated for the expected sample sizes according to the equations given in Hedayat, Rao, and Stufken (1988). The relative efficiency of the estimators were calculated as $R[T_{Bi}] = var[\bar{Y}_{SRS}]/var[T_{Bi}]$ where $i = 1, 2$ depending on the numbering scheme used for the quadrats.

3.3 Adaptive Sampling Excluding Contiguous Units

A final sampling design we consider is a modified adaptive cluster sampling design in which the neighborhood is composed of the four rook neighbors and the initial sample is taken sequentially according to a without replacement strategy. If a unit selected in the initial sample does not satisfy the adaptive condition C, the neighborhood of the selected unit is excluded from subsequently being selected for the initial sample. Conversely, if a unit selected in the initial sample does satisfy C, then adaptive sampling of the neighborhood is initiated and continues until the network and all edge units are sampled. The network and edge units are then excluded from reentering the sample through selection via the initial sample. Initial sampling continues sequentially until either there are no units left that can be sampled or the fixed initial sample size n_1 is reached.

Denote a sample as the set $s = \{u_{k_1}, u_{k_2}, ..., u_{k_n}\}$ where u_{k_i} is the ith sampled unit and k_i is the population label for that unit. Let m_{k_i} be the number of units in the network associated with the ith unit where $m_{k_i} = 1$ if $Y_{k_i} \notin C$ and $m_{k_i} \geq 1$ otherwise. Let e_{k_i} be the number of edge units for the network associated with unit u_{k_i} if $Y_{k_i} \in C$ or the number of units to be excluded from sampling if $Y_{k_i} \notin C$. Then, the probability of unit u_i being included in the final sample is given by

$$P(u_i \in s) = \pi_i^E = \sum_{S^*} \sum_{R^*} \prod_{j=1}^{n_1} \frac{m_{k_j}}{N - \sum_{l=1}^{j-1}(m_{k_l} + e_{k_l})}$$

where S^* is the set of all ordered samples s that contain unit u_i, i.e. $S^* = \{s = \{u_{k_1}, u_{k_2}, ..., u_{k_n}\} : u_i \in s\}$, and R^* is the set of all permutations of the ordering of the samples in S^*.

An unbiased estimator of the population mean is the usual Horvitz-Thompson estimator using the first-order inclusion probabilities π_i^E, denoted here as T_E. The variance of the estimator is obtained using the first-order inclusion probabilities given above and the second-order inclusion probabilities given by

$$P(u_i, u_j \in s) = \pi_{ij}^E = \sum_{S^*} \sum_{R^*} \prod_{t=1}^{n_1} \frac{m_{k_t}}{N - \sum_{l=1}^{t-1}(m_{k_l} + e_{k_l})}$$

where S^* is the set of all ordered samples s that contain units u_i and u_j, i.e. $S^* = \{s = \{u_{k_1}, u_{k_2}, ..., u_{k_n}\} : u_i, u_j \in s\}$ and R^* is as above.

For any given population, the inclusion probabilities are difficult to calculate since, for any reasonable sample size, the number of permutations involved is extremely large. A simple alternative estimator which does not involve the inclusion probabilities is the sample mean, $\bar{Y}_E = \sum Y_i/n$, where n is the random final sample size. This estimator is easily shown to be biased but has relatively small variance because of the restrictive form of without replacement sampling.

To calculate the means and variances of these two estimators, we first ran 3000 Monte Carlo simulations of AESRS sampling to obtain approximate first-order inclusion probabilities, $\pi_i^E, i = 1, ..., N$. We then ran a second set of 1000 simulations in which the estimators' values were obtained using the inclusion probabilities approximated in the first set of simulations. Then., the means and variances of the two estimators T_E and $\bar{Y}_E$ were approximated using the simulated values. The relative efficiency of the estimators were calculated by comparing the approximate variance or MSE (for $\bar{Y}_E$) to the variance of the SRS sample mean from a sample of the expected sample size.

4 Results

In the following, we compare the sampling strategies for the different populations using the relative efficiencies of the estimators rather than the

TABLE 1. Expected total sample size (E[ν]) for an initial SRS of size n_1 =10, number of Black-White joins (#BW) in the population, and the ratio of the within network variance to the total variance (σ_W/σ). The last two columns list the variance of the Horvitz-Thompson estimator of μ (V[T_{HT}]) and the relative efficiency of the estimator (R[T_{HT}] = V[$\bar{Y}_{SRS}$]/V[T_{HT}]) for *ASRS* with the adaptive sampling criterion $C = \{Y_i \geq 1\}$. The populations are indicated by the expected number of parents λ_P and the variability, τ, of the children about the parents.

λ_P	τ	E[ν]	#BW	σ_W/σ	V[T_{HT}]	R[T_{HT}]
1	3	13.52	8	0.33	0.270	1.238
1	5	19.15	13	0.40	0.224	1.140
1	8	29.80	18	0.57	0.122	1.320
5	1	13.48	14	0.35	3.744	1.200
5	2.5	25.59	21	0.62	2.162	1.150
5	5	53.20	35	0.60	0.395	0.682
5	10	78.67	31	0.64	0.004	11.070
10	1	25.30	52	0.29	20.013	0.497
10	2.5	75.19	53	0.66	1.957	0.271

variances. This was done since the different designs tend to have different expected sample sizes. Consequently, the variances are not directly comparable.

For an initial sample size of 10 and the rook neighborhood, the ASRS strategy has approximately the same relative efficiency as the AESRS strategy with the Horvitz-Thompson estimator ($AESRS$; T_E) for most of the populations studied (see Tables 1 and 2). There are a few populations for which ($AESRS$; T_E) is slightly more efficient, notably the populations with small numbers of clusters which are somewhat dispersed ($\lambda_P = 1$, $\tau = 5$ or 8). This is likely due to the fact that the final expected sample sizes are larger for AESRS than for ASRS.

For both sampling strategies, there is no clear indication of the type of population for which the adaptive sampling effort is most appropriate. Thompson (1990, 1994) surmised that it would be those populations for which the expected and initial sample sizes are close and where the within-network variance is a high proportion of the total variance. As came be seen in Table 1, this is not quite the case. It does appear that the smaller the number of black-white joins the more efficient T_{HT} is relative to $\bar{Y}_{SRS}$ but other factors we considered here do not provide clear evidence as to when the adaptive designs are more useful. The

number of black-white joins is indicative of the rarity and size of networks in the population where small numbers imply highly aggregated small clusters.

The very large relative efficiencies under all three sampling strategies for

TABLE 2. Approximate expected sample sizes and relative efficiencies for two estimators for *AESRS* with the rook neighborhood. The estimators are the Horvitz-Thompson estimator (T_E) and the sample mean ($\bar{Y}_E$). The relative bias of the sample mean estimator ($RB[\bar{Y}_E] = E[\bar{Y}_E]/\mu$) is given and its relative efficiency is calculated as $R[\bar{Y}_E] = V[\bar{Y}_{SRS}]/MSE[\bar{Y}_E]$).

λ_P	τ	$E[\nu]$	$V[\bar{Y}_{SRS}]$	$R[T_E]$	$RB[\bar{Y}_E]$	$MSE[\bar{Y}_E]$	$R[\bar{Y}_E]$
1	3	13.89	0.324	1.20	0.37	0.091	3.57
1	5	20.43	0.235	1.23	0.65	0.111	2.11
1	8	32.78	0.141	1.55	0.84	0.077	1.82
5	1	13.96	4.311	1.17	0.25	1.562	2.76
5	2.5	27.75	2.234	1.16	0.59	1.368	1.63
5	5	59.58	0.208	0.88	0.91	0.198	1.05
5	10	85.45	0.030	21.30	1.00	2.8e-4	107.21
10	1	28.63	8.404	0.42	0.31	30.59	0.28
10	2.5	89.32	0.192	0.79	0.97	0.236	0.81

the one population ($\lambda_P = 5$; $\tau = 10$) are unusual. In a separate study, Christman (1996b) showed that for some populations, notably those with a small to intermediate number of networks which spread out over a large proportion of the population, the ($ASRS$; T_{HT}) strategy has unusually small variance compared to SRS sampling.

An interesting result is that the sample mean when used with the AESRS design has very small MSE relative to the variance of the SRS sample mean. Hence, as can be seen from Tables 1 and 2, $\bar{Y}_E$ has the highest relative efficiencies compared to the other strategies for all populations except one. Unfortunately, this comes at the cost of a large negative bias in the estimator (see Table 2 for the relative bias of the estimator with respect to μ). Another problem is that an estimate of the variance of $\bar{Y}_E$ is not currently available for the same reasons that T_E is not a useful estimator: there is no simple way of estimating the probabilities π_i^E and π_{ij}^E. A conservative approach would be to use the usual SRS estimator of the variance which effectively ignores that the sampling is AESRS.

When the populations are re-indexed so that the two-dimensional spatial aspect is ignored, one possible effect on the spatial arrangement in the population is that more clusters are created since a point cluster that covers quadrats in both the north-south and east-west directions will be effectively sub-divided when the units are relabelled. Hence, such a renumbering might lower the relative efficiency of ($ASRS$; T_{HT}) since the population has been modified to be less rare/less clustered. On the other hand, the renumbering is most appropriate when one is interested in two-unit neighborhoods such as the north-south or east-west units. For these types of neighborhoods, the expected sample size tends to be smaller so that the relative efficiency tends to be larger. In fact, both results are seen when comparing the relative

TABLE 3. Expected sample sizes and relative efficiencies for the Horvitz-Thompson estimator from *ASRS* (T_{HT}) from *ASRS* sampling and from *BSEC* sampling (T_B) for two different neighborhoods. The neighborhoods are based on two separate numbering schemes for identifying the population units (see text).

		BSEC-1			*BSEC-2*		
λ_P	τ	$\mathbf{E}[\nu]$	$\mathbf{R}[\mathbf{T}_{HT1}]$	$\mathbf{R}[\mathbf{T}_{B1}]$	$\mathbf{E}[\nu]$	$\mathbf{R}[\mathbf{T}_{HT2}]$	$\mathbf{R}[\mathbf{T}_{B2}]$
1	3	11.057	0.933	1.132	11.057	0.933	0.993
1	5	12.825	1.256	1.181	12.825	1.256	0.994
1	8	15.508	1.252	1.243	15.508	1.252	0.996
5	1	11.239	1.237	0.994	11.239	1.237	0.993
5	2.5	13.786	1.684	0.993	13.802	1.682	0.995
5	5	24.293	0.646	1.530	22.804	0.622	0.994
5	10	43.182	0.373	–	37.728	0.345	–
10	1	14.817	0.759	0.996	14.644	0.760	0.987
10	2.5	32.556	0.539	1.018	31.061	0.503	0.999

efficiencies of ($ASRS$; T_{HT}) for the rook neighborhood to the two one-dimensional neighborhoods BSEC-1 and BSEC-2 (Tables 1 and 3). The relative efficiencies for T_{HT} for three of the study populations is higher for the rook neighborhood than for either of the singly-indexed neighborhoods ($\lambda_P = 1, \tau = 3$; $\lambda_P = 1, \tau = 8$; and $\lambda_P = 5, \tau = 10$).On the other hand, the two singly-indexed neighborhoods outperform the rook neighborhood in almost all of the other populations.

For the two singly-indexed neighborhoods, the BSEC sampling strategy is at least as efficient as SRS for every population studied. This same result was found for other populations, other samples sizes and re-indexing schemes (Christman, 1996a). In the case of the BSEC-2 numbering scheme (indexing each column from top to bottom), the BSEC strategy had the same variance as the (SRS; $\bar{Y}_{SRS}$) strategy for every population and therefore was less efficient than ($ASRS$; T_{HT}) for some of the populations studied (Table 3). On the other hand, when the renumbering was done in a serpentine fashion (BSEC-1), ($BSEC$; T_{B1}) was more efficient than SRS for half of the populations. It also had higher relative efficiencies than the ($ASRS$; T_{HT}) strategy for some of the populations, notably the populations that are less clustered.

5 Conclusions

In this paper, we explored the behavior of the adaptive sampling strategy ($ASRS$; T_{HT}) as compared to (SRS; $\bar{Y}_{SRS}$) for a variety of populations and to other sampling strategies. We showed that the Horvitz-Thompson estimators of the mean for the two BSEC designs are always at least as efficient as $(SRS;\ \bar{Y}_{SRS})$ for all populations considered and that they were sometimes more efficient than a $(ASRS; T_{HT})$ strategy that uses a neighborhood of two adjacent units. On the other hand, the $(ASRS; T_{HT})$ design with a neighborhood of two adjacent neighbors was found to be more efficient than $(SRS;\ \bar{Y}_{SRS})$ for only some of the same populations as the $(ASRS;\ T_{HT})$ strategy using the rook neighborhood. A final sampling strategy that we considered is a sequential adaptive procedure in which neighborhoods around units that do not satisfy C are deliberately excluded from entering the final sample $(AESRS)$. Two possible estimators were considered, a Horvitz-Thompson type of estimator (T_E) and the sample mean $(\bar{Y}_E)$. The relative efficiencies of T_E are about the same or higher than those for T_{HT} for each population in the study. Interestingly, $\bar{Y}_E$ is biased but has very low MSE relative to $(SRS; \bar{Y}_{SRS})$ and hence has a higher relative efficiency than T_E for all but one population studied.

6 References

[1] Biernacki, P. and Waldorf, D. (1981). Snowball sampling: problems and techniques in chain referral sampling. *Sociol. Methods and Research,* **10**, 141-163.

[2] Christman, M. C. (1996a). Efficiency of adaptive sampling designs for spatially clustered populations. To appear in *Environmetrics.*

[3] Christman, M. C. (1996b). Comparison of Efficiency of Adaptive Sampling in Some Spatially Clustered Populations. To appear in the American Statistical Association *1996 Proceedings of the Section on Statistics and the Environment,* American Statistical Association, Alexandria, VA.

[4] Hedayat, A. S., Rao, C. R., and Stufken, J. (1988). Sampling designs excluding contiguous units. *Journal of Statistical Planning and Inference,* **19,** 159-170.

[5] Hedayat, A. S. and Stufken, J. (1995). Sampling designs to control selection probabilities of contiguous units. *Preprint No. 95-22,* Statistical Laboratory, Department of Statistics, Iowa State University, Ames, IA.

[6] Kalton, G. and Anderson, D. W. (1986). Sampling rare populations. *J. R. Statist. Soc. A*, **149**, *Part 1*, 65-82.

[7] Pontius, J. S. (1996). Probability proportional to size selection in strip adaptive sampling. Technical Report II-96-1 in Series II, Theory and Methods, Department of Statistics, Kansas State University, Manhattan, KS.

[8] Roesch, F. A., Jr. (1993). Adaptive cluster sampling for forest inventories. *Forest Science*, **39,** 655-669.

[9] Smith, D. R., Conroy, M. J., and Brakhage, D. H. (1995). Efficiency of adaptive cluster sampling for estimating density of wintering waterfowl. *Biometrics*, **51,** 777-788.

[10] Sudman, S. (1985). Efficient screening methods for the sampling of geographically clustered special populations. *Journal of Marketing Research*, **22**, 20-29.

[11] Thompson, S. K. (1990). Adaptive cluster sampling. *Jour. of the Amer. Statistical Assoc.*, **85,** 1050-1059.

[12] Thompson, S. K. (1992). *Sampling.* John Wiley & Sons, Inc., New York, NY.

[13] Thompson, S. K. (1994). Factors influencing the efficiency of adaptive cluster sampling. Technical Report 94-0301, Technical Reports and Reprint Series, Center for Statistical Ecology and Environmental Statistics, The Pennsylvania State University, University Park, PA.

[14] Thompson, S. K. and Seber, G. A. F. (1996). *Adaptive Sampling.* John Wiley & Sons, Inc., New York, NY.

[15] Upton, G. and Fingleton, B. (1985). *Spatial Data Analysis by Example, Volume I. Point Patterns and Quantitative Data.* John Wiley & Sons, Inc., New York, NY.

Using Geostatistical Techniques to Map the Distribution of Tree Species from Ground Inventory Data

Rachel Riemann Hershey*,
Martin A. Ramirez, and David A. Drake

U. S. D. A. Forest Service
United States

ABSTRACT Some kinds of information on biodiversity can only be collected from on-the-ground surveys, providing information complementary to that gained by remote sensing. But a ground inventory, particularly over large areas, is expensive and labor intensive. Using geostatistical techniques, we can use known values at sample points to estimate the values of unsurveyed areas in between. By exploring characteristics such as the spatial pattern and variation in the sample data collected, additional information about the unsurveyed areas can be spatially modeled and estimated. From these estimates, a modeled map and dataset of the resource can be created, complete with understandable parameters of accuracy and uncertainty. The importance of identifying the objectives, understanding the phenomena, choosing the appropriate interpolation method and assessing the results is discussed, and some of the tools available to address each of these areas are presented. Ecological subregions are suggested as appropriate units for identifying species subpopulations for modeling and interpolation. Tree-species composition in Pennsylvania is used as the example, using data from the U.S. Department of Agriculture national forest inventory. The resulting modeled dataset provides a picture of individual tree-species distribution and relative abundance across the entire region.

Keywords and phrases Species distribution, uncertainty, conditional simulation, indicator kriging.

---

*Corresponding author address: U.S.D.A. Forest Service, 5 Radnor Corporate Center, Radnor, PA 19087-4585 U.S.A.

1 Introduction

On-the-ground inventory can be the only way some kinds of information on forest composition can be collected. But a ground inventory is an expensive and intensive process. This presents a formidable problem when forestry management or research is conducted over large areas. An alternative approach is to "map" values by interpolation from sample locations. Geostatistical techniques such as ordinary kriging, indicator kriging, multigaussian kriging, conditional simulation, and a host of spatial data exploratory methods are existing tools that can be used for this purpose. Although much of their use and development has applied in the earth sciences, geostatistical techniques are being increasingly applied wherever such spatial tools are required for understanding and estimating the resource at unsampled locations, and for understanding the spatial characteristics of a phenomenon. Given the interest in knowing where various natural resources occur, and the uncertainty of those estimates, forestry and the analysis of terrestrial vegetation resources is a growing application area for geostatistics.

In this study we were interested in creating a "map" depicting the current distribution of individual tree species over broad areas, such as the entire state of Pennsylvania. We were interested in estimates of where each species occurred, in what densities it occurred relative to the other species in that area, and in the uncertainty associated with those estimates. Of significant interest, too, were the variability and the spatial character of each species' occurrence, and whether this reflected a known natural pattern of that species, or affected our ability to estimate it. In addition, we wanted to capture this information in a form that could be used in conjunction with other datasets and further analyses.

2 Approach

With each type of kriging or simulation, the assumptions are different, the results are different, and the data types can be different, making each most useful in different situations. Which technique is most appropriate depends heavily on the phenomena being examined, the sample data being used, and the kind(s) of output desired.

2.1 Phenomena

How tree species are distributed across the landscape is affected by many factors, including environmental conditions and direct human influence via harvesting and other land-use histories. And each factor may occur at several different scales. Over large areas, large-scale geographic and environmental factors such as latitude, climate, mountain ranges, and other large topographic features all have an effect. In Pennsylvania, for example, sugar maple is found along with the other northern hardwoods predominantly across the northern part of the state, where both the higher latitudes and the higher elevations of the Allegheny mountains and the Allegheny Plateau coincide (Alerich 1993). At a different scale, over much smaller distances, moisture, soil type, local topography, and local disturbances can have a distinct effect on the occurrence of tree species. And all of those factors can frequently occur at spatial scales less than that resolved by the forest inventory (FIA) plots used in this study. It was expected that the influences of these small-scale factors would be expressed simply as noise in any spatial exploration of the data, but that much of the variation in tree species resulting from the broad-scale factors probably would be picked up by the FIA plot data because of the better matching of scales at which they occur.

2.2 Data

The sample data were collected by the Northeastern Forest Experiment Station's Forest Inventory and Analysis (FIA) unit in the 1988-1990 inventory of Pennsylvania. Basal area–the summed cross-sectional area at breast height–was calculated for all live trees 1.0 inches or larger on the plot (Hansen et al. 1992). The data were for individual tree species, by basal area (ba) per acre as a proportion of the total basal area (% ba/acre). The data were accessed from individual tree records in the Forest Service's Eastwide Tree-Level Database and summarized as %ba/acre for each species by plot. In Pennsylvania, there were 5,100 plots. After some initial investigation, nonforested plots and those with total ba/acre equal to zero (due to missing data) were removed, leaving 2,905 plots. The fine-scale forest/nonforest detail is not resolvable at this scale of sampling, and including the nonforest points in the analysis only added noise to the underlying spatial structure associated with each species' distribution. Although there was no fixed spacing, this sampling intensity and selection of points results in a distribution of plots averaging 2.5 km apart and spread fairly evenly throughout the state.

2.3 Desired output

The study objective was to create, using geostatistical techniques, a spatial dataset of individual tree-species distribution. This general objective could be broken down into three more specific objectives. First, we were interested in a dataset that for each species provided a picture of the spatial distribution and spatial pattern of that species to add to our understanding of that resource. Second, we were interested in providing datasets for individual species distributions that could be queried and combined to create a dataset of an individual forest cover type specific to a user's definition. Third, we were interested in these methods and dataset(s) as a possible way to make the FIA sample data more easily available in a spatial context. Using sugar maple as the example, these objectives could all be translated into more specific desires as:

- providing an estimate of sugar maple occurrence,
- providing an estimate of sugar maple "importance" in terms of %ba/acre,
- providing a measure of uncertainty associated with the two estimates,
- maintaining local variability,
- maintaining the characteristics of the original sample data, and
- handling sample data with highly skewed distributions.

Maintaining the variation inherent in the sample data was considered a critical goal, for that variation is essential to reminding us, when we use any modeled dataset, that there are processes occurring in the landscape for which our present source of information (i.e. the sample plots) and/or present knowledge are insufficient. This information on variation can be described in the form of an uncertainty about the estimate at each location, and in the form of retaining the local spatial variation in the sample data. Both forms are reflected in two of the criteria listed previously.

3 Methods

3.1 Data exploration

Exploring the sample data is a critical first step prior to any interpolation. It is important not only for checking the data for possible errors, but also for understanding the characteristics of the sample data that may bias the results. Those characteristics, along with what is desired for output, will affect what interpolation methods are most applicable.

Examination of the basic **univariate statistics** revealed that each species exhibited extremely skewed distributions, frequently with more than 50% of the plots containing less than 1% ba/acre. Although expected from what we know of tree-species distributions, this situation can create a bias in the estimates of some interpolation methods. In this study, the data were transformed to a normal distribution for use in conjunction with the conditional simulation. The normal-score transform used was a nonlinear transform, but it provided a 1–to–1 mapping of values to allow for an accurate back transformation to %ba/acre values (Deutsch and Journel 1992).

The **variogram**, covariance, and correlogram, three functions for summarizing spatial continuity, each essentially depict the variation between sample data values at increasing distances from each other (Isaaks and Srivastava 1989). If there is recognizable spatial dependence or structure in the variogram, a model can be fitted to that structure. It is this model of how that species' %ba/acre values vary (on average) with distance away from any single point that is used in the kriging and simulation routines. When the data have strong univariate characteristics, that can mask the data's spatial characteristics as depicted in the variogram. In such cases, as was true for every species examined here, the variogram of the normal-scored data often reveals considerably more spatial dependence and structure than that of the raw data. In this study, a variogram was calculated for both the raw sample data and for a normal-score transform of the sample data, using a lag distance of 500 m with no directional component. An indicator variogram also was calculated and modeled for use in the indicator kriging.

To assess how areas of "local" variability change across the region, descriptive statistics of mean and standard deviation were calculated for each 3000×3000 m cell using a 15×15 km area as the window describing the "local" area. The resulting dataset provided a picture of how variable the data were over small distances and how that variation differed in different areas of the region under study. All species exhibited a proportional effect, with areas of high local means corresponding to areas of high local standard deviation, indicating a lack of stationarity. This situation was not entirely unexpected but posed a potential problem as stationarity is an important assumption of all of the interpolation methods used here. Using normal-scored data largely eliminated this situation.

3.2 Choosing appropriate areas/regions

When subpopulations of a species have a significantly different pattern of spatial distribution, treating the populations separately in the interpolation will improve the final estimates. Essentially, by capturing more than one population within a single variogram, the resulting model is frequently appropriate to neither. These subpopulations may be described by geographic area or by some other defining characteristic such as stand age (e.g., hemlock in Pennsylvania) (Riemann Hershey 1996). Evidence from the data exploration, and/or any previous knowledge about the ecology or land-use history of the phenomena, can indicate that there may be several subpopulations of the same species that could be separated. In the case of tree species, where the spatial pattern and distribution of individual tree species is still more influenced by latitude and large topographic features than by human administrative boundaries such as states, it was suspected that ecological subregions might provide a better default area of investigation than states. These ecological units, part of the Forest Service's national hierarchical framework of ecological units, are classified and mapped based on "associations of those biotic and environmental factors that directly affect or indirectly express energy, moisture, and nutrient gradients which regulate the structure and function of ecosystems. These factors include climate, physiography, water, soils, air, hydrology, and potential natural communities" (McNab and Avers 1994). Several ecosubregions in Pennsylvania and New York were investigated separately and their statistical characteristics compared with each other and with the state summaries.

3.3 Interpolation methods

Kriging and the related routines of conditional simulation offer a way of creating a relatively continuous surface of estimated values which take advantage of (and can retain in some cases) the local spatial variation inherent in the sample dataset. There are several types of kriging and conditional simulation, and each is useful in different situations. The following are only highlights of three of the methods chosen as most appropriate, including some of the most distinctive features of each that affected its applicability here. The importance of each of these features depends on what we are interested in from the estimation.

Kriging estimates are essentially weighted moving averages of the original data values—taking the distance, direction, and redundancy of neighboring points into account using the model defined from the variogram. **Ordinary kriging** (**OK**) does honor the overall (global) mean and the sample data values. However, the averaging process results in output that is distinctly smoothed, and pockets of one or two high sample values can have a substantial effect on the surrounding estimates–undesirable characteristics for our objectives. OK does report an estimation variance, but when the sample data are not multivariate normal, its use as a measure of estimate reliability is probably erroneous because it is dependent on the data location and redundancy of the sample points and variogram model type used in the estimate. Kriging estimation variance is not dependent on data values (Deutsch and Journel 1992).

An indicator transform divides the data into two classes— above or below a designated cutoff value. **Indicator kriging** (**IK**) provides an estimate of the probability, for each estimated cell, that it falls above or below that cutoff value. The output dataset thus indicated the probability that sugar maple occurred at each location. In this study, the cutoff chosen was 0%ba/acre, indicating the presence or absence of that species. Indicator kriging, unlike OK, does not assume that the data have a particular distribution.

A third method investigated was sequential gaussian **conditional simulation** (**sgCS**) (Deutsch and Journel 1992; Rossi et al. 1993). Rather than determining a single "best" estimate, conditional simulation determines multiple estimates for each cell. All are equally probable and yet alternative realizations of the data determined from multiple simulation runs. This set of estimates can be used to build an entire distribution for each cell, that represents the range of possible values. A summary statistic

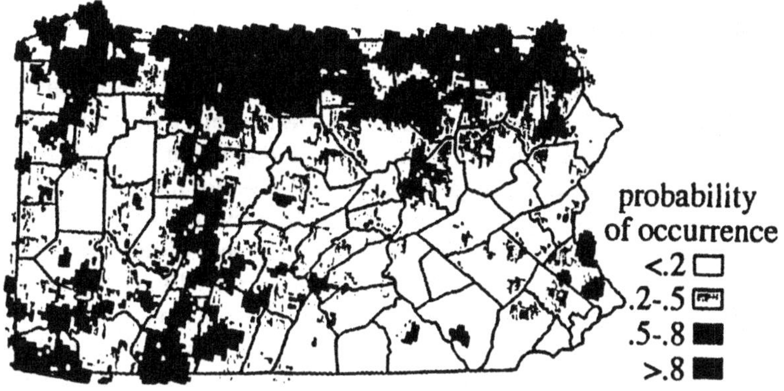

FIGURE 1. One of the four estimated datasets describing the distribution of sugar maple in Pennsylvania: the probability that sugar maple is present.

such as the mean or median of this distribution can then be chosen and used as the modeled "estimate" of %ba/acre for that cell,[1] and another value such as the standard deviation or inter-quartile range as the expression of uncertainty or "range of uncertainty." In this study, the median and a percentile range capturing approximately two-thirds of the distribution ($17th$ and $83rd$ percentiles) were chosen as representative of each cell's distribution. Unlike OK, sgCS does honor in each realization both the sample histogram (and the univariate statistics of the sample data) and the sample variogram/covariance. In addition, spatial variability is an integral component, and sgCS is effective in preserving local spatial means. It also retains much more local variability, a characteristic of the resource at this scale that we were particularly interested in retaining. The disadvantage of sgCS is that it assumes that the sample data are univariate normal, bivariate normal, and higher moment normal. In this case, we could make the data univariate normal with a normal-score transform and check it against the behavior of a bivariate normal dataset. In the likely scenario that all criteria are not fully satisfied, as was assumed to be the case here, the user should be aware that the results may be affected (Rossi et al. 1993). To determine whether there was substantial bias in the results, we chose to check independently the charactistics of an individual realization against the characteristics of the sample data.

[1]The methods used in this study are described in detail in Rossi et al. (1993) and Isaaks and Srivastava (1989); the analysis was performed using GSLIB routines (Deutsch and Journel 1992) with some additional routines written by R.E. Rossi.

4 Results

The objective of this study was slightly unusual compared to applications in earth sciences in one respect—a dataset was desired not to answer a specific question (e.g., where is the best location for a sugarbush or a mill), but to provide a resource dataset(s) that could be called on for many uses—ideally, wherever spatial information about species distribution and occurrence is required. Thus, there are four datasets, or four pieces of data for each cell location, that have been chosen here as final output. First, the results of the indicator kriging run, the probability that there is sugar maple present in a particular cell, is a valuable dataset (Fig. 1). This method makes few requirements of the data and, therefore, outputs robust results. If a user is interested only in where sugar maple occurs, then the probability output from IK is the most useful, and, therefore, was chosen as one of the critical output datasets to be maintained here. The next three output datasets chosen, an estimate of %ba/acre and the plus and minus uncertainty associated with that estimate, address the interest in knowing how much sugar maple occurs. For this, the results of the conditional simulation method were chosen. Although its demands on the normality of the sample data were great, in this case there appeared to be little bias when the characteristics of the predicted estimates were compared with what was expected of them. Although this may not be true for all species, and would have to be checked in each case, this method is most desirable because of its capacity to retain the local spatial variation inherent in the sample data. The summary datasets created from the conditional simulation runs (sgCS-median, sgCS-17 and sgCS-83) provide both an estimate and a measure of uncertainty, retain the most local variability, and maintain the characteristics of the sample data fairly well. The median "estimate" of %ba/acre values alone did not maintain the FIA summary statistics at the state and unit level, but those statistics did fall within the calculated uncertainty–between the 17th and 83rd percentiles (capturing 66% of the estimate distribution at each cell).

Dividing and modeling the data by ecoregion did reveal a different spatial structure in each. Adjacent ecosubregions had substantially different variograms, indicating the probability of different subpopulations of sugar maple in each, as least in terms of their spatial distribution patterns (Fig. 2). Given this evidence, future investigation and interpolation of individual tree species in the Northeast will be by ecosubregions.

The accuracy of the results from any model is important information for users of those data. How well does the output dataset portray the characteristics of the phenomena it was designed to capture? If it was intended to estimate current landcover as observed on the ground, how well does it do that? If it was intended to capture local variability, how well does it do that? Whether the resulting estimated dataset actually describes the occurrence and density of sugar maple involves two assumptions: 1) that

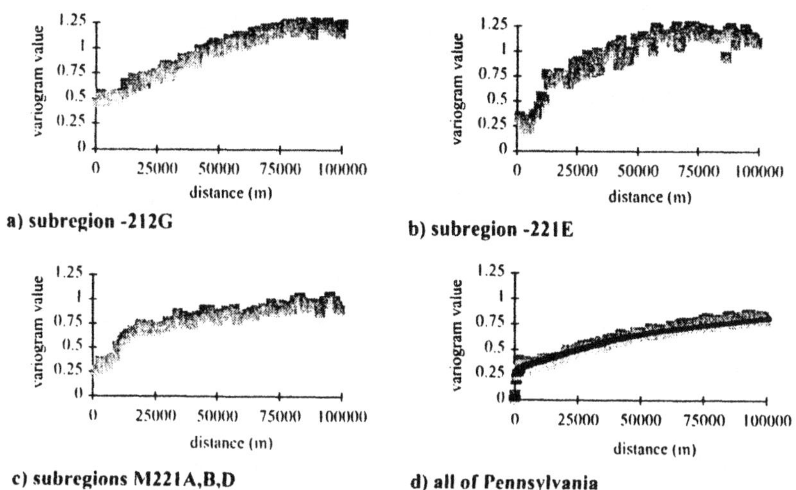

FIGURE 2. Comparison of sugar maple variograms calculated for four different areas in Pennsylvania. The variograms for each of the three ecosubregions (a, b, c) are substantially different from each other and from the variogram calculated for the state as a whole (d) in range, shape, and sill. This indicates that there are, at least in terms of spatial distribution patterns, several subpopulations that should be modeled separately.

the modeled dataset is representative of the sample data, and 2) that the sample data are representative of the phenomena. The first item can be checked by comparing the characteristics of the field data to those of the model predictions at as many scales as are appropriate given the data. The second item is determined largely by the sample design and our understanding of the phenomena, but we also can check the results against other independent sources of individual tree-species distribution–ideally of higher accuracy–where they exist. In this case, the lack of independent datasets of sufficient detail and describing the information we were trying to capture left us concentrating primarily on checking the first assumption. In this study, the univariate, variogram/covariance, and local statistics of each of the estimated datasets were compared to those of the original sample data (Fig. 3).

5 Discussion/Conclusions

The estimated datasets that are output by indicator kriging and sgCS have the potential to be very useful. Most tree species in the area examined exhibit substantial spatial dependence in the variograms of the normal-scored data, suggesting that there is considerable potential for the estimation of such datasets from FIA data. Each species exhibited some variety in spatial

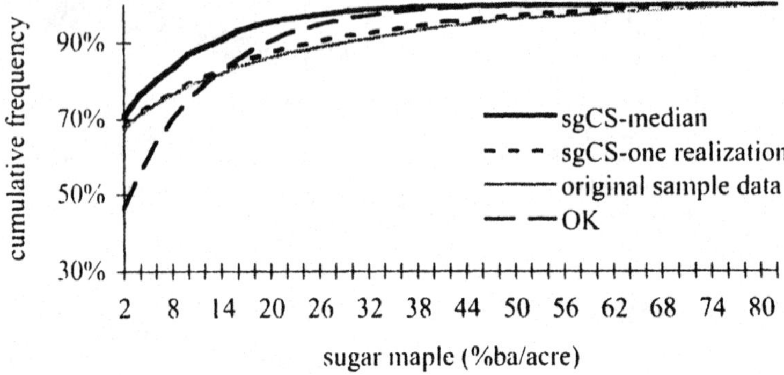

FIGURE 3. One way of assessing the resulting estimated datasets is to check how well each retain the characteristics of the original sample data. Shown here is a comparison of the univariate statistics of the original and modeled datasets.

patterns, spatial dependence, and resulting uncertainty of the estimates, and each may therefore require different levels of additional fine tuning depending on the objectives of the specific analysis and the time and expertise available.

These techniques make explicit the uncertainties associated with an estimate in a form that can be incorporated when the data are used. This feature adds considerable utility and flexibility in the use of the resulting estimates, as the risk of errors of commission or omission can be specifically determined and manipulated to suit the current objectives.

There is a high level of variance associated with these estimates of %ba/acre–in many locations this variance can be as much as the estimate itself. The dataset nevertheless provides a descriptive picture of species distribution at the state level. Compared to previous depictions of current species distribution from FIA data summarized at the county level, this method provides a much more detailed picture of species occurrence and distribution. Although estimates probably could be improved and variances diminished by additional investigation into each species, such as further dividing subpopulations or collecting additional data where the uncertainty is too high, the current estimates are informative and provide a useful basis from which to proceed.

These datasets of individual species distribution do not contain any of the fine-scale forest/nonforest detail. If such information is desired, more detailed datasets describing the forest/nonforest land cover would have to be derived from a more intense point sample [2] or the continuous but aver-

[2]Riemann Hershey, Rachel, D.A. Drake, and M.A. Ramirez. Producing a forest/nonforest map from the FIA photointerpretation data using Indicator Kriging. Un-

aged data available from satellite imagery. Such detailed datasets could be used as a "mask" and overlaid on any of the datasets of species distribution.

Maintaining information on individual species separately allows considerable flexibility in the use of species distribution data. Instead of being limited to previously defined fixed classes, forest cover types can be uniquely defined to capture more accurately the habitat required for a particular study. The potential also exists to use one or more of the species datasets as a decision layer in the interpretation of satellite imagery. The two datasets offer complementary information about the actual species composition on the ground. There are more possibilities for applying geostatistical techniques than have been investigated here. For example, some species may exhibit a spatial correlation with a particular soil, climate, topography, or reflectance data from satellite imagery. Indicator kriging and sgCS, in particular, allow such ancillary or "soft" information to be incorporated into the estimation process.

6 References

[1] Alerich, C.L. (1993) Forest Statistics for Pennsylvania–1978 and 1989. Resource Bulletin. NE-126. Radnor, PA. USDA Forest Service, Northeastern Forest Experiment Station.

[2] Biondi, F., D.E. Myers, and C.C. Avery. (1994) Geostatistically modeling stem size and increment in an old growth forest. *Canadian Journal of Forest Research*, **24**, 1354-1368.

[3] Deutsch, C.V. and A.G. Journel. (1992). *GSLIB: Geostatistical Software Library and User's Guide.* Oxford University Press, New York.

[4] Ghosh, M. and J.N.K. Rao. (1994) Small Area Estimation: An Appraisal. *Statistical Sciences*, **9**, 55-93.

[5] Hansen M.H., T. Frieswyk, J.F. Glover, and J.F. Kelly. (1992) The Eastwide Forest Inventory Data Base: Users Manual. General Technical Report NC-151. USDA Forest Service, North Central Experiment Station. St. Paul, MN.

[6] Isaaks, E.H. and R.M. Srivastava. (1989) *An Introduction to Applied Geostatistics.* Oxford University Press, New York.

[7] McNab, W.H. and P.E. Avers. (1984) Ecological Subregions of the United States: Section Descriptions. Administrative Publication WO-WSA-5. USDA Forest Service, Washington, DC.

published report on file at USDA Forest Service, Northeastern Forest Experiment Station, Forest Inventory and Analysis Unit, Radnor, PA.

[8] Riemann Hershey, R. (1996) Understanding the spatial distribution of tree species in Pennsylvania. pp. 73-82. In: Mowrer, H.T. et al. (tech coords). Spatial Accuracy Assessment in Natural Resources and Environmental Sciences. Second International Symposium. May 21-23. 1996. General Technical Report. RM-GTR-277. Fort Collins, CO. USDA Forest Service, Rocky Mountain Forest and Range Experiment Station.

[9] Rossi, R.E., D.J. Mulla, A.G. Journel, and E.H. Franz. (1992) Geostatistical tools for modeling and interpreting ecological spatial dependence. *Ecological Monographs*, **62**, 277-314.

[10] Rossi, R.E., P.W. Borth, and J.J. Tollefson. (1993) Stochastic simulation for characterizing ecological spatial patterns and appraising risk. *Ecological Applications*, **3**, 719-735.

Global Analysis of Ozone Data Based on Spherical Splines

Meng Jie
Yunnan University
People's Republic of China

Dominique Haughton and Nicholas Teebagy
Bentley College
United States

ABSTRACT In this paper, we present an analysis of satellite ozone data based on spherical splines (Wahba, 1990). This gives us the possibility of examining trends in smoothed ozone levels averaged over the earth, taking into account the noise in measurements of ozone levels. We also use our estimated splines to examine trends in the variability of ozone levels accross the earth: our measure of variability is based on a chi-square distance between the estimated spline and a uniform distribution of ozone. A decreasing trend emerges for averaged smoothed ozone levels, while the variability of ozone levels seems to be stationary.

To fit spherical splines to ozone data, we use techniques of Wahba (1990). We propose a simple but effective graphical method to select the number of spherical harmonics to include in the spline and the coefficient of smoothing λ.

1 Introduction

The possibility of a decrease in stratospheric ozone content has become a matter of wide-spread concern because of the important role of ozone in the earth environment. To observe and describe the trend in the amount of stratospheric ozone, both ground and satellite methods have been developed; satellite ozone data have received more and more attention because of their global coverage. Since 1979, a daily observation on each portion of earth covering 1° latitude and 1.25^o longitude has been collected by the Nimbus 7/Toms, Meteor 3/Toms and the Gome satellites.

Several methods have been used to attempt to assess the trend in ozone levels via the analysis of satellite data. Such efforts include the study of the time series of minimum measured ozone levels, or of weighted averages (see Stolarski et al., 1986, Guo et al., 1988, Bojkov et al., 1990, and Herman et al., 1995). Ozone levels are measured in Dobson Units (DU), and the area within the 220DU contour zone has been investigated (Herman et al., 1995). For each latitude, Niu and Tiao (1995) have used a space-time model to describe ozone data.

Two quantities at least are of interest in attempting to assess a global ozone trend: a measure of overall ozone content, but also a measure of the variability over the earth of ozone contents. Indeed, if such a variability were to increase over time, that would be a matter for serious concern. In this paper, we propose a spherical spline to fit satellite ozone data and then assess the trend in overall ozone content and in the variability of the distribution of ozone over the earth based on this spline model.

2 Spherical Splines

Spline models have received a lot of attention in statistics because of their flexibility and distribution-free nature (Wegman and Wright, 1983). We show below how a spherical spline can be fitted to ozone data.

Consider the following model for n observations on ozone levels at different points P_i on the earth:

$$y_i = f(P_i) + \epsilon_i \qquad i = 1, \ldots, n \tag{1}$$

where the ϵ_i are independent identically distributed (i.i.d.) $N(0, \sigma^2)$, $P = (\theta, \phi)$,where θ is the longitude ($0 \leq \theta \leq 2\pi$) and ϕ is the latitude $-\frac{\pi}{2} \leq \phi \leq \frac{\pi}{2}$ at the location P. A fitted spherical spline for the y_i is a function f on the sphere (such that f and its first derivatives are absolutely continuous and its second derivatives are square integrable) which minimizes:

$$\frac{1}{n}\sum_{i=1}^{n}(f(P_i) - y_i)^2 + \lambda \int_S (\Delta f)^2, \tag{2}$$

where Δ denotes the Laplacian operator on the sphere. Note that the first term in (2) is a least squares term, and the second term controls the smoothness of f.

Following Wahba (1990) section 2.2, we consider a spline of the form:

$$f(P) = \sum_{l=0}^{\infty}\sum_{s=-l}^{l} f_{l,s}F_{l,s}(P), \tag{3}$$

where the

$$F_{l,s}(\theta,\phi) = \begin{cases} \theta_{ls}\sin(s\theta)P_l^{|s|}(\sin(\phi)) & -l \le s < 0 \\ \theta_{l0}P_l(\sin(\phi)) & s = 0 \\ \theta_{ls}\cos(s\theta)P_l^s(\sin(\phi)) & 0 < s \le l \end{cases}$$

are eigenfunctions (often referred to as spherical harmonics) of the Laplacian operator on the sphere (see Wahba (1990) p. 25), with

$$\theta_{ls} = \begin{cases} \sqrt{2}\sqrt{\frac{2l+1}{4\pi}\frac{(l-|s|)!}{(l+|s|)!}} & s \neq 0 \\ \sqrt{\frac{2l+1}{4\pi}} & s = 0 \end{cases}$$

Here, the P_l and P_l^s are the Legendre polynomials and Legendre functions respectively, defined as:

$$P_l(z) = \frac{1}{2^l l!}\frac{\partial^l (z^2-1)^l}{\partial z^l} \qquad l = 0, 1, ... \tag{4}$$

$$P_l^s(z) = (1-z^2)^{s/2}\frac{\partial^s P_l(z)}{\partial z^s} \qquad l = 1, ..., s = -l, ..., l. \tag{5}$$

Note that the $F_{l,s}$ form an orthonormal system, that is: $\int_S F_{l,s}F_{l',s'} = 0$ for $(l,s) \neq (l',s')$ and $\int_S F_{l,s}^2 = 1$. We then have (see Wahba (1990) p. 26):

$$\Delta f = \sum_{l=1}^{\infty}\sum_{s=-l}^{l} f_{l,s}\Delta F_{l,s}(\theta,\phi) = -[l(l+1)]\sum_{l=1}^{\infty}\sum_{s=-l}^{l} f_{l,s}F_{ls}(\theta,\phi)$$

So, since the $F_{l,s}$ form an orthonormal system,

$$\int_S (\Delta f)^2 dP = \sum_{l=1}^{\infty}\sum_{s=-l}^{l}[l(l+1)]^2 f_{ls}^2 \tag{6}$$

In order to obain an approximate spline for the y_i, we will then choose f_{ls} to minimize:

$$\frac{1}{n}\sum_{i=1}^{n}(y_i - \sum_{l=0}^{N}\sum_{s=-l}^{l} f_{l,s}F_{l,s}(P_i))^2 + \lambda\sum_{l=0}^{N}\sum_{s=-l}^{l}[l(l+1)]^2 f_{l,s}^2 \tag{7}$$

In section 4, we will describe a procedure to select suitable values of N and λ.

3 Fitting the Model

3.1 Data

Our monthly satellite ozone data, in Dobson Units (DU), was obtained from the Internet (jwocky.gsfc.nasa.gov). One observation is given for each

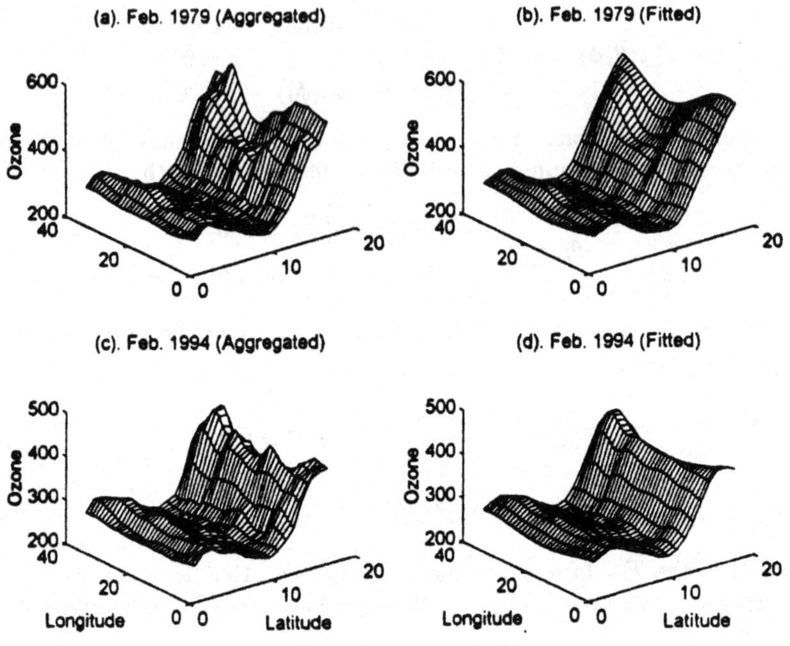

FIGURE 1 a-d

the form $\{y_{ij}, i = 1, ..., 36, j = 1, ...18\}$, where the index i corresponds to longitude positions and the index j to latitude positions. Figure 1 a,c, Figure 2 a,c and Figure 3 a,c show plots of aggregated ozone data in terms of latitude and longitude indices for February 1979 and 1994 (Fig. 1 a,c), for October 1979 and 1994 (Fig. 2 a,c), and for 1979 and 1994 as a whole (Fig. 3 a,c).

3.2 Fitting the Model

Let us define a matrix X as follows:

$$X = \begin{pmatrix} F_{0,0}(P_1) & F_{1,-1}(P_1) & F_{1,0}(P_1) & F_{1,1}(P_1) & \cdots & F_{N,N}(P_1) \\ \cdots & \cdots & \cdots & \cdots & \cdots & \cdots \\ \cdots & \cdots & \cdots & \cdots & \cdots & \cdots \\ \cdots & \cdots & \cdots & \cdots & \cdots & \cdots \\ F_{0,0}(P_n) & F_{1,-1}(P_n) & F_{1,0}(P_n) & F_{1,1}(P_n) & \cdots & F_{N,N}(P_n) \end{pmatrix}.$$

and let

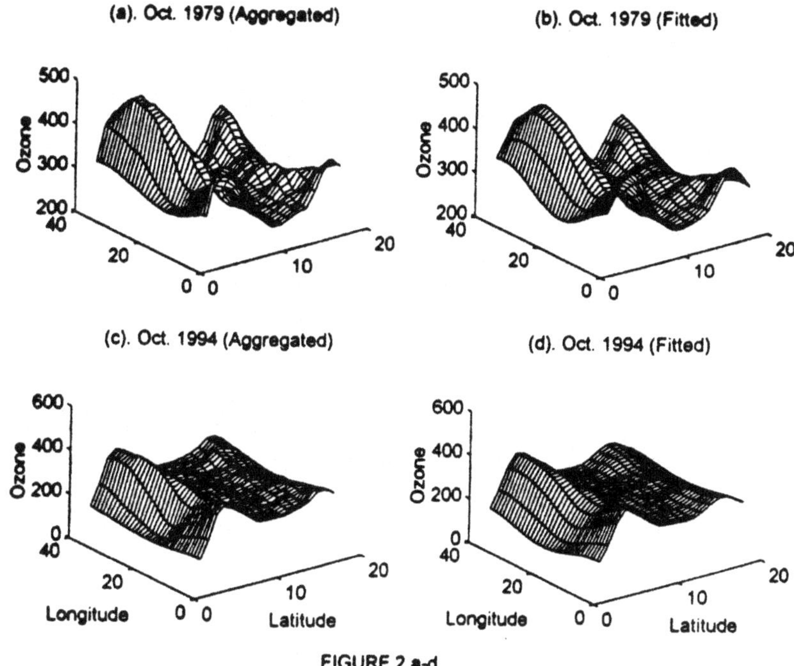

FIGURE 2 a-d

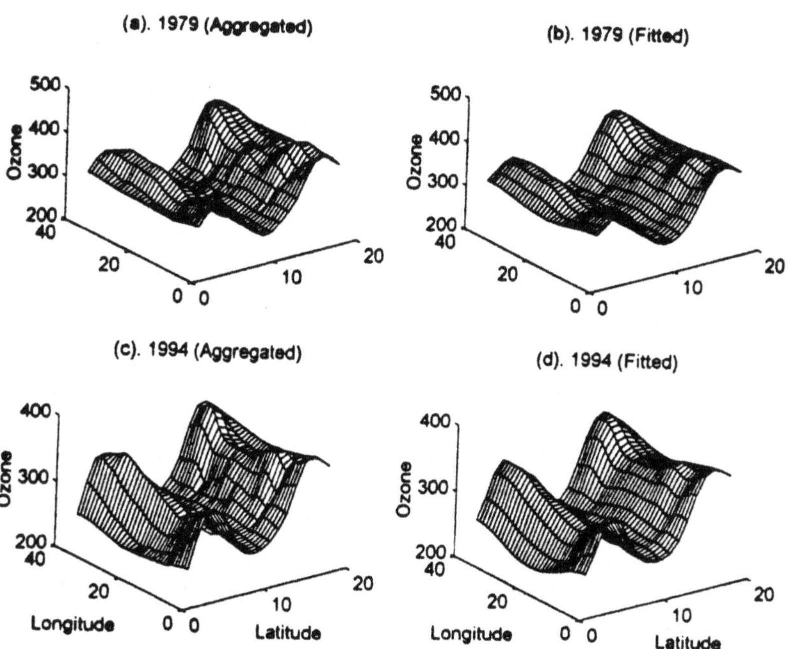

FIGURE 3 a-d

$$Y = (y_1, ..., y_n)^T$$

and

$$f_\beta = (f_{0,0}, f_{1,-1}, ..., f_{N,N})^T.$$

Let also D be the diagonal matrix with (l, l) entry $[l(l+1)]^2$. Equation (7) can then be rewritten as:

$$\frac{1}{n}(Y - Xf_\beta)^T(Y - Xf_\beta) + \lambda f_\beta^T D f_\beta \tag{8}$$

The minimizing solution $\hat{f}_\beta$ can be calculated as:

$$\hat{f}_\beta = (X^T X + n\lambda D)^{-1} X^T Y \tag{9}$$

By way of illustration, we give expressions for a few of the base functions $F_{l,s}$ and estimated values for the corresponding $f_{l,s}$ for October 1994:

$$[F_{l,s}] = \begin{bmatrix} \cdots & \cdots & \cdots & \cdots \\ & & F_{2,-2} & \cdots \\ & F_{1,-1} & F_{2,-1} & \cdots \\ F_{0,0} & F_{1,0} & F_{2,0} & \cdots \\ & F_{1,1} & F_{2,1} & \cdots \\ & & F_{2,2} & \cdots \\ \cdots & \cdots & \cdots & \cdots \end{bmatrix}$$

so

$$[F_{l,s}] = \begin{bmatrix} \cdots & \cdots & \cdots & \cdots \\ & & -\sqrt{\frac{15}{16\pi}}\sin 2\theta\cos^2\phi & \cdots \\ & -\sqrt{\frac{3}{4\pi}}\sin\theta\cos\phi & -\sqrt{\frac{15}{4\pi}}\sin\theta\cos\phi\sin\phi & \cdots \\ \sqrt{\frac{1}{4\pi}} & \sqrt{\frac{3}{4\pi}}\sin\phi & \sqrt{\frac{5}{16\pi}}(3\sin^2\phi - 1) & \cdots \\ & \sqrt{\frac{3}{4\pi}}\cos\theta\cos\phi & \sqrt{\frac{15}{4\pi}}\cos\theta\cos\phi\sin\phi & \cdots \\ & & \sqrt{\frac{15}{16\pi}}\cos 2\theta\cos^2\phi & \cdots \\ \cdots & \cdots & \cdots & \cdots \end{bmatrix}$$

$$[\hat{f}_{l,s}] = \begin{bmatrix} \cdots & \cdots & \cdots & \cdots \\ & & \hat{f}_{2,-2} & \cdots \\ & \hat{f}_{1,-1} & \hat{f}_{2,-1} & \cdots \\ \hat{f}_{0,0} & \hat{f}_{1,0} & \hat{f}_{2,0} & \cdots \\ & \hat{f}_{1,1} & \hat{f}_{2,1} & \cdots \\ & & \hat{f}_{2,2} & \cdots \\ \cdots & \cdots & \cdots & \cdots \end{bmatrix} = \begin{bmatrix} \cdots & \cdots & \cdots & \cdots \\ & & -1.016 & \cdots \\ & -8.429 & 12.333 & \cdots \\ 1032.260 & -36.696 & 22.327 & \cdots \\ & -0.207 & 5.040 & \cdots \\ & & 1.706 & \cdots \\ \cdots & \cdots & \cdots & \cdots \end{bmatrix}$$

Note that the constant $\hat{f}_{0,0}F_{0,0}$ (approximately equal to 291.195 for October 1994) is a constant approximation to the function f, and that the terms involving $\{F_{1,-1}, F_{1,0}, F_{1,1}\}$ (a system of spherical coordinates on the sphere) provide with a first order approximation of the function f. Interestingly, the estimated $\hat{f}_{l,0}$ is usually greater than the other estimated $\hat{f}_{ls}$, $(s \neq 0)$. The corresponding function $F_{l,0} = \theta_{l0}P_l(\sin\phi)$, depends on the latitude ϕ only. That means that ozone values depend more strongly on latitude. This is typical of all the models we fitted.

3.3 Analysis of results

3.3.1 Remarks on global plots of ozone levels

Based on a cross-validation method to be presented in section 4, we chose $N = 9$ and $\lambda = 10^{-5}$. The fitted surfaces are given in Figure 1 b,d, Figure 2 b,d and Figure 3 b,d. Visible directly from the graphs are the lower ozone values for Antarctica (latitude index of 1), but also for the heavily populated regions in the mid Northern latitudes. The graphs also show that in the same month of different years (1979 and 1994), the surfaces have a similar shape, but the shift downward from 1979 to 1994 appears to affect essentially the entire surfaces. In February, a relatively large downward shift occurs at the north pole (latitude index of 16), from about 580DU to about 400DU. In October, the graphs indicate the downward shift of ozone values in Antarctica, from about 270-340DU to about 120-170DU, as documented elsewhere. Note that the ozone values at the North and South poles seem to decrease at about the same rate in February and October respectively, so conceivably an ozone hole could form in February above the North pole in the future.

3.3.2 Trends in the mean and variablity of the distribution of ozone over the earth

In order to obtain an overall average $OZAV$ for the ozone distribution which takes into account the noise in the observations, we propose to use our fitted spline $\sum_{l=0}^{N}\sum_{s=-l}^{l}\hat{f}_{ls}F_{ls}(\theta,\phi)$, integrated as follows over the unit sphere S:

$$OZAV = \int_S \sum_{l=0}^{N}\sum_{s=-l}^{l}\hat{f}_{l,s}F_{l,s}(\theta,\phi)/4\pi$$

It is easy to check that:

$$OZAV = \hat{f}_{0,0}F_{0,0}.$$

So the first term in our fitted spline is an estimator of average ozone levels. We could get an estimator of average ozone levels in any particular region by integrating over this region.

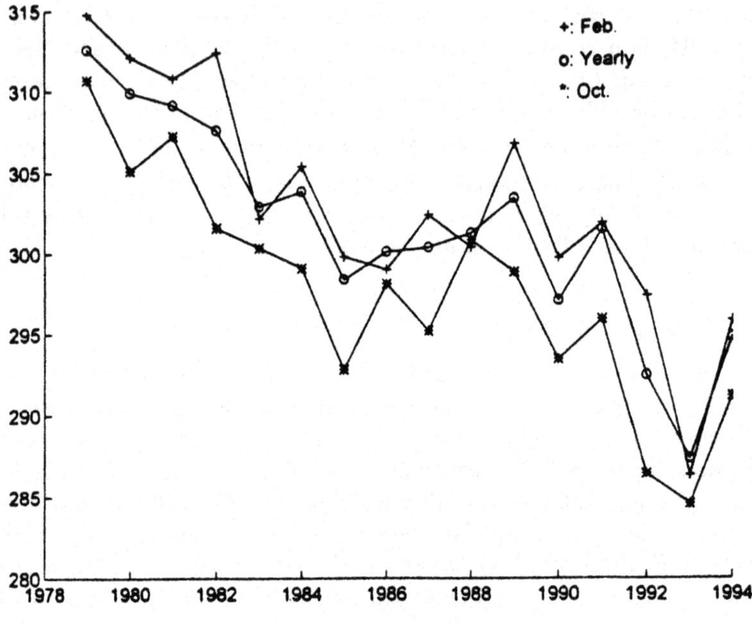

FIGURE 4 AVERAGE OZONE LEVELS

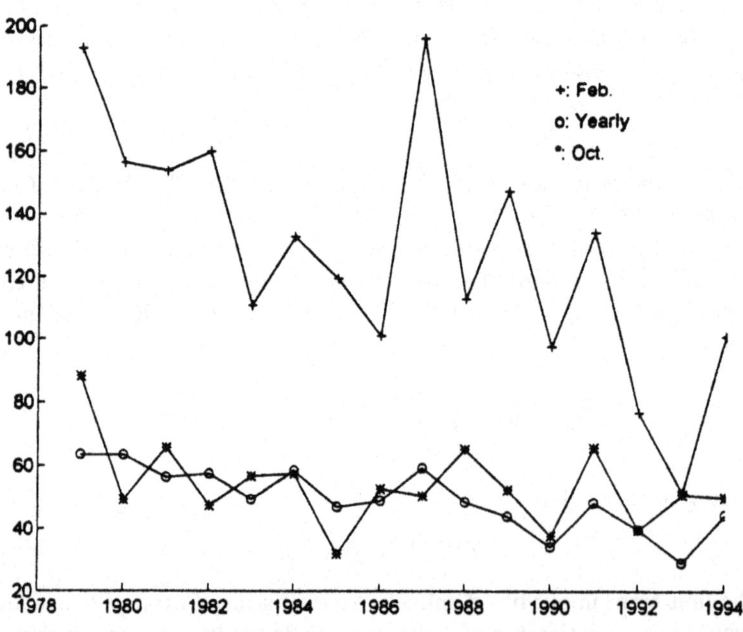

FIGURE 5 VARIABILITY OF OZONE LEVELS

Values of estimated ozone averages are given in Figure 4 for splines fitted to February data, to October data, and to yearly (averaged) data, for 1979-1994. Figure 4 does open the possibility of a decreasing trend for overall ozone averages, particularly when compared to the trend in variabilities which we now present.

As a measure of the variability $OZVAR$ of the distribution of ozone, we propose a "chi-square" distance between the ozone distribution and the uniform distribution, defined as follows:

$$OZVAR = \int_S [\sum_{l=0}^{N} \sum_{s=-l}^{l} \hat{f}_{l,s} F_{l,s}(\theta,\phi) - \hat{f}_{0,0} F_{0,0}]^2 / \hat{f}_{0,0} F_{0,0}$$

Since the $F_{l,s}$ form an orthonormal system, we have:

$$OZVAR = \sum_{l=1}^{N} \sum_{s=-l}^{l} \hat{f}^2_{l,s} / \hat{f}_{0,0} F_{0,0}. \qquad (10)$$

The values of $OZVAR$ for the months of October, February, and for the whole year are given for 1979-1994 in Figure 5. No obvious trend emerges for the overall variability of the ozone distribution; the variability tends to be higher in February as can also be seen from the surface plots in Figures 1-3.

4 Choice of N and of the smoothing parameters λ.

The ordinary cross-validation function is defined as

$$V_0(\lambda, N) = \frac{1}{n} \sum_{k=1}^{n} (y_i - X \hat{f}_\beta^{[k]}(\lambda, N))^2 \qquad (11)$$

where $\hat{f}_\beta^{[k]}(\lambda, N)$ minimizes

$$\frac{1}{n} \sum_{\substack{i=1 \\ i \neq k}}^{n} (y_i - X f_\beta)^2 + \lambda \sum_{l=1}^{\infty} \sum_{s=-l}^{l} [l(l+1)]^2 f_{ls}^2$$

Based on the October 1994 data (the most recent available data), we calculate $V_0(\lambda, N)$. Figure 6a gives plots of the square root of $V_0(N, \lambda)$ in terms of the (base 10) logarithm of λ for different values of N (N decreases as one moves up the graph), and Figure 6b gives plots of the square root of $V_0(N, \lambda)$ in terms of N for different values of the base 10 logarithm of λ (λ increases as one moves up the graph). In order to use these plots to

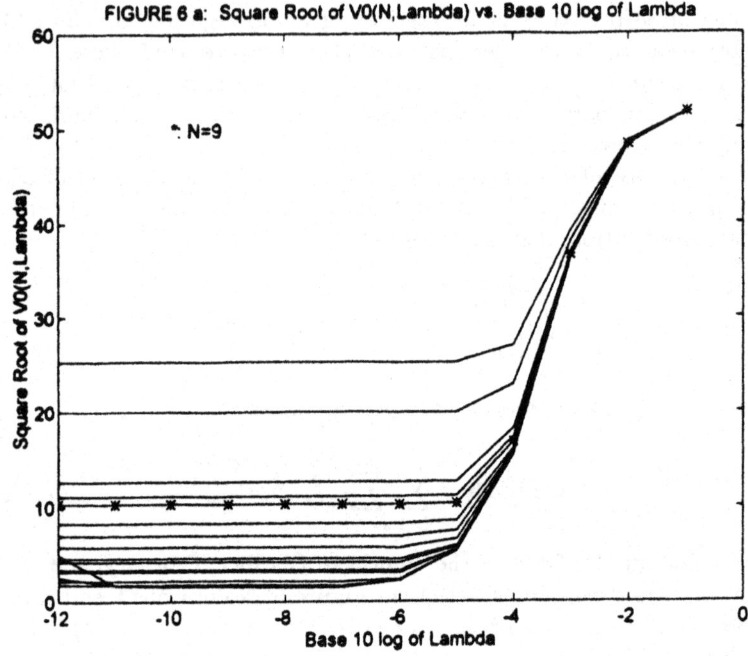
FIGURE 6 a: Square Root of V0(N,Lambda) vs. Base 10 log of Lambda
*: N=9
Square Root of V0(N,Lambda)
Base 10 log of Lambda
60
50
40
30
20
10
0
-12
-10
-8
-6
-4
-2
0

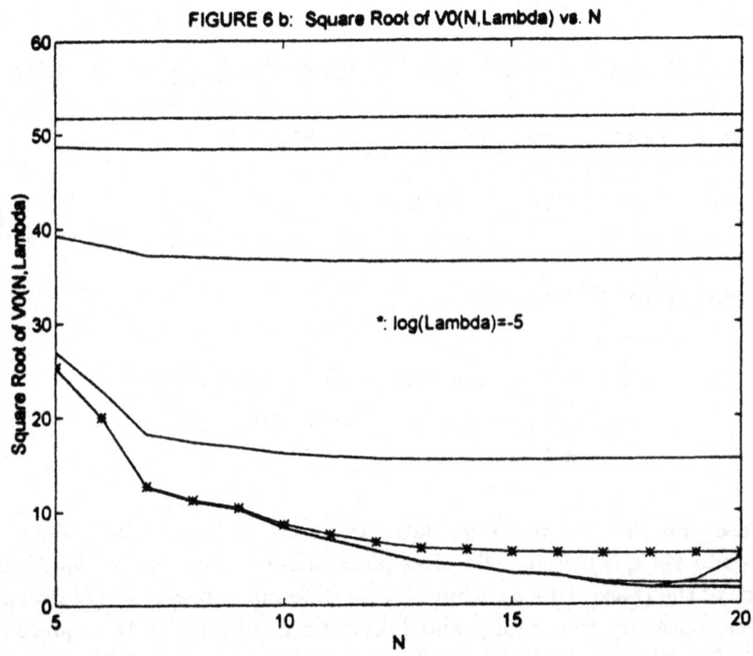
FIGURE 6 b: Square Root of V0(N,Lambda) vs. N
*: log(Lambda)=-5
Square Root of V0(N,Lambda)
N
60
50
40
30
20
10
0
5
10
15
20

select suitable values for N and λ, we take into account the fact that the random error due to the measurement of satellite ozone data is no less than about 6 (Kelly Chance, Smithsonian Institute, Harvard University, personal communication). So choices of λ and N resulting in values of the square root of $V_0(N, \lambda)$ of less than 6 are likely to overfit the data. Allowing for the fact that other sources of errors are likely to be present let us select N and λ to allow for a possible random error of about 10. Looking at Figure 6a, 6b, it appears that a choice of $N = 9$ yields quite a few values of λ satisfying this requirement and that a value of λ of 10^{-5} (smaller values would be possible too) is satisfactory.

5 References

[1] Bojkov, R. D., L. Bishop, W. J. Hill, G. C. Reinsel, and G. C. Tiao (1990). A Statistical Trend Analysis of Revised Dobson Total Ozone Data Over the Northern Hemisphere, *Journal of Geophysical Research*, **95**, 9795-9807.

[2] Davis, Harry F. (1963). *Fourier Series and Orthogonal Functions*, Allyn and Bacon, pp. 191-233.

[3] Guo Shichang and Wei Dingwen (1988). Characteristics of the Temporal-Spatial Variation in Atmospheric Ozonosphere over the North Hemisphere During the Period of 1963-1985, *Advances in Atmospheric Science*, **5**, 361-368.

[4] Herman, J. R., P. A. Newman, R. McPeters, A. J. Krueger, P. K. Bhartia, C. J. Seftor, O. Torres, G. Jaross, R. P. Cebula, D. Larko and C. Wellemeyer (1995). Meteor3/total ozone mapping spectometer observations of the 1993 ozone hole, *Journal of Geophysical Research*, **100**, 2973-2983.

[5] Stolarski, R. S., A. J. Krueger, M. R. Schoeberl, R. D. Peters, P. A. Newman, and J. C. Alert (1986). Nimbus 7 Satellite Measurements of the Springtime Antarctic Ozone Decrease, *Nature*, **322**, 808-811.

[6] Wahba, G. (1990). *Spline Models for Observational Data*, CBMS-NSF Regional Conference Series in Applied Mathematics, SIAM, Philadelphia.

[7] Wegman, E. J. and I. W. Wright (1983). Splines in Statistics, *Journal of the American Statistical Association*, **78**, 351-365.

[8] Xufeng Niu and George C. Tiao (1995). Modelling Satellite Ozone Data, *Journal of the American Statistical Association*, **90**, 969-983.

Bounded Influence Estimation in a Spatial Linear Mixed Model

Ana F. Militino and M. Dolores Ugarte *

Departamento de Estadística e Investigación Operativa
Universidad Pública de Navarra

ABSTRACT Kriging is an interpolation method that consists of finding a predictor linear function of the observations, minimizing the mean squared prediction error or kriging variance. Under multivariate normality assumptions, the given predictor is the best linear unbiased predictor, but if the underlying distribution is not normal, the estimator shall not be unbiased and shall be vulnerable to outliers. In the spatial context, it is not only the presence of outliers that may spoil the predictions, but also the boundary sites, usually corners, that tend to have high leverage. Therefore, kriging predictions are very sensitive on these corners, giving rise to values extremely vulnerable to small changes in the data. To overcome this situation, a spatial linear mixed model is proposed, deriving a bounded influence estimator of the location parameters. To illustrate the results, an application to Davis topographic data is presented.

Key words and phrases: kriging; Dirichlet tessellation; random effects; generalized M estimator.

1 Introduction

The fit of a spatial linear model is a necessary task in precipitation, hydrology, mining statistics and more generally in geostatistics and environmental studies. It can be accomplished by a regression procedure known as kriging. The procedure has been extensively used in the literature (Ripley, 1981; Cressie, 1991), giving predictors of unobserved values of a spatially distributed variable and providing an estimate of the variance of the predictor error as well. Under multivariate normality assumptions, the given predictor is the best linear unbiased predictor, but if the underlying distribution is not normal, the estimator shall not be unbiased and shall be

*Address: Universidad Pública de Navarra, Campus Arrosadía, 31006 Pamplona, Spain. E-mail: militino@upna.es and lola@upna.es

vulnerable to outliers. Two robust kriging proposals have been given by Hawkins and Cressie (1984). However, as the authors themselves recognize, one variant may be computationally prohibitive, whereas the other produces inaccurate estimates. Militino (1996) proposes an M-estimator of the spatial linear model that is easy to compute, but robust against outlying responses cases only.

Rather than assuming that outliers may reflect an unexpected degree of freedom of inherent variability, we may admit the possibility that the sample reflects low-level contamination from a population other than that represented by the basic model. A common theoretical model for this occurrence of outliers in a single sample is a two component normal mixture. One of the components, with a large prior probability, represents the good observations and the other, with small probability, represents the bad observations. The idea, easily extended to a finite number of components may be accomplished with finite mixture models. Militino and Ugarte (1996) propose the use of a spatial linear mixed model and give an M-estimator of the location parameters.

In the spatial context, however, it is not only the presence of outliers that may spoil the predictions, but also the boundary sites, usually corners, that tend to have high leverage. That is why we concentrate our attention on using bounded influence estimators in a spatial linear mixed model. These estimators limit the influence that any small subset of the data has on the estimated coefficients while minimizing the asymptotic variance at the normal model. The bounded influence estimators achieve a breakdown point of roughly .50, a bounded influence function and a high efficiency versus least squares when the underlying distribution function is Gaussian. The breakdown point is simply the smallest contamination that may completely ruin an estimator. The influence function gives the amount of change in the estimator that can be wrought by an infinitesimal amount of contamination. Then, the purpose of the bounded influence estimators is to bound both the influence of residuals and the influence of position.

This paper is organized in 6 sections. Section two recalls the spatial linear model. Section three examines mixed models. Section four is devoted to bounded influence estimators and the transformations needed to apply them in the spatial context. Section five is dedicated to construct the bounded influence estimator in a spatial linear mixed model, and the last section gives an example based on Davis topographic data.

2 The Spatial Linear Model

Let us introduce the usual way of expressing the spatial linear model $Z(\mathbf{x}) = \mu(\mathbf{x}) + \epsilon(\mathbf{x})$, where $\mathbf{x}$ is the location at which an observation is taken, $\mu(\mathbf{x})$ is the mean function of the stochastic process $Z(\mathbf{x})$ and $\epsilon(\mathbf{x})$ is a zero mean error process or fluctuation with $\text{var}(\epsilon(\mathbf{x})) = \text{var}(Z(\mathbf{x})) = \sigma^2$. Note that $\mu(\mathbf{x})$ represents the "trend" or "drift" and is usually given through a

polynomial surface by $\mu(\mathbf{x}) = \sum_{i=1}^{p} f_i(\mathbf{x})\beta_i = \mathbf{f}(\mathbf{x})^T\beta$, where T indicates transpose. In addition, the procedure requires a knowledge of the covariance function satisfying $\mathbf{K}(\mathbf{x}_i, \mathbf{x}_j) = \mathrm{Cov}(Z(\mathbf{x}_i), Z(\mathbf{x}_j)) = C(d)$ for all $\mathbf{x}_i, \mathbf{x}_j \in R^2$, where d is the Euclidean distance between $\mathbf{x}_i$ and $\mathbf{x}_j$.
Under this assumption, kriging gives an estimate of β using generalized least squares (GLS) and minimizing the mean squared error or kriging variance. The natural estimator of the trend surface parameters $\beta = (\beta_1, \cdots, \beta_p)^T$ is the GLS estimator given by

$$\hat{\beta}_{GLS} = [\mathbf{F}^T\mathbf{K}^{-1}\mathbf{F}]^{-1}\mathbf{F}^T\mathbf{K}^{-1}\mathbf{Z}, \tag{1}$$

where $\mathbf{Z} = (z_1, \cdots, z_n)^T$ is the vector of the given observations, $\mathbf{K}$ is its covariance matrix and $\mathbf{F}$ is the design matrix

$$\mathbf{F} = \begin{bmatrix} f_1(\mathbf{x}_1) & \dots & f_p(\mathbf{x}_1) \\ \vdots & \dots & \vdots \\ f_1(\mathbf{x}_n) & \dots & f_p(\mathbf{x}_n) \end{bmatrix} = \begin{bmatrix} \mathbf{f}(\mathbf{x}_1)^T \\ \vdots \\ \mathbf{f}(\mathbf{x}_n)^T \end{bmatrix}.$$

This is the best linear unbiased estimator under the assumption of normality. However, the GLS estimator as well as other linear estimators lack robustness in the presence of atypical values (Cressie, 1991; Hawkins and Cressie, 1984).

3 Mixed Models

As far as the different uses of the mixed models are concerned, they include the identification of outliers and the investigation of robustness of certain statistics to departures from normality. Here, we shall give a brief review of these models before using them in the spatial context. The common idea underlying these models is that the data arise from two or more groups all with common distributional form but different parameters.
The EM algorithm (Dempster et al., 1977) is a basic tool for the estimation of the parameters by maximum likelihood in mixed models. Dempster et al. considered the mixture problem as one of many examples in which the data can be viewed as incomplete. They interpreted the mixture data as incomplete data by regarding an observation on the mixture as missing its component (or category) of origin. The components correspond to the random effects.
A disadvantage of any approach using a specified parametric form (e. g. normal) for the mixing distribution of the random effects is the possible hypothesis dependency on the conclusions. The influential paper of Heckman and Singer (1984) showed substantial changes in estimating the parameters of variance component models with quite small changes in mixing distribution specification. This difficulty can be avoided by nonparametric maximum likelihood estimation of the mixing distribution. In this work we propose a spatial linear mixed model, for which a robust nonparametric maximum likelihood estimation of the mixing distribution is derived.

4 The Bounded-Influence Estimator

Consider a linear model of the form $\mathbf{Y} = \mathbf{X}\beta + \mathbf{e}$, where $\mathbf{X}$ is a full column rank $n \times p$ matrix of known constants, β is a $p \times 1$ vector of parameters, and $\mathbf{e}$ is an $n \times 1$ vector of random errors that are independent and identically distributed. Let σ^2 denote the variance of e_i and $\mathbf{x}_i$ the ith row of $\mathbf{X}$. The first column of $\mathbf{X}$ is a column of 1s. The M estimate of β is the solution to the estimating equation

$$\sum_{i=1}^{n} \psi\left(\frac{y_i - \mathbf{x}_i^T \beta}{\sigma}\right)\mathbf{x}_i = \mathbf{0},$$

where ψ is an odd and bounded function. In principle, we have broad latitude in choosing the function ψ. The properties of the M-estimator are essentially determined by this function. One important issue in choosing ψ is the balance between robustness and efficiency. To achieve this purpose different functions have been given in the literature, such as Huber-psi function, Andrews function or biweight function (see Hoaglin et al., 1985). The effect of these functions is to cut the influence of anomalous residuals. In practice, σ is replaced by an estimate based on an initial set of the residuals. It is common to consider the median absolute deviation.

M-estimators are efficient and highly robust to unusual values of y_i, but one rogue leverage point can break them down completely. In order to produce stable results under these circumstances, the bounded-influence estimators or generalized M (GM) estimators have been developed with different proposals (see, for instance Mallows, 1975 and Simpson et al., 1992). The class of Mallows or Schweppe GM estimates of β are given by the solution to the estimating equation

$$\sum_{i=1}^{n} \psi\left(\frac{y_i - \mathbf{x}_i^T \beta}{u_i \sigma}\right) w_i \mathbf{x}_i = \mathbf{0},$$

where Mallows type corresponds to $u_i = 1$ and Schweppe type corresponds to $u_i = w_i$. As with the M estimates, in practice σ is replaced by an initial robust estimate of scale. The weights $w_i = w(\mathbf{x}_i), i = 1, \cdots, n$ depending on the design points, might be suitable choices so that the GM estimates are bounded both in the y and $\mathbf{x}$ spaces.

For example, Mallows (1975) weights $\{w_1, \cdots, w_n\}$ given by

$$w_i = \min\left\{1, \left\{\frac{d}{(\mathbf{x} - \hat{\mu}_x)^T \hat{C}_x^{-1} (\mathbf{x} - \hat{\mu}_x)}\right\}^{\alpha/2}\right\} \tag{2}$$

are appropriate, where $\hat{C}_x^{-1}$ and $\hat{\mu}_x$ are high-breakdown robust estimates of the scatter and location of the $\mathbf{x}$ variables, respectively. A possible choice for $(\hat{\mu}_x, \hat{C}_x^{-1})$ is given by the center and the covariance of the smallest ellipsoid containing at least $[(n+p+1)/2]$ points (minimum volume ellipsoid estimator); d can be taken to be the square root of the 95th percentile of a χ^2 random variable with p degrees of freedom (Rousseeuw and van Zomeren, 1990). Recommendations on the exponent parameter α were discussed by Simpson et al. (1992), giving the case $\alpha = 1$ as usual.

Nevertheless, the GM estimators are obtained from a model with independent errors whereas in the spatial model this assumption is not available. To solve this, we propose the use of a transformation based on case-deletion idea. With this 1-1 transformation we preserve normality and obtain a heteroskedastic model instead of a model where the errors have a non-diagonal covariance matrix (Militino and Ugarte, 1996). The heteroskedastic model takes the form

$$\tilde{\mathbf{Z}} = \tilde{\mathbf{F}}\beta + \tilde{\varepsilon}, \tag{3}$$

where $\tilde{\mathbf{Z}} = (\tilde{z}_1, \cdots, \tilde{z}_n)^T$, $\tilde{z}_i = z_i - \mathbf{Z}_{(i)}^T \mathbf{K}_{(i)}^{-1} \mathbf{k}_i$, $z_i = z(\mathbf{x}_i)$, $i = 1, \cdots, n$, is the observation at the ith location $\mathbf{x}_i$, $\mathbf{Z}_{(i)} = (z_1, \cdots, z_{i-1}, z_{i+1}, \cdots, z_n)^T$ is the vector of observations except the ith observation, $\mathbf{k}_i = \mathrm{Cov}(z_i, \mathbf{Z}_{(i)})$, $\mathbf{K}_{(i)}^{-1}$ is the inverse of $\mathbf{K}$ after leaving the ith observation out, and

$$\tilde{\mathbf{F}} = \begin{bmatrix} \tilde{f}_1(\mathbf{x}_1) & \dots & \tilde{f}_p(\mathbf{x}_1) \\ \vdots & \dots & \vdots \\ \tilde{f}_1(\mathbf{x}_n) & \dots & \tilde{f}_p(\mathbf{x}_n) \end{bmatrix} = \begin{bmatrix} \tilde{\mathbf{f}}(\mathbf{x}_1)^T \\ \vdots \\ \tilde{\mathbf{f}}(\mathbf{x}_n)^T \end{bmatrix}$$

is the design matrix with $\tilde{\mathbf{f}}(\mathbf{x}_i) = \mathbf{f}(\mathbf{x}_i) - \mathbf{F}_{(i)}^T \mathbf{K}_{(i)}^{-1} \mathbf{k}_i$. Moreover, $\mathrm{var}(\tilde{z}_i) = \sigma^2 s_i^2$.

If the data are irregularly spaced, it also could be appropriate to introduce a weight each time we leave an observation out. This may be done through the tile areas of the Dirichlet tessellation which is based on associating a polygon D_i with each point of a sample inside D, the region of interest. Each one of the points inside this polygon, also called Dirichlet cell or tile, is nearer to the referred sampled point than to any other. These areas allow us to balance the consequences we have in the likelihood maximization process each time we leave an observation out.

5 Bounded-Influence Estimator of the Spatial Linear Mixed Model

After transforming the original data z_i into $\tilde{z}_i$, a finite mixture model is proposed:

$$\tilde{\mathbf{Z}} = \tilde{\mathbf{F}}\beta + \mathbf{b}\alpha + e, \tag{4}$$

where the random effect α is an intercept parameter with K components, $\mathbf{b}$ is the design matrix of its coefficients and the error e is assumed to have a normal distribution.

If the distribution of the random effect is unspecified, the nonparametric maximum likelihood (NPML) estimate of the mixing distribution may be used. The NPML estimate of the mixing distribution is a discrete distribution on a finite number K of mass-points (Laird, 1978). The likelihood function of $\tilde{\mathbf{Z}}$ is given by

$$L(\tilde{\mathbf{Z}}|\beta,\sigma) = \prod_{i=1}^{n}\sum_{k=1}^{K} p_k h(\tilde{z}_i|\beta_k,\alpha_k,\sigma) = \prod_{i=1}^{n}\sum_{k=1}^{K} p_k h_{ik},$$

where p_k are the probability masses at known mass-points $\tilde{z}_k$ and h_{ik} is the likelihood function of the ith observation in the kth component. The procedure has been implemented in GLIM4 by Aitkin and Francis (1995) using the EM algorithm. This algorithm implies the following estimation scheme: (1) The E-step calculates the posterior probability that observation $\tilde{z}_i$ comes from component k

$$W_{ik} = \frac{p_k h_{ik}}{\sum_{l=1}^{K} p_l h_{il}}, \tag{5}$$

and (2) the M-step computes the conditional expectation solving

$$\sum_{k=1}^{K}\sum_{i=1}^{n} W_{ik} e_{ik} \tilde{\mathbf{f}}(\mathbf{x}_{ik}) = 0. \tag{6}$$

Several choices of w and ψ are possible to bound the influence of estimates obtained from (5) and (6). For example, Mallows weights and logistic function are suitable.

The algorithm starts with a robust weighted estimation of the location parameters and a robust estimate of the scale parameter given by the median absolute deviation. The weights are $a_i w_i / s_i^2$, where a_i, $i = 1, \cdots, n$, are the surrounding area of the Dirichlet tessellation. The algorithm is an iterative procedure for the E-step and the M-step. Thus, at the mth-iteration the E-step calculates

$$\tilde{W}_{ik}^{(m)} = \frac{p_k^{(m)} \tilde{h}_{ik}^{(m)}}{\sum_{l=1}^{K} p_l^{(m)} \tilde{h}_{il}^{(m)}},$$

where $\tilde{h}_{ik}^{(m)} = f(\tilde{z}_{ik}/\gamma^{(m)}, \sigma_i, s_i^2, a_i, w_i)$ and $\gamma = (\beta, \alpha)$. The M-step solves

$$\sum_{k=1}^{K}\sum_{i=1}^{n} \tilde{W}_{ik} \frac{a_i w_i}{s_i^2} \psi\left(\frac{e_{ik}}{\sigma}\right) \tilde{\mathbf{f}}(\mathbf{x}_{ik}) = 0. \tag{7}$$

6 Example

In this section we are going to illustrate the proposed procedure and we shall compare it with the NPML approach introduced by Aitkin and Francis

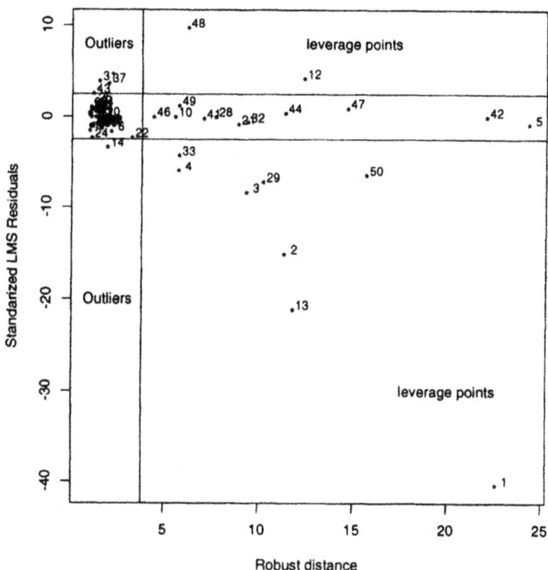

FIGURE 1. Plot of robust residuals versus robust distances for Davis data.

(1995). The example corresponds to 52 topographic data cited in Davis (1986), which consist of measurements of the earth's surface within a 310-square foot area. They are topological elevations over a small area on the northern side of a hill. Due to the fact that Davis was interested in the analysis of maps, he used the survey to produce contours of the region. In this example we fit a quadratic trend and estimate $r_0 = 1$ as range parameter of the chosen exponential covariance function. Not surprisingly, this range parameter has also been obtained through robust procedures (Cressie and Hawkins, 1980). Further, $\tilde{z}_i, \tilde{\mathbf{f}}_i$ and s_i^2 are derived.

To illustrate the behavior of the bounded influence estimator we have detected leverage points and outliers using the procedure introduced by Rousseeuw and van Zomeren (1990). They classify the data into regular observations, vertical outliers, good leverage points and bad leverage points. The identification is based on a display in which the robust residuals are plotted versus robust distances. Points to the right side of the vertical borderline through $\sqrt{\chi^2_{p;0.975}}$ are leverage points, whereas points outside the horizontal tolerance band $[-2.5, 2.5]$ are regression outliers. Figure 1 shows the leverage points of the topographic data set. Although the cutoff values are to some extent arbitrary, the observations 1, 5 and 42 may be considered leverage points. Besides, points with large robust distances are also regression outliers.

To decide the appropriate number of components is an important issue, for which several tests have been proposed. Unfortunately they are still lacking a fundamental mathematical foundation. In the context of general mixed models, the improvement of them is not a simple task (McLachlan and Basford, 1988). We propose to check the correct number of components using the previous plot. From this criterion, the optimal number is not more than 4. The cases are classified into the component to which they have the highest probability of belonging.

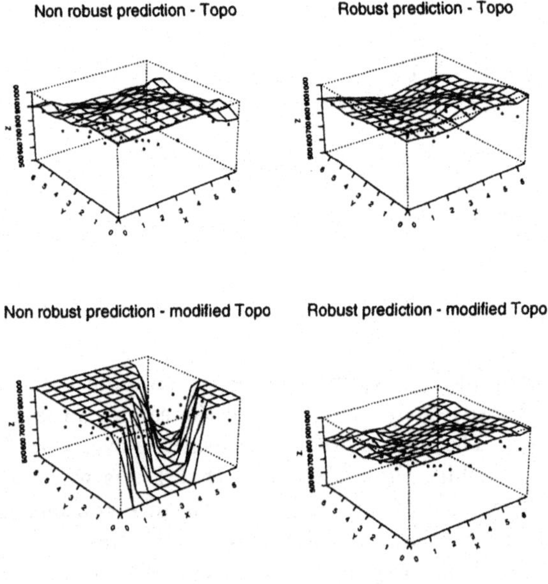

FIGURE 2. Prediction surfaces for Davis data.

The next step is to estimate Mallows weights and to run the iterative procedure in order to obtain the bounded influence estimates of the location parameters of model (4). In the present example, the randomness of the intercept is considered, although it is plausible to randomize other terms in the model. The scaled logistic function has been selected as function ψ although other choices are also possible. The bounded influence nonparametric maximum likelihood (BI-NPML) approach provides an optimal fit in 3 components based on the deviance, whereas the NPML approach tends

to use a larger number of components. However, both methods give similar estimations in three components.
Robustness signifies insensitivity to small deviations from the assumptions. The occurrence of gross errors in a small fraction of the observations has to be regarded as a small deviation. However, it is not trivial to deduce the resistant properties of the new BI estimator in a three dimensional plot. To achieve this, we provoke a small deviation in the model by adding 10,000 units to the first observation, which is located on the left upper corner of D. Now, it seems appropriate to compare the efficiency of the BI-NPML estimate versus the NPML. The selection of 10,000 units is completely arbitrary, but it shows the behavior of both estimations in an easy way.
Figure 2 summarizes the results showing four prediction surfaces in three components. The two upper figures show the prediction surfaces obtained for the original data set. The left one with the NPML procedure and the right one with the BI-NPML. By contrast, the lower figures show the prediction surfaces in the modified topo data set. It is clearly seen that the prediction surfaces for the original data set are quite similar, whereas in the modified topo, the prediction surfaces have a different behavior. The non robust version, on the left lower corner, becomes completely spoiled. However, the robust version of the prediction surface remains unchanged in spite of the modification made in the data set.
Implementation of the iterative procedure written in S-Plus is avalaible from the authors.

Conclusions

It is by now well known that the method of least squares is a nonresistant fitting procedure. A small proportion of the data cases can strongly influence the fitted model. Accommodation and identification are the major approaches for dealing with aberrant cases. Then, it seems that a combination of both things could be fruitful. In this paper, the NPML approach of the finite mixture model is a convenient step in the identification process, allowing the separation of the atypical observations in different components. Furthermore, the accommodation process is accomplished by a bounded influence estimation, correcting not only outlying responses but leverage points as well.

References

Aitkin, M. and Francis B. J. (1995). Fitting overdispersed generalized linear models by nonparametric maximum likelihood. *GLIM Newsletter*, **25**, 37-45.

Cressie, N. A. C. (1991). *Statistics for Spatial Data*. Wiley Series in Probability and Mathematical Statistics.

Cressie, N. and Hawkins, D. M. (1980). Robust estimation of the variogram. *Mathematical Geology*, **12**, 115-125.

Davis, J. C. (1986). *Statistics and Data Analysis in Geology*. 2nd ed. John Wiley and Sons, New York.

Dempster, A. P., Laird, N. M. and Rubin, D. B. (1977). Maximum likelihood from incomplete data via the EM-algorithm. *Journal of the Royal Statistical Society, Series B*, **39**, 1-38.

Hawkins, D. M. and Cressie, N. A. C. (1984). Robust kriging: A proposal. *Mathematical Geology*, **16**, 3-18.

Heckman, J. J. and Singer, B. (1984). A method for minimizing the impact of distributional assumptions in econometric models of duration. *Econometrica*, **52**, 271-320.

Hoaglin, D. C., Mosteller, F. and Tukey, J. W. (1985). *Exploring Data Tables, Trends, and Shapes*. Wiley Series in Probability and Statistics.

Laird, N. M. (1978). Nonparametric maximum likelihood estimation of a mixing distribution. *Journal of the American Statistical Association*, **73**, 805-811.

Mallows, C. L. (1975). *On some topics in Robustness*. Technical memorandum, Bell Telephone Laboratories, Murray Hill, NJ.

McLachlan, G. J. and Basford, K. E. (1988). *Mixture Models. Inference and Applications to clustering*. Marcel Dekker.

Militino, A. F. (1996). M-estimation of the drift coefficients of a spatial linear model. *Mathematical Geology*, in press.

Militino, A. F. and Ugarte, M. D. (1996). Robust estimation of the location parameters of a spatial linear model via random effects, in *Statistical Modelling*, 275-282, edited by G.M. Marchetti, A. Forcina, R. Hatzinger and G. Galmacci. Published in Graphos, Citta' di Castello, Italy.

Ripley, B. D. (1981). *Spatial Statistics*. Wiley Series in Probability and Mathematical Statistics.

Rousseeuw, P. J. and van Zomeren, B. C. (1990). Unmasking multivariate outliers and leverage points (with discussion). *Journal of the American Statistical Association*, **85**, 633-651.

Simpson, D. G., Ruppert, D. and Carroll, R. J. (1992). On one-step GM estimates and stability of inferences in linear regression. *Journal of the American Statistical Association*, **87**, 439-450.

Spatial Correlation Models as Applied to Evolutionary Biology

Mary C. Christman and Robert W. Jernigan*

American University
United States

ABSTRACT One of the keys to comparative analyses in evolutionary biology is the ability to model phylogenetic influence on trait variation among related taxa. In recent years spatial autocorrelation models have become more popular in such analyses. In the context of evolutionary biology, spatially correlated is akin to "phylogenetically related". We consider two of the current methods for "controlling" or "subtracting out" the effects due to phylogeny. The methods of interest are a mixed MANOVA model (Lynch, 1991, Evolution) and a spatial autocorrelation model with a fixed, known weight matrix (Ord, 1975, JASA). In the MANOVA model, the phylogeny is included via an $n \times n$ matrix of phylogenetic relationships, G, that is incorporated into the variance-covariance matrix of the random effects. In the univariate spatial autocorrelation model, the phylogenetic information enters into the analysis via a weight matrix **W**. We compare the two models using data on several morphometric traits among four populations of an amphipod, *Gammarus minus*. DNA sequence data is employed as the measure of relatedness. The models have been modified to allow for replicate observations in each trait and population combination. We show that these two models are substantively different in that the quantities remaining after subtraction do not contain the same information about the trait. The spatial autocorrelation model partitions the trait values into two components, P, the phylogenetic effect, and (S+E) the site-specific plus noise effects. Conversely, Lynch's mixed model partitions the effects as (P+S), a "heritable" value, and E, the random noise. These differences have important implications for evolutionary comparative studies.

Key words and phrases: Spatial autocorrelation model, multivariate ANOVA model, EM algorithm.

---

*We thank David Culver and Daniel Fong for the data and discussions of the data and Justin Chang and Thomas Kane for the sequence data. This work was supported in part by a University Senate Research grant from American University.

1 Introduction

The dependence of random processes and data on their spatial arrangement and pattern has been widely studied in recent years. Methods have been developed to exploit the knowledge of spatial patterns and correlations to provide greater understanding and predictive success. But there are settings in which the spatial patterns are to be expected and often then not of primary interest. Indeed, it is the residuals, after the spatial correlation has been "controlled" or "subtracted out", that can be suggestive of other underlying causes or processes.

Evolutionary biology is one application that both extends the scope of and "subtracts out" spatial correlations. For example, in evolutionary biology spatially correlated can be extended to represent species that are "phylogenetically related". Such spatial autocorrelation models have become quite useful to comparative analyses in evolutionary biology in which the goal is to establish the generality of evolutionary observations. The approach that we will consider is one that attempts to model phylogenetic influence on trait variation among related taxa. In particular we will consider two of the current methods for modeling and then "controlling" or "subtracting out" the effects due to phylogeny.

The methods of interest are a mixed MANOVA model (Lynch, 1991) and a spatial autocorrelation model with a fixed, known weight matrix (Ord, 1975). Both models are considered variance apportioning methods in that they are purported to determine the proportion of variation of a trait that is attributable to phylogeny and the proportion due to taxon specific effects, e.g. natural selection or genetic drift (Miles and Dunham 1993, Losos and Miles 1994, Harvey and Pagel 1991). This partitioning of trait variation allows for separate analysis of the information remaining after phylogenetic influences have been eliminated. This remaining information can be analyzed further to study adaptive patterns among the taxa.

We show that these two models are substantively different in that the quantities remaining after subtraction do not contain the same information. The spatial autocorrelation model will be shown to partition the trait values into two components, P, the phylogenetic effect, and (S+E) the site-specific plus noise effects. Conversely, Lynch's mixed model partitions the effects as (P+S), a "heritable" value, and E, the random noise. These differences have important implications for evolutionary comparative studies.

2 The Models

2.1 Spatial Autocorrelation Model

Cheverud and Dow (1985, Cheverud, Dow and Leutenegger 1985) proposed the use of spatial network or autocorrelation models (Ord 1975, Cressie

1993) to partition morphometric trait values into a phylogenetic component and a "specific" component free of phylogenetic influence. They model the average trait values for the taxa as

$$\mathbf{y} = \rho\mathbf{W}\mathbf{y} + \varepsilon \tag{1}$$

where $\mathbf{y}$ is a $n \times 1$ vector of mean trait values for n taxa, ρ is the phylogenetic correlation coefficient $\in$[-1,1], $\mathbf{W}$ is a $n \times n$ "phylogenetic connectivity matrix", and ε, the vector of residual values. Here, $\rho\mathbf{W}\mathbf{y}$ represents the phylogenetic component of the trait values and is the vector of expected values of the traits for each taxon calculated as weighted averages of the trait values of the other phylogenetically related taxa in the sample. The residuals, $\varepsilon = \mathbf{y} - \rho\mathbf{W}\mathbf{y}$, represent the taxon specific effects and are assumed to be $\mathrm{MVN}(0, \sigma^2\mathbf{I})$. Maximum likelihood estimates of the parameters, ρ and σ^2, are obtained using Ord's (1975) direct search procedure which replaces the determinant of $(\mathbf{I} - \rho\mathbf{W})$ with $\prod_{i=1}^{n}(1 - \rho\lambda_i)$ where the λ_i, $i = 1, ..., n$ are the eigenvalues of $\mathbf{W}$.

In this model, the phylogenetic information enters into the analysis via the weight matrix $\mathbf{W}$ where each element of the matrix quantifies the phylogenetic relatedness between two taxa. Large weights imply closely related taxa and the weights decline as a function of the relatedness distance between two groups. In the example which follows we employ DNA sequence data to obtain a measure of distance based on branch lengths. That is, w_{ij} represents the branch length between the ith and j^{th} taxa so that $w_{ij} > 0$ for $i \neq j$ and $w_{ij} = 0$ for $i = j$. The $\mathbf{W}$ matrix is usually scaled so that each row sums to 1; this allows for the interpretation of ρ as a correlation coefficient (Ord, 1975).

As just described, in phylogenetic studies it is often assumed that the mean morphometric trait value is known and hence there exists for the ith taxon only one value of Y, y_i. In reality, this mean is based on a sample from the taxon (population) and the sampling error is ignored in the analyses. In fact, a computer simulation study by Martins (1996) , focusing mainly on Type I and II error rates, concludes that more than 15 taxa are required for good performance of this model. We overcome this problem by extending the model given in (1) to allow for replicate observations of the morphometric trait for the ith taxon and incorporate the sampling error into the model as part of the error term.

Let n_i be the number of observations of the morphometric trait for the ith taxon such that $\sum_{i=1}^{n} n_i = N$, let $\mathbf{y}_i = [y_{i1}, y_{i2}, ..., y_{in_i}]'$ be the $n_i \times 1$ vector of observed values, and let $\varepsilon_i = [\varepsilon_{i1}, \varepsilon_{i2}, ..., \varepsilon_{in_i}]'$ be the vector of error terms associated with the observed values for the replicates in the ith taxon. Further, let $\mathbf{y} = [\mathbf{y}_1', \mathbf{y}_2', ..., \mathbf{y}_n']'$ and $\varepsilon = [\varepsilon_1', \varepsilon_2', ..., \varepsilon_n']'$. Finally, let $\mathbf{W}_{ij}^*$ be the $n_i \times n_j$ matrix composed solely of the element w_{ij}/n_j and let $\mathbf{0}_{n_i \times n_i}$ be a matrix of zeroes. Then, model (1) can be extended to the following:

$$\begin{bmatrix} \mathbf{y}_1 \\ \mathbf{y}_2 \\ \cdot \\ \cdot \\ \cdot \\ \mathbf{y}_n \end{bmatrix} = \rho \begin{bmatrix} \mathbf{0}_{n_1 \times n_1} & \mathbf{W}^*_{12} & \cdots & \mathbf{W}^*_{1n} \\ \mathbf{W}^*_{21} & \mathbf{0}_{n_2 \times n_2} & \cdots & \mathbf{W}^*_{2n} \\ \mathbf{W}^*_{31} & \mathbf{W}^*_{32} & \cdots & \mathbf{W}^*_{3n} \\ \cdots & \cdots & \cdots & \cdots \\ \mathbf{W}^*_{n1} & \mathbf{W}^*_{n2} & \cdots & \mathbf{0}_{n_n \times n_n} \end{bmatrix} \mathbf{y} + \begin{bmatrix} \varepsilon_1 \\ \varepsilon_2 \\ \cdot \\ \cdot \\ \cdot \\ \varepsilon_n \end{bmatrix} = \rho \mathbf{W}^* \mathbf{y} + \varepsilon \tag{2}$$

Since $\mathbf{W}^*$ has exactly n distinct eigenvalues, the maximum likelihood estimators of the parameters are obtained using essentially the same computational procedure described above.

The spatial autocorrelation models given above are univariate only, i.e. only one morphometric trait is analyzed. The mixed model in the next section is a multivariate model in which several traits are analyzed simultaneously and are allowed to be correlated.

2.2 Lynch's Mixed Model

In the mixed analysis of variance model proposed by Lynch (1991) for phylogenetic studies, the average value of the jth trait in the ith taxon, denoted $\bar{y}_{ij}$, is partitioned into a linear combination of three components:

$$\bar{y}_{ij} = \mu_j + a_{ij} + \varepsilon_{ij} \tag{3}$$

where μ_j is the grand mean for the jth trait that is common to all n taxa; a_{ij} is a random effect considered to be a "heritable additive value" for the jth trait in the ith taxon; and, ε_{ij} is the associated error term. The predicted value for the jth trait, $(\mu_j + a_{ij})$, is interpreted to be the phylogenetically heritable component of the mean of the jth trait for the ith taxon and according to Lynch is the phylogenetic effect in the model of Cheverud *et al.* (1985) (Lynch, 1991, p.1066). The rationale for the separation is similar to that of the spatial autocorrelation model in that both models attempt to separate the effects of phylogenetic and non-phylogenetic factors; the two methods of partitioning are quite different though.

In matrix formulation the model for k traits is

$$\bar{\mathbf{y}} = \mathbf{X}\mu + \mathbf{a} + \varepsilon$$

where $\bar{\mathbf{y}} = [\bar{y}_{11}, \bar{y}_{21}, \cdots, \bar{y}_{n1}, \bar{y}_{12}, \cdots, \bar{y}_{nk}]'$ is the $nk \times 1$ vector of mean values, $\mu = [\mu_1, \mu_2, \cdots, \mu_k]'$ is the $k \times 1$ vector of trait means, $\mathbf{X}$ is an $nk \times 1$ incidence matrix containing k ones vectors, $\mathbf{1}_{n \times 1}$, on the diagonal, and $\mathbf{a}$ and ε are the $nk \times 1$ vectors of additive and residual effects, respectively. The error terms are assumed to be MVN$(\mathbf{0}_{nk \times 1}, \mathbf{R})$ where the variance-covariance matrix is the Kronecker product $\mathbf{R} = \mathbf{E} \otimes \mathbf{I}$. Here, $\mathbf{E}$ is the $k \times k$ matrix containing $\tau(j, j\prime) = \tau^2(j)$ if $j = j\prime$ and $\tau(j, j\prime) > 0$ if $j \neq j\prime$ and $\mathbf{I}$ the

$n \times n$ identity matrix. Similarly, the additive values $\mathbf{a}$ are assumed to be random multivariate normals with mean $\mathbf{0}_{nk\times 1}$ and $\text{Var}(\mathbf{a}) = \mathbf{D} = \mathbf{A} \otimes \mathbf{G}$ where $\mathbf{G}$ is a fixed $n \times n$ matrix of phylogenetic relationships, and $\mathbf{A}$ is the matrix containing the variances of each of the traits' additive values, $\sigma_a^2(j)$, on the diagonals and the covariances between random effects of the jth and $(j\prime)^{th}$ traits, $\sigma_a(j, j\prime)$, in the off-diagonal positions. The two random terms, $\mathbf{a}$ and ε, are assumed to be independent. As can be seen, in this approach, incorporation of the phylogenetic effects is accomplished through the variance-covariance structure induced by the $\mathbf{G}$ matrix.

The parameters in the model are estimated (predicted) using the expectation-maximization (EM) algorithm which produces maximum likelihood estimates of the quantities of interest (Dempster *et al.*, 1977; Thompson and Shaw, 1990 and 1992; Lynch, 1991; Searle et al., 1992). This technique for estimating (predicting) the phylogenetic effects requires that the $\mathbf{G}$ matrix of phylogenetic relationships be non-singular, i.e. that $\mathbf{G}^{-1}$ exist.

Once again, the model described in (3) assumes that the population mean values for the traits under study are known when in reality the values used in the analyses are sample estimates. Just as was done for the spatial autocorrelation model, we can extend the mixed MANOVA model to include replicates for the jth trait in the ith taxon and incorporate the sampling error into the error term.

Let $\mathbf{y}_{ij} = [y_{ij1}, y_{ij2}, \cdots, y_{ijn_i}]'$ be the vector of replicate values for the jth trait in the ith taxon and let $\varepsilon_{ij} = [\varepsilon_{ij1}, \varepsilon_{ij2}, \cdots, \varepsilon_{ijn_i}]'$ be the associated vector of error terms. Then, the extended model is given by:

$$\mathbf{y} = \mathbf{X}\mu + \mathbf{Z}\mathbf{a} + \varepsilon$$

where $\mathbf{y} = [\mathbf{y}_{11}, \mathbf{y}_{21}, \cdots, \mathbf{y}_{1k}, \mathbf{y}_{21}, \cdots, \mathbf{y}_{nk}]'$ is the $Nk \times 1$ vector of observed trait values; $\mathbf{X}$ is the $Nk \times k$ incidence matrix with k ones vectors, $1_{N\times 1}$, along the diagonal; μ is as above; $\mathbf{Z}$ is the $Nk \times nk$ incidence matrix with the matrix $Diag\{1_{n_i \times 1}\}_{i=1}^{n}$ repeated k times along the diagonal; $\mathbf{a}$ is the $nk \times 1$ vector of random effects; and, ε the $Nk \times 1$ vector of error terms is given by $\varepsilon = [\varepsilon_{11}, \varepsilon_{21}, \cdots, \varepsilon_{1k}, \varepsilon_{21}, \cdots, \varepsilon_{nk}]'$.

In this formulation, the random effects vector $\mathbf{a}$ is still $\text{MVN}(\mathbf{0}_{nk\times 1}, \mathbf{D})$ but the error terms are assumed now to be $\text{MVN}(\mathbf{0}_{Nk\times 1}, \mathbf{R})$ where $\mathbf{R} = \mathbf{E} \otimes \mathbf{I}$ is now an $Nk \times Nk$ matrix with $\mathbf{E}$ the same as above and $\mathbf{I}$ an $N \times N$ identity matrix. Finally, as above, $\text{cov}(\mathbf{a}, \varepsilon) = \mathbf{0}$.

The expectation-maximization algorithm is again used to find maximum likelihood estimates of the parameters, the only difference being that the algorithm allows for replicates in place of single values. We refer the reader to Lynch (1991), and Cheverud, Dow and Leutenegger (1985) for details on implementing and estimating various parameters of the models. We implemented the programs in MATLAB (Moler 1993).

3 Methods

3.1 The Models

In the models of interest there are actually three components to the average trait value. Following Cheverud *et al.* (1985), we can conceptually divide a trait value (T) into a phylogenetic component (P), taxon specific component (S) and a random noise component (E), i.e. T=P+S+E. This last term includes variability that is otherwise unaccounted for, such as sampling error.

Using the above partitioning we show that the spatial autocorrelation model partitions the trait values into two components, P, the phylogenetic effect, and (S+E) the site-specific plus noise effects. Conversely, Lynch's mixed model partitions the effects as (P+S), a "heritable" value, and E, the random noise.

3.2 The Dataset

The data are morphological measurements for four populations of amphipods, *Gammarus minus*, found in caves and springs located in West Virginia (Fong 1989, Jernigan *et al.* 1994). There are two cave populations (Benedict and Organ Caves) and two spring populations (Davis and Organ Springs). Benedict Cave and Davis Spring are hydrologically connected and distinct from Organ Cave and Organ Spring which are themselves hydrologically connected.

The variables used in this study are i) head length (in mm $\times 100$), ii) eye shape as (eye area)$^{1/2}$/(head length), and iii) antennal shape as (peduncle 1 length)/(head length). Each variable was measured on one individual from each of 197 full-sib groups of 60-day old individuals grown under identical conditions. The resultant data include 51 replicates from the Davis Spring population, 40 replicates from the Benedict cave population, 75 replicates from the Organ Spring population, and 31 replicates from the Organ Cave population. All data were standardized prior to analyses.

3.3 The Phylogeny

The phylogenetic relationships among the four populations were based on a 400 base pair mitochondrial DNA sequence from different animals (Chang, 1995). A geographically and hydrologically distant spring population, Bone Norman Resurgence, was used as the outgroup. The phylogeny was estimated using maximum likelihood techniques (Felsenstein 1981) on the mtDNA data in which transversions are weighted twice that of transitions.

For the mixed model, we used a **G** matrix in which the elements are calculated as one minus the proportion of total branch length between two populations. For the spatial autocorrelation model, the **W** connectivity matrix was based on $\mathbf{G}$. First the diagonals were set to zero and then the matrix was row normalized so that the elements within a row sum to one.

4 Results

The results of the analyses on head length, eye shape and antennal shape are given in Table 1 and Figure 1. The Table lists the estimated (predicted) values of the model components for partitioning the effects. The average values of the residuals for each trait and each population were calculated and are also given in the Table.

For all three traits the estimated autocorrelation coefficients ($\hat{\rho}$) are not significantly different than zero. For example, the autocorrelation coefficient for head length is estimated at -0.10 with a standard error of 0.57 (Table 1). Similar analyses using Lynch's mixed effects model yield the same results regarding the contribution of phylogeny to trait variation. While these results imply that phylogeny does not contribute to trait variation, we believe that this adds emphasis to our findings of the differences between the two methods. As is described below the partitioning by the spatial autocorrelation model supports the lack of phylogenetic contribution to the trait variation (by similarity of the predicted values) whereas the mixed model does not.

What is distinctive between the two models are the magnitudes of the partitions of the trait values in the two components. In the mixed effects model, the variation attributed to phylogeny, $\mu + \mathbf{a}$, is the same order of magnitude and has the same sign as the average residual effect, $\mathbf{e}$, in the spatial autocorrelation model. This pattern is evident in all three traits. For example, for eye shape, the predicted phylogenetic effect for each of the four populations is virtually identical in value to the residual effect in the spatial autocorrelation model (see Table 1).

To further examine the differences in partitioning between the two models, we plot their residuals. Figure 1 shows notched box plots of the residuals for the four populations for a given model and trait. As is clearly demonstrated in the graphs, the residuals from the mixed effects model do not differ among the four populations for any of the traits. This occurs only if the model components $\mu + \mathbf{a}$ capture all of the variability of the traits and populations so that the residuals contain only the sampling variability among individual animals. That is exactly what happens in the mixed model when applied to the *Gammarus minus* dataset. Hence, we interpret this to mean that the non-phylogenetic component, as well as the phylogenetic component, is captured in the $\mu + \mathbf{a}$ term in the model.

Conversely, the spatial autocorrelation model does not ascribe all trait variation to a phylogenetic effect since the residuals are demonstrably different in location among the four populations for some of the traits, notably

A. Headlength

	Mixed Effects Model		Spatial Autocor. Model	
Site	$(\mu + a)$	$\bar{e}$	$\hat{y}$	$\bar{e}$
Davis Spring (n=51)	-0.2155	-0.0760	0.0085	-0.2297
Benedict Cave(n=40)	-0.0823	0.0077	0.0069	-0.0812
Organ Spr. (n=75)	0.3416	0.0554	0.0251	0.3732
Organ Cave (n=31)	-0.3657	-0.0207	-0.0104	-0.3757

B. Eye Shape

	Mixed Effects Model		Spatial Autocor. Model	
Site	$(\mu + a)$	$\bar{e}$	$\hat{y}$	$\bar{e}$
Davis Spring	0.8155	0.0067	0.3601	0.4620
Benedict Cv.	-1.2731	0.0039	0.0751	-1.3440
Organ Spr.	0.6510	-0.0027	0.4536	0.1945
Organ Cave	-1.2737	-0.0088	0.0559	-1.3385

C. Antennal Shape

	Mixed Effects Model		Spatial Autocor. Model	
Site	$(\mu + a)$	$\bar{e}$	$\hat{y}$	$\bar{e}$
Davis Spring	-0.1548	-0.0268	-0.0125	-0.1691
Benedict Cv.	0.7355	0.0400	0.1122	0.6632
Organ Spr.	0.0233	0.0224	0.0324	0.0132
Organ Cave	-0.7506	-0.0615	-0.0962	-0.7159

TABLE 1. Results of analyses of morphometric traits in four populations of *Gammarus* minus using the two variance apportioning models. The phylogenetic information was incorporated using the MLE phylogeny based on mtDNA analyses as described in the text. In the spatial autocorrelation model, r is estimated to be -0.10 (s.e.=0.570) for headlength; -0.42 (s.e.= 0.613) for eye shape calculated as (eye area)$^{1/2}$/(head length); and, -0.30 (s.e.=0.606) for antennal shape calculated as (peduncle 1 length)/(head length).

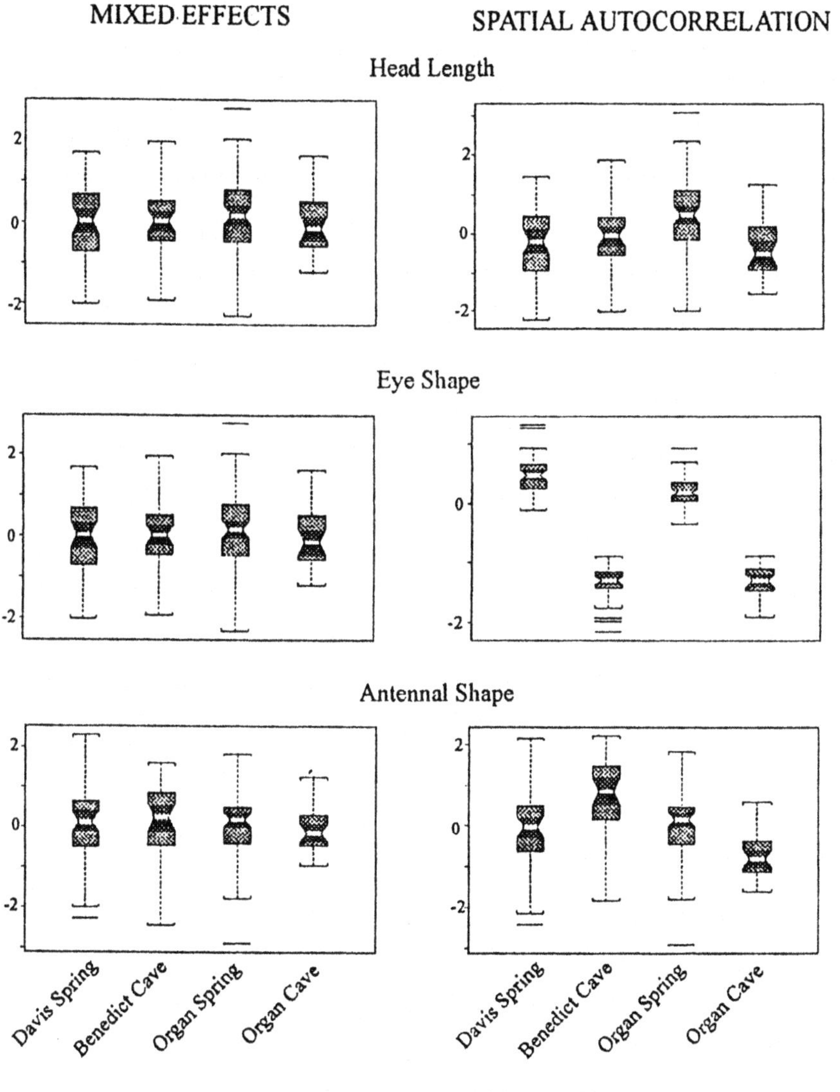

MIXED EFFECTS

SPATIAL AUTOCORRELATION

Head Length

Eye Shape

Antennal Shape

Davis Spring Benedict Cave Organ Spring Organ Cave

Davis Spring Benedict Cave Organ Spring Organ Cave

FIGURE 1. Box plots of the residuals for each of the three traits for each of the two models.

eye area and antennal shape. In the case of eye shape, residuals correspond to the pattern expected if eyes are reduced in cave populations due to natural selection and genetic drift relative to spring populations (Culver, Kane, and Fong 1995). In the case of antennal shape, the pattern for Benedict Cave (relatively larger antennae) corresponds to the result expected if natural selection were acting to increase extra-optic sensory structures in cave populations.

It is clear from our analyses (Christman, Jernigan, and Culver, 1996) that the mixed effects model does partition "heritable" effects but does not distinguish between phylogenetic and non-phylogenetic effects, i.e. the $\mu + \mathbf{a}$ model term captures both the phylogenetic and taxon specific (P+S) components. This is seen in the fact that the residual terms all appear to contain only random noise, i.e. $\mathbf{e}$ captures the noise (E). On the other hand, the spatial autocorrelation model partitions the trait variation into two components, one due to phylogeny and the other due to site-specific (plus noise) effects. That is, it appears that $\hat{\rho}\mathbf{Wy}$ contains the phylogenetic component (P) and the residuals, $\mathbf{e}$, contain the taxon specific and noise terms (S+E). The lack of congruence in the partitioning of the two models may stem from the different uses of the phylogenetic information. The spatial autocorrelation model includes this information in the W matrix which has a direct effect on and functionally predicts the measured trait (Y). In contrast, the mixed effects model includes the phylogenetic information in a second-order covariance and thus the effect on the measured trait is more indirect. This situation might be further clarified with a dataset in which there is a significant phylogenetic effect. We are expanding this research to consider how the two models behave with simulated data based on evolution and natural selection models.

5 References

[1] Chang, J. C. 1995. *Phylogenetic Analysis of Adaptation in the Crustacean Gammarus minus.* M.S.Thesis, University of Cincinnati, Cincinnati, Ohio.

[2] Cheverud, J. M. and Dow, M. M. 1985. An autocorrelation analysis of the effect of lineal fission on genetic variation among social groups. *American Journal of Physical Anthropology* **67**:113-121.

[3] Cheverud, J. M., Dow, M. M. and Leutenegger, W. 1985. The quantitative assessment of phylogenetic constraints in comparative analyses: sexual dimorphism in body weight among primates. *Evolution* **39**:1335-1351.

[4] Christman, M. C., Jernigan, R. W. and Culver, D. C. 1996. A comparison of two models for estimating phylogenetic effect on trait variation. To appear in *Evolution.*

[5] Cressie, N. A. C. 1993. *Statistics for Spatial Data, revised edition.* John Wiley and Sons, Inc., New York, New York.

[6] Culver, D.C., T. C. Kane and D. W. Fong. 1995. *Adaptation and Natural Selection in Caves. The Evolution of Gammarus minus.* Harvard University Press, Cambridge, Massachusetts.

[7] Dempster, A. P, N. M. Laird, and D. B. Rubin. 1977. Maximum Likelihood from incomplete data via the EM algorithm. *Journal of the Royal Statistical Society Series B* **39**:1-38.

[8] Felsenstein, J. 1981. Evolutionary trees from DNA sequences: a maximum likelihood approach. *Journal of Molecular Evolution* **17**:368-376.

[9] Fong, D. W. 1989. Morphological evolution of the amphipod Gammarus minus in caves: quantitative genetic analysis. *American Midland Naturalist* **121**:361-378.

[10] Harvey, P. H. and Pagel, M. D.. 1991. *The Comparative Method in Evolutionary Biology.* Oxford University Press, New York, New York.

[11] Jernigan R. W., Culver, D. C., and Fong, D. W. 1994. The dual role of selection and evolutionary history as reflected in genetic correlations. *Evolution* **48**: 587-596.

[12] Losos, J. B. and Miles D. B. 1994. Adaptation, constraint, and the comparative method: phylogenetic issues and methods, in *Ecological Morphology: Integrative Organismal Biology,* ed. by P.C. Wainwright and S. T. Reilly. University of Chicago Press, Chicago, Illinois.

[13] Lynch, M. 1991. Methods for the analysis of comparative data in evolutionary biology. *Evolution* **45**:1065-1080.

[14] Martins, E. P. 1996. Phylogenies, spatial autoregression, and the comparative method: a computer simulation test. *Evolution* **50**:1750-1765.

[15] Miles, D. B. and Dunham, A. E. 1992. Comparative analyses of phylogenetic effects in the life-history patterns of iguanid reptiles. *American Naturalist* **139**:848-869.

[16] Miles, D. B. and Dunham, A. E. 1993. Historical perspectives in ecology and evolutionary biology: the use of phylogenetic comparisons. *Annual Review of Ecology and Systematics* **24**:587-619.

[17] Moler, C. 1993. *The MATLAB Reference Guide.* The Mathworks, Natick, Massachusetts.

[18] Ord, K. 1975. Estimation methods for models of spatial interaction. *Journal of the American Statistical Association* **70**:120-126.

[19] Searle, S. R., Casella, G., and McCulloch, C. E. 1992. *Variance Components.* John Wiley and Sons, Inc. New York, NY.

[20] Thompson, E. A. and Shaw, R. G. 1990. Pedigree analysis for quantitative traits: variance components without matrix inversion. *Biometrics* **46**:399-413.

[21] Thompson, E. A. and Shaw, R. G. 1992. Estimating polygenic models for multivariate data in large pedigrees. *Genetics* **131**:971-978.

Rainfall Modelling Using a Latent Gaussian Variable

C.A. Glasbey and I.M. Nevison

Biomathematics and Statistics Scotland
United Kingdom

ABSTRACT A monotonic transformation is applied to hourly rainfall data to achieve marginal normality. This defines a latent Gaussian variable, with zero rainfall corresponding to censored values below a threshold. Autocorrelations of the latent variable are estimated by maximum likelihood. The goodness of fit of the model to Edinburgh rainfall data is comparable with that of existing point process models. Gibbs sampling is used to disaggregate daily rainfall data, to generate typical hourly data conditional on daily totals.

Key words and phrases: Gibbs sampling, normalising transformation, rainfall disaggregation, time series.

1 Introduction

Temporal and spatio-temporal models of rainfall, either univariate or in combination with other climatic variables, are needed for many reasons, including simulation, forecasting and disaggregation. Monthly rainfall data are often modelled as Gaussian processes, but daily and hourly rainfall data typically have distributions with a singularity at zero and a long upper tail. Many models have been proposed, based either on point processes [9, 11] or constructed in two stages – first a binary rain/no-rain process and then a rainfall distribution applied to the wet periods [8, 13]. These models are far more difficult than Gaussian ones to study analytically, to combine with models of other weather variables [10], or to make use of in forecasting or disaggregation [6]. In particular, the need for disaggregation arises if rainfall estimates are required at a finer temporal or spatial resolution than are available in recorded data.

In this paper we develop an alternative approach, previously considered by Bell [2] and Hutchinson [7]: we apply a monotonic transformation to hourly rainfall data to achieve marginal normality, an approach akin to trans-Gaussian kriging [4]. This defines a latent Gaussian variable, with

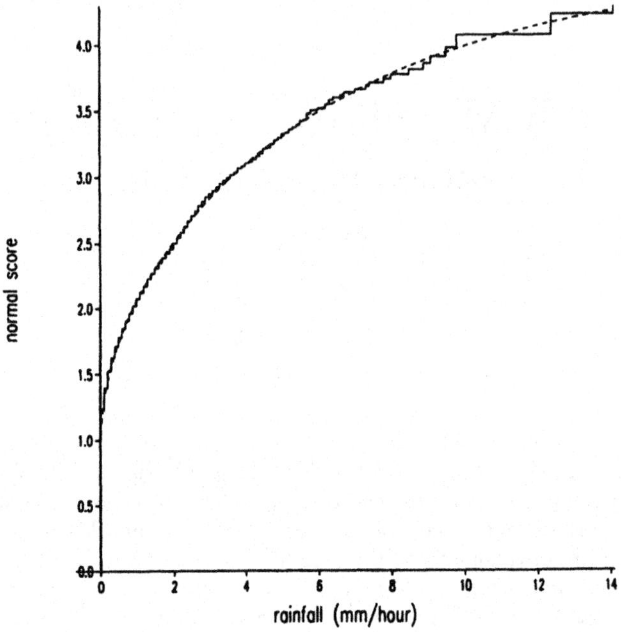

FIGURE 1. *Normal probability plot for 10 years of hourly rainfall data (—), and the fitted curve, a quadratic function of power-transformed rainfall (- - -).*

zero rainfall corresponding to censored values below a threshold, which we summarise by its autocorrelation function. Latent variable models are well established in categorical data analysis [1]. In §2, we identify and estimate the parameters in this model, using data from Edinburgh for illustration. Then, in §3 we check the validity of the model by comparing summary statistics from the data with those from simulations of the model and of a point process model [6, 11]. In §4, we show how Gibbs sampling can be used to disaggregate rainfall data. Finally, in §5 we critically evaluate the model.

2 Estimation

Fig 1 shows, as a continuous line, the normal probability plot for 10 years of hourly rainfall data from Turnhouse airport, Edinburgh. Note, all normal scores exceed 1.0 because 89% of hours were dry. An analytically-invertible monotonic fit to the plot was sought, to transform the rainfall data to marginal normality (with zero mean, unit variance). A power-transformation alone was not quite adequate, but a quadratic in power-transformed rainfall,

$$y = \beta_0 + \beta_1 r^\gamma + \beta_2 r^{2\gamma} \qquad \text{for} \quad r > 0,$$

gave a good fit, where r denotes hourly rainfall and y denotes the latent variable. Parameters were estimated by non-linear least squares, giving $\beta = (1.05, 1.10, -0.09)$ and $\gamma = 0.6$. (With these parameter values, the function is monotonic only for $r < 20.3$mm, which places an upper limit of 4.4 on y, but this has a very small probability of 6×10^{-6} of being exceeded, i.e. once in 19 years.) The estimated transformation is displayed as the dashed line in Fig 1.

The autocorrelation function is sufficient to characterise fully a stationary Gaussian process. Autocorrelation coefficients of the latent variable cannot be estimated directly because, although y is known when $r > 0$, in rain-free hours y is censored, we know only that $y < 1.05$. However, it is relatively straightforward to estimate the autocorrelation coefficient at a particular time lag, by numerically maximising the likelihood of the observed bivariate histogram of the censored latent variable. Autocorrelations for lags up to twenty days were each estimated separately, and are shown as the plotted points in Fig 2. The rate of decay is not exponential: both short-term effects of a few hours duration, and persistent correlations lasting several days, typical of cyclonic weather systems, are apparent. No diurnal pattern was found (although this could easily be included in this model), so the fluctuations in autocorrelation were attributed to sampling variation. To smooth out these fluctuations and estimate the autocorrelation function, mixtures of exponential curves,

$$\text{cor}(y_t, y_{t+l}) = \sum_{i=1}^{m} \alpha_i e^{-\lambda |l|} \qquad \text{subject to} \quad \sum_{i=1}^{m} \alpha_i = 1,$$

were fitted by non-linear least squares. The constraint that all coefficients are positive is sufficient for the function to be valid. A mixture of four exponentials, with $\alpha = (0.21, 0.51, 0.20, 0.08)$, $\lambda = (0.48, 0.17, 0.049, 0.0077)$ hour^{-1}, was judged to be adequate and is plotted as the line in Fig 2. One way to interpret this function is that the latent variable is a weighted sum of four Markov processes, and therefore the rainfall model is a hidden-Markov process. More sophisticated methods, such as Markov chain Monte Carlo [12], could have been used to estimate the autocorrelation function, perhaps simultaneously with parameters in the normalising transformation. However, because the number of observations is in excess of 87000, we do not think that efficiency of estimation is of critical consideration in this application.

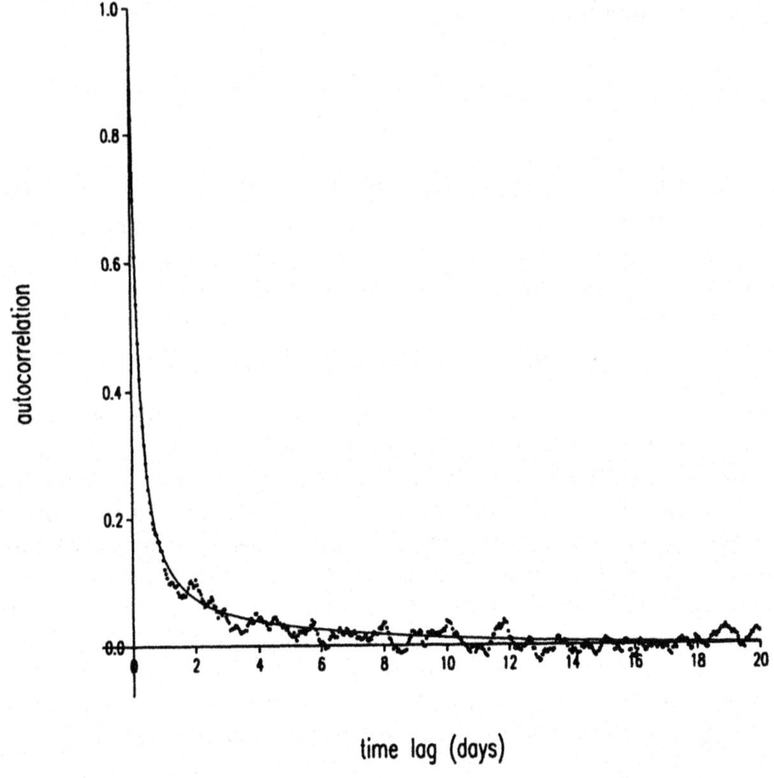

FIGURE 2. *Autocorrelations of latent variable at a range of time lags, estimated from censored data (·) and a fitted mixture of four exponentials (—).*

3 Validation

To check the adequacy of the model, 100 years of data were simulated, using an autoregressive process derived from the estimated autocorrelation function, with lag terms up to twenty days and y truncated at 4.4. Partial autocorrelations beyond this lag were assumed to be negligible. (Alternatively, an exact representations of the autocorrelation function could have been achieved using a fourth-order autoregressive third-order moving-average process.) A large number of summary statistics were compared with those from the data. The most critical of these statistics are given in Table 1, together with results from a particular clustered-point-process model [11] fitted by the method of moments [6]. (Some analytic results are available for both models, but for simplicity we have relied on simulations.) There

	Edinburgh data	Latent Gaussian model	Point process model [11]
Hourly data			
proportion wet	0.11	0.11	0.11
mean rainfall (mm)	0.068	0.070	0.067
standard deviation	0.33	0.34	0.32
autocorrelation lag 1	0.55	0.66	0.53
lag 2	0.38	0.46	0.31
lag 3	0.28	0.34	0.23
mean duration of dry run	22.	21.	28.
standard deviation	43.	33.	35.
mean duration of wet run	2.7	2.6	3.4
standard deviation	3.1	2.7	2.9
Aggregated daily data			
proportion wet	0.53	0.58	0.52
mean rainfall (mm)	1.6	1.7	1.6
standard deviation	3.6	4.0	3.4
autocorrelation lag 1	0.19	0.21	0.20
lag 2	0.08	0.08	0.06
lag 3	0.02	0.04	0.03
mean duration of dry run	2.8	2.2	2.1
standard deviation	2.9	1.7	1.5
mean duration of wet run	3.1	3.0	2.3
standard deviation	2.7	2.7	1.8

TABLE 1. *Summary statistics for 10 years of Edinburgh's rainfall data and 100 years of simulated data for two models.*

is close agreement in the first three statistics because of the estimation procedures. Agreement for other statistics is not quite so good, but is still reasonable. The point process model produces a closer match to hourly and daily autocorrelations, whereas the latent Gaussian model agrees better with observed run-lengths of dry and wet periods.

To explore further the discrepancies in rainfall autocorrelations, the bivariate distributions of rainfall in two hours, a fixed time lag apart, were examined. Fig 3(a) shows the bivariate histogram of observed rainfall at lag one hour, with counts displayed as shades of grey. The symmetry in Fig 3(a) about the main diagonal supports the assumption of time reversibility which is implicit in the latent Gaussian model. Fig 3(b) shows the expected counts, at lag one hour, from the latent Gaussian model. To compare the distributions, standardised residuals ({observed count − predicted count}/sqrt{predicted count}) are shown in Fig 3(c). Groups of positive and negative residuals can be seen in the bottom-left of Fig 3(c),

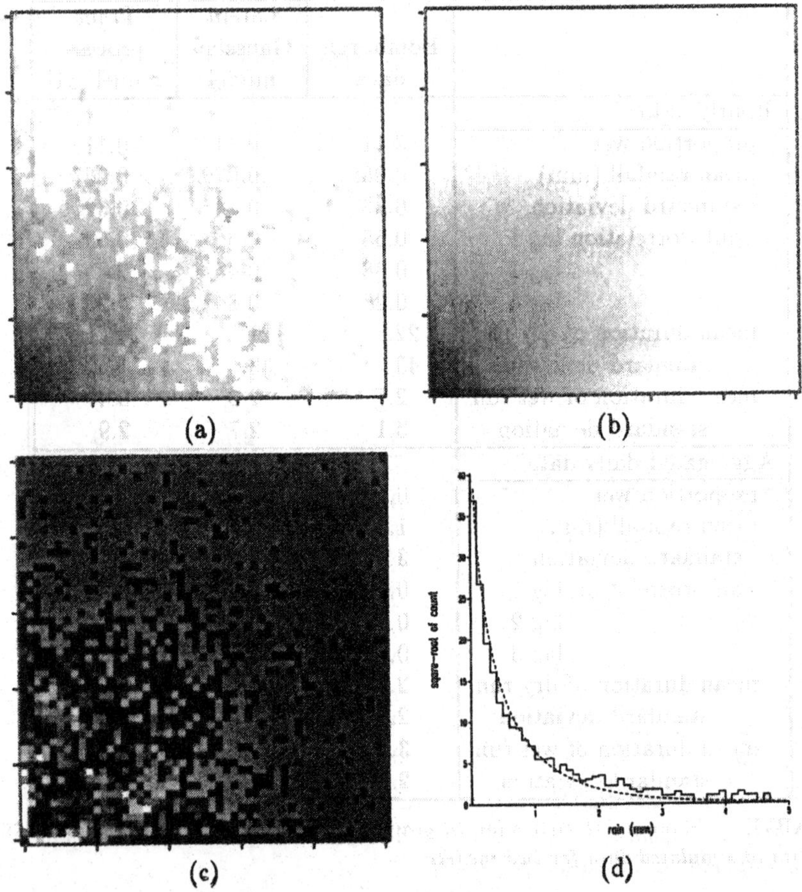

FIGURE 3. *Bivariate distribution of rainfall in consecutive hours (for rainfall in the range 0 - 5 mm):* **(a)** *histogram of observed data (zero counts are displayed as white squares, and progressively darker squares denote larger counts,* **(b)** *predicted counts from Latent Gaussian model,* **(c)** *standardised residuals (zeroes are displayed as mid-greys, negative residuals as lighter shades of grey and positive residuals as darker shades of grey,* **(d)** *histogram of rainfall in one hour when the previous hour was rain-free (observed: —, fitted: - - -).*

showing lack of fit of the model. In particular, there is a sequence of negative then positive residuals in both the first column and last row of the display. These are pairs of hours, one of which is rain-free and the other wet. Fig 3(d) shows the histogram for the last row of Figs 3(a), together with predicted values from the latent Gaussian model. Some lack of fit is evident, particularly for rainfall 2–5mm, but it represents very few hours. A similar pattern was observed in bivariate distributions at other short time lags.

We conclude that the latent Gaussian model fits the data reasonably well in comparison with the clustered-point-process model. The worst fit occurs in the rainfall autocorrelations, but examination of bivariate distributions at a range of time lags has shown this to be small. If, in a particular application, a discrepancy in the autocorrelations was thought to be critical, this could be overcome by choosing values of the autocorrelation coefficients of the latent variable to give an exact match [7], which is easy to do because there is a 1-1 correspondence between the autocorrelations in the two variables. Discrepancies in the bivariate histograms would still exist, of course. In §5, we discuss possible ways to overcome these.

4 Disaggregation

A particular strength of the latent Gaussian approach to rainfall modelling is that it is relatively easy to either disaggregate or forecast, using the Gibbs sampler. We will illustrate this by considering disaggregation of daily Edinburgh data, i.e. simulation of stochastically-representative hourly data, conditional on daily totals. In practice, we would not usually know the appropriate parameter values at a site if rainfall were only recorded daily, but we could use estimates from the nearest hourly site, or spatially interpolate over several sites.

We initially allocate rainfall uniformly over each 24 hour period, to match the daily data, transform to latent variables, and set $y = 0$ on rain-free days. Then, the Gibbs sampler simulates in turn each day's set of latent variables, conditional on the latent variables on all other days. Initialising this simulation involves solving 24 sets of 960 simultaneous linear equations. By repeating this procedure over the full time series many times, a Markov chain of rainfall sequences is simulated from the appropriate distribution.

The hourly values of the latent variable on a single day, conditional on latent variables on all other days, are multivariate normally distributed. It is a standard result that their variances are derivable from the autocorrelation function (we used 20 days before and after the day under consideration, and assumed that partial autocorrelations were negligible outside this range), and their means also depend on the past and future latent variables. For disaggregation, we need to simulate from this distribution, subject to the constraint that, after transforming to the rainfall scale, the total amount of rain for that day matches the known value. There are many possible ways to achieve this, such as adaptive rejection sampling [5], but we took the simple approach of repeated sampling from the multivariate normal distribution until the rainfall total fell within either 0.05mm or 1% of the target. We then rescaled the latent variable in order to get an exact match for that day. This method proved to be efficient enough, requiring an average of 170 simulations per day, although considerably larger numbers were sometimes needed on very wet days.

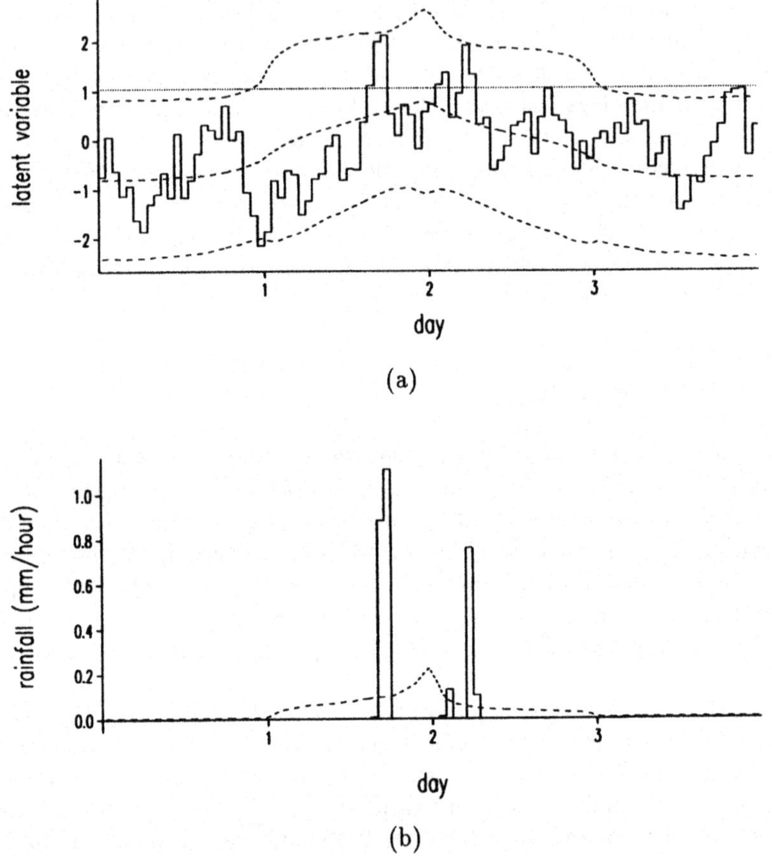

FIGURE 4. *Illustration of disaggregation, when day 1 has a total of 2mm of rain, day 2 has 1mm of rain, and all preceding and succeeding days are rain-free.* **(a)** *A single realisation of the latent variable (—), and expected values and 95% confidence envelopes (- - -) estimated from 10000 simulations. (The threshold of 1.05, above which rainfall occurs, is also shown (···).)* **(b)** *The single realisation of rainfall resulting from (a) (—), and expected rainfall (- - -).*

The Markov chain appears to converge rapidly and to have good mixing properties: summary statistics converged to stable values within five iterations, and the average correlation between consecutive simulations was only 8%. However, correlations were as high as 55% at the beginning and end of very wet days. Therefore, after a burn-in period of ten iterations, we took every tenth sequence as an independent disaggregation. Summary statistics (not presented) agree well with those in Table 1. Fig 4 illustrates the results obtained for two wet days during a long dry period. Note that the expected values and variances of the latent variable are not constant within a day. Perhaps surprisingly, we see that the expected rainfall reaches a clear peak on the final hour of day one. However, a similar pattern was subsequently found in the data themselves.

The latent Gaussian model can be used in a similar way for forecasting from hourly data. In this case, the Gibbs sampler is used to simulate values of the latent variable for rain-free hours in the past, and then to simulate the latent variable into the future. Alternatively, an analytic approach may be possible.

5 Discussion

One inelegant feature of the latent Gaussian model is that, unlike point process models [11], it is not scale independent. For example, if hourly data arise from such a model, then daily data cannot also do so, although it may be possible to formulate the model in continuous time. Also, we share some of Sir David Cox's reservations, expressed in a review of time series in 1981 [3], that 'by pointwise transformation of a Gaussian series it is possible to produce series with any required marginal distribution. Such a construction will, however, often be artificial, especially for discrete distributions.' However, others maintain that point processes are themselves unnatural models for rainfall and many of the processes in the high atmosphere which generate rainfall are Gaussian. A further drawback of the latent Gaussian model is that it is difficult to see how to embed it in a broader class of models, so as to be able to generalise the basic model in situations where multivariate normality is not satisfied. It may be possible to model the latent variable as a probabilistic mixture of two or more Gaussian processes, or to simultaneously transform two or more consecutive rainfalls to multivariate normality, but both these approaches seem to encounter technical difficulties.

On the positive side, the model is simple to understand and to fit to data, it agrees well with Edinburgh's rainfall data, and is comparatively easy to use for simulation, disaggregation and forecasting. Also, the latent Gaussian model generalises elegantly to encompass both spatio-temporal data and multivariate situations involving other climatic variables, provided that distributional assumptions prove to be reasonable. We would expect both forecasting and disaggregation to be more appropriate in a multivariate, spatial setting. We are pursuing these ideas further, together with improving the estimation procedure and disaggregation algorithm.

ACKNOWLEDGEMENTS

The work was supported by funds from the Scottish Office Agriculture, Environment and Fisheries Department.

6 References

[1] Andersen, E.B. (1990). *The Statistical Analysis of Categorical Data.* Springer-Verlag, Berlin.

[2] Bell, T.L. (1987). A space-time stochastic model of rainfall for satellite remote-sensing studies. *Journal of Geophysical Research*, **92**, 9631-9643.

[3] Cox, D.R. (1981). Statistical analysis of time series: some recent developments. *Scandinavian Journal of Statistics*, **8**, 93-115.

[4] Cressie, N.A.C. (1991). *Statistics for Spatial Data.* Wiley, New York.

[5] Gilks, W.R., Best, N.G., Tan, K.K.C. (1995). Adaptive rejection Metropolis sampling within Gibbs sampling. *Applied Statistics*, **44**, 455-472.

[6] Glasbey, C.A., Cooper, G., McGechan, M.B. (1995). Disaggregation of daily rainfall by conditional simulation from a point-process model. *Journal of Hydrology*, **165**, 1-9.

[7] Hutchinson, M.F. (1995). Stochastic space-time weather models from ground-based data. *Agricultural and Forest Meteorology*, **73**, 237-264.

[8] Katz, R.W., Parlange, M.B. (1995). Generalizations of chain-dependent processes: applications to hourly precipitation. *Water Resources Research*, **31**, 1331-1341.

[9] Le Cam, L. (1961). A stochastic description of precipitation. In *Proceedings of the Fourth Berkeley Symposium on Mathematical Statistics and Probability* (ed. J. Neyman) **3**, 165-186.

[10] Richardson, C.W. (1981). Stochastic simulation of daily precipitation, temperature, and solar radiation. *Water Resources Research*, **17**, 182-190.

[11] Rodriguez-Iturbe, I., Cox, D.R., Isham, V. (1988). A point process model for rainfall: further developments. *Proceedings of the Royal Society, London, Series A*, **417**, 283-298.

[12] Sanso, B., Guenni, L. (1997). Venezualan rainfall data analysed using a Bayesian space-time model. *Applied Statistics*, (in press).

[13] Stern, R.D., Coe, R. (1984). A model fitting analysis of daily rainfall data (with discussion). *Journal of the Royal Statistical Society, Series A*, **147**, 1-34.

Estimation of Individual Exposure Following a Chemical Spill in Superior, Wisconsin

Elena N. Naumova*, Timothy C. Haas, and Robert D. Morris

Medical College of Wisconsin
United States

ABSTRACT The goal of this study was to evaluate the use of self-reported survey data as an indication of exposure. Parametric and nonparametric statistical models and functions including Generalized Linear Models, Cumulative Logit link models, and the quasi-likelihood function, were used to fit the possibly nonlinear relationship between self-reported exposure and spatial location. Because the errors in estimates of exposure based on self-reported data are different from the errors in estimates from deterministic simulations, the similarities between these estimates should reflect the underlying spatial stochastic processes corresponding to the true exposure. This is demonstrated using data from a chemical spill in Superior, Wisconsin.

Key words and phrases: generalized linear model; cumulative logit link model; quasi-likelihood; exposure; health; survey data; spatial.

1 Introduction

Environmental health professionals often face the problem of retrospective assessment of exposure following a short term release of toxic chemicals. More often than not, few if any quantitative environmental measurements are available. The common way to evaluate individual exposures when it is

---

*The authors gratefully thank Dr. William G. Warren and Dr. David R. Brillinger for their helpful comments and suggestions. For correspondence: Center for Environmental Epidemiology, Department of Family and Community Medicine, Medical College of Wisconsin, 8701 Watertown Plank Road, Milwaukee, WI, 53226-0509, or e-mail: enaumova@post.its.mcw.edu

impractical or impossible to measure exposures of an individual is to estimate using modeling (EPA, 1995). The survey-research methods can also provide important information about individual exposure (e.g. distance to source, time spent in the contaminated area, experience of toxic symptoms). Very little is known about the use of human neuro-physiological responses to low concentrations of gaseous chemicals (e.g. odor intensity; nasal, eye, or throat irritation) as an indicator of exposure, except that the human ability to detect odor can vary and can have a nonlinear relationship with concentration (Dunn, 1996).

In this paper we examine a relationship between the exposure evaluated from survey data and the exposure simulated by a deterministic model. For this purposed we used the original data sets as a part of the analysis of environmental and health effects of a chemical spill in Superior, Wisconsin (Morris et al, 1996). The organization of the article is as follows. After a brief overview of a chemical spill of aromatic distillates, in Section 2 the description of the original data sets is given in detail with the emphasis on the procedure for forming an ordered response variable which reflects the reported individual exposure, on the potential for bias associated with self-reported data, and on the inaccuracies in determining the respondents locations. In Section 3 a brief description of the cumulative logit link model for ordered response and an alternative logistic model for dichotomized self-reported response is given. These models were used to obtain reliable individual exposure estimates by fitting the possibly nonlinear relationship between self-reported exposure and spatial location. The procedure for constructing the linear predictors which allowed for estimating the exposure at fixed locations with respect to the reported response in the local neighborhood is presented. An outline of the "model-based residuals" construction, to describe the differences between statistical models and the "true" value, is given in Section 4. Because no physical monitors were available, the deterministic model of the chemical cloud movement was used in place of actual measurements. In Section 5 of this paper, the results of the study are discussed. Section 6 summarizes the findings and concludes the paper.

2 Data

Early on the morning of June 30, 1992, a train derailment in Superior, Wisconsin resulted in the spill of more than 20,000 gallons of aromatic distillates into the Nemadji river. Most of the contents of the tank car released into the Nemadji River evaporated from the water surface while being carried downstream to Lake Superior. A visible cloud with an unpleasant, irritating odor formed by the spilled material drifted over residential areas, requiring the evacuation of 40,000 people. People near the spill site experienced immediate symptoms such as burning eyes, coughing, breathing difficulties, burning throat, and irritation of their mucous membranes and some reported to nearby emergency rooms. In 1995, a telephone survey was conducted to evaluate possible associations between the spill and the incidence of disease in Superior.

The survey of the residents of the contaminated and surrounding areas provided information from 565 residents including addresses at the time of the spill, their reported intensity of smell, the time of the evacuation from the contaminated area and individual concerns about health effects. Survey subjects were asked if they smelled the spill. Those who could smell the spill (n=352) were asked, "How strong was the smell from the chemical spill? Would you say it was very strong, somewhat strong, not very strong or not at all strong?" We assumed that the self-reported smell intensity reflected the strongest detected concentration of chemicals over time spent in the contaminated area. The answers to these questions were converted to ordered response variables with four categories. For each respondent, the ordered response had either "high exposure" (if smell intensity was reported as "very strong", n=155), "moderate exposure" (if smell intensity was reported as "somewhat strong", n=136), "low exposure" (if smell intensity was reported as "not very strong", n=52; "not at all strong", n=6; "don't know/not sure", n=3), or "no exposure", n=213. These four categories were viewed as an underlying ordinal variable reflecting the reported individual exposure. As an additional measure of the reported individual exposure, the binary outcome was also suggested. The dichotomization was performed between the "exposed" residents with "high exposure" and "-moderate exposure" on one hand, and the "non exposed" residents with "low exposure" and "no exposure" on the other.

Because the reported smell intensity is subjective, it might have been biased due to the respondents' high sensitivity to chemicals or odor, or their belief that the spill had caused a health problem. To reduce such bias, a binary covariate reflecting a high sensitivity to chemicals or odor was suggested. This covariate was recorded as "non sensitive" if the respondent reported that he was never told by the doctor that he "is highly sensitive to chemicals or odor"; and as "sensitive" if the respondent reported that he was told by the doctor or considered himself to be highly sensitive to chemicals or odor.

Survey respondents were asked the address of their primary residence at the time of the spill. These addresses were converted to latitude and longitude by an address matching procedure available in the MapINFO Geographic Information System (GIS) software package. For various reasons, some addresses could not be geocoded automatically. To the greatest extent possible, these addresses were geocoded manually by locating them on a street map of Douglas County. To do this, the closest address was found and the residence was placed at that location. When this was not possible, the address was placed at intersection of the two closest streets.

The error in the specification of residence location by the street address matching procedure was greater for rural areas than for urban areas. For those addresses giving only a route number, the closest street intersection was taken as the residents location. As a consequence, one point in the map of the rural area often represented more then one respondent. In the city area one point might also represent more than one person in an area with multi-unit buildings, but this did not indicate an error introduced by geocoding.

3 Model descriptions and initial assumptions

To evaluate the individual levels of exposure due to the chemical spill, we assumed a linear relationship between exposure level and distance from exposure source. One approach used a standard generalized linear model for prediction of exposure at a fixed location on the basis of self-reported smell intensity and respondent residency obtained from the survey. Let Y be the ordered response of individuals in the study and be restricted to one of a fixed set of possible values. The $k-$ possible values of Y form $k-$ response categories. Agresti (1990, p.318) discussed three types of logits for ordered response categories: adjacent-categories logits, continuation ratio logits, and cumulative logits. For cumulative logits, the ordered response categories form logits of cumulative response probabilities γ_j (McCullagh and Nelder, 1989, p.149) such as $\gamma_1 = \pi_1,\ \gamma_2 = \pi_1 + \pi_2, ...,\ \gamma_k \equiv 1$.

The simplest model in this class involves parallel regressions on the chosen scale (McCullagh and Nelder, 1989), such as $\log\{\gamma_j(s)/(1-\gamma_j(s))\} = \theta_j - \beta^T s,\ j = 1, ..., k-1$; where $\gamma_j(s) = \Pr(Y \leq j|s)$ is the cumulative probability up to and including category j, when the covariate vector is s; θ and β are treated as unknown and θ must satisfy $\theta_1 \leq \theta_2 \leq ... \leq \theta_{k-1}$ to ensure that the probabilities are non-negative.

Let Z be an underlying unobserved continuous random variable, such that $Z - \beta^T s$ has the standard logistic distribution. If this variable lies in the interval $\theta_{j-1} < Z \leq \theta_j$, then $y = j$ is recorded. Let Z have the logistic distribution with mean $\beta^T s$ and scale parameter $\exp(\tau^T s)$, then according to McCullagh and Nelder (1989, p.154) $\operatorname{logit}\gamma_j(s) = (\theta_j - \beta^T s)/\exp(\tau^T s)$ or $z_j \equiv (\theta_j - \beta^T s)/\sigma$.

The standardized variable, z, has mean 0 and variance $\pi^2/3$. Let $\omega = \exp(z)$, then the standard logistic distribution is defined by $F(z) = \omega/(1+\omega)$ and the log-likelihood for γ_j is $L = \sum g(z_j) - \log(\sigma)$, where $g = z - 2\log(1+\omega)$. For identifiability, $\beta \equiv 0$. The vector β that maximized this function is the estimate of the models parameters. The values of Y predicted at s-location can be recovered as $\exp(\theta|s)$. The cumulative logit model was implemented using the "survreg"-function in Splus.

In an alternative model, the ordered response was converted to a binary response by ignoring information concerning self-reported intensity, or in other words, by dichotomization of the self-reported response. In this case we express the logistic regression model as $\log\{\pi(s)/(1-\pi(s))\} = \beta s$ (Agresti, 1990). In this formulation the prediction was performed using a class of GLM.

We assumed that the chemical cloud was continuous, low lying to the northeast of the spill site (as demonstrated by a videotape taken from a civilian aircraft), and was approximately shaped as an ellipse. Following the geometric property of an ellipse, the distances from two fixed points, named foci, in the plane have a constant sum (Thomas and Finney, 1990, p.528). If one the ellipse foci - F_1 is fixed at spill site location, another foci - F_2, is assumed to be located downstream on Nemadji River close to the river mouth. So, the sum of the Euclidean distances between the respondents' location and both foci for each respondent formed a linear predictor. To keep a positive association, the inverse of the sum of the distances (ISD) was suggested.

Another way for making predictions using the assumption about continuous properties of the cloud, was to model a more sophisticated (and less developed) location transformation such as an interaction (Hastie and Tibshirani, 1990, p.264), which is convenient in Generalized Additive Modeling (GAM). Using the same assumption about the ellipsoid shape of the diffusion of the chemical cloud, the interaction should include linear and quadratic terms (Chambers and Hastie, 1993). Modeling interaction with an orthogonal polynomial of fourth degree was selected (Venables and Ripley, 1994).

Use of described predictors allowed for estimating the exposure at fixed locations with respect to the reported response in the local neighborhood.

4 The baseline for comparison of exposure estimates

For purposes of comparison, the baseline was defined to be the individual cumulative relative exposure from the air dispersion model recommended by EPA (EPA, 1995). To predict airborne chemical transport the Industrial Source Complex 3 (ISC3), a steady-state Gaussian plume model, was used. The ISC3 model required real-time hourly surface weather data such as temperature, wind direction, wind speed, mixing height, and stability class, and assumed that all the pollutants were vaporized within the first hour of the spill. The ISC3 model outcomes were the relative concentration for six time points (hourly from 3AM to 8AM) at 6560 locations arranged in a non-orthogonal non-collinear evenly spaced grid. This study was limited to the cumulative relative concentration obtained by summing all six time points.

To assign cumulative relative exposure for each respondent and to make the ISC3-model data available for comparison, the cumulative concentration values from the deterministic ISC3-model were converted to an orthogonal regular evenly spaced grid using a linear interpolation with the triangulation scheme (Akima, 1978). The cumulative concentration values for points outside the models area were assigned zero and then re-scaled from 0 to 3. The cumulative concentration had a highly skewed, multimodal, continuous distribution with high concentrations limited to a very small area. Given the highly skewed nature of the data, a logit transformation was applied giving an additional scale for comparison.

For exposure estimates at a fixed location, an average of the cumulative concentration (scale 1) and an average of the logit-transformation (scale 2) in a rectangular window with the twelve nearest grid values were taken. Each of these two scales formed matrices of estimates - $\mathbf{M}_1$ and $\mathbf{M}_2$ with 20x20 cells. The $\mathbf{M}_1$ was created based on the cumulative concentration, and $\mathbf{M}_2$ was created based on the logit-transformation of the cumulative concentration.

"Model-based residuals" were taken as the difference between the exposure that was predicted based on self-reported data and each exposure estimate - $\mathbf{M}_1$ and $\mathbf{M}_2$. The descriptive statistics of these residuals were treated as indicators of an agreement between the statistical model and the "true" value. The residuals between $\mathbf{M}_1$ and $\mathbf{M}_2$ reflected the agreement between the bases for comparison.

5 Results

The map of Superior shown in Figure 1 indicates the location of the respondents residences along with the location of the Nemadji River. This map also shows the dichotomizated self-reported smell intensity data: the "exposed" (shown as a solid diamond on map, n=191) versus the "non exposed" (shown as an empty circle, n=374). Since one point in the map of rural area due to geocoding inaccuracy often represented more then one respondent, points were separated for plotting by using a jittering-procedure (Akima, 1978). Under the simple assumption that the river was the source of exposure, this plot shows that the relationship between the self-reported intensity and the distance to spill source was not linear. To check for a monotonic spatial trend in outcome in relation to location, the reported smell intensity was modeled as a smoothed function of longitude and latitude with the "loess"- nonparametric local robust smoother (Cleveland, 1979). The highest values of exposure for the reported smell intensity appeared to be northeast of the spill site, diminishing close to the river mouth. The spill site location was taken as the intersection of the Nemadji river and the Burlington Northern railway. The coordinates

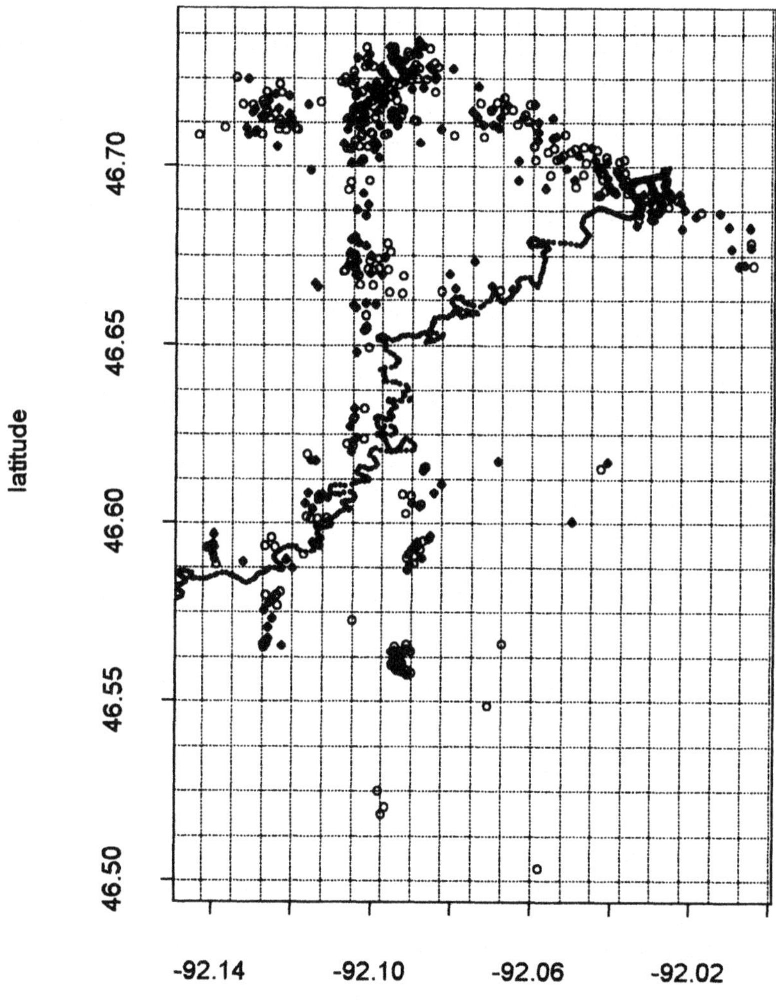

Figure 1. The locations of the Superior respondents' residences along the Nemadji River and the regular grid of rectangular cells. Two types of marks indicate the exposure binary response: 'non exposed' (an empty circle) and 'exposed' (a solid diamond).

of the spill site, F_1={-92.1208, 46.5939}, and the river mouth, F_2={-92.02, 46.7}, were used for constructing the ISD-predictor. To check for linearity in modeling the reported smell intensity as a function of the ISD, the GAM with the "loess" smoother was conducted. The additive contribution decayed with decreasing ISD, hence the ellipsoid linearized the relationship between the exposure level and the distance from the spill cloud.

The mean-variance relationship for the self-reported smell intensity was evaluated in a set of rectangular windows. Interpretation of this relationship required some caution because of the widely different degrees of freedom on which each variance is based (Venables and Ripley, 1994). The mean-variance relationship was bell-shaped. The non-linear approximation of this relationship supported the assumption that the variance of an outcome can be dependent on the mean. The variance was small for the extremes and high for the intermediate values of outcome. Those assumptions supported a prediction based on quasi-likelihood. Modeling based on quasi-likelihood was performed for both predictors. Having in general good fitting properties (residual deviance: 828.0 on 562 degrees of freedom; coefficient for ISD: 0.2274; std. error: 0.0471), the model had difficulties in fitting the extremes.

Two types of models: the cumulative logit link model (L) and the logit model for binary response (B); with two types of linear predictors: the inverse of the distances sum (I) and interaction term (P); were performed with and without an additional covariate reflecting chemical sensitivity (S and O respectively). The model-based residuals between predicted exposure from eight models and matrices $\mathbf{M}_1$ and $\mathbf{M}_2$ described above (computed on the set of rectangular cells shown in Figure 1) were evaluated.

The descriptive statistics for the model-based residuals are shown in Table 1. In general, the binomial model gave the smallest variance in residuals for the original scale deterministic model - $\mathbf{M}_1$ and the cumulative logit model gave the smallest mean in residuals for the logit-transform scale deterministic model - $\mathbf{M}_2$. The best agreement was reached between the cumulative logit model with the interaction term adjusted for chemical sensitivity, LPS-model, and the logit-transformation of the cumulative concentration - $\mathbf{M}_2$ (mean = 0.01, var =0.132). A dichotomization of self-reported intensity (B) agreed well with original scale deterministic model - $\mathbf{M}_1$, but consistently overestimated the exposure in comparison with $\mathbf{M}_2$. Both predictor types had good fitting characteristics, but modeling interaction with an orthogonal polynomial of fourth degree (P) gave less mean in residuals than the inverse distance sum predictor (I). At the same time the inverse distance sum predictor for all of the model gave a smaller variance than an orthogonal polynomial predictor. For most of the models the inclusion of an additional covariate reflecting chemical sensitivity tended to reduce the residuals in term of their mean and variance.

The residuals between $\mathbf{M}_1$ and $\mathbf{M}_2$ which reflected the agreement between the comparison bases had very small variation and high correlation (var=0.29, r = 0.89).

Table 1. The descriptive statistics for the model-based residuals

	$\mathbf{M}_1$ -	(original)	$\mathbf{M}_2$ -	(logit-transform)
*Model abbreviation**	*Mean*	*Variance*	*Mean*	*Variance*
L P S	0.243	(0.208)	0.010	(0.132)
L P O	0.256	(0.226)	0.022	(0.132)
L I S	0.265	(0.234)	0.032	(0.117)
L I O	0.275	(0.250)	0.042	(0.119)
B P S	0.090	(0.077)	-0.143	(0.218)
B P O	0.103	(0.082)	-0.130	(0.204)
B I S	0.110	(0.071)	-0.123	(0.156)
B I O	0.122	(0.078)	-0.111	(0.149)

* L="logit", B="binomial", P="polynomial", I="inverse distanse", S/O=with/without an adjustment for chemical sensitivity.

The spatial distribution of the cumulative concentrations, obtained from deterministic models, and the predicted exposure, based on self-reported smell intensity, is displayed as an image-plot (Figure 2) along with the locations of the spill site on the Nemadji River. Following the image-plot of the cumulative concentrations (a) and the logit - transformation of the cumulative concentrations (b), the most contaminated area appears to be southeast of the Nemadji River.

Figure 2c demonstrates the spatial distribution of the predicted exposure obtained from logit models for the BIS-model; and Figure 2d shows the image of the predicted exposure obtained from the LPS-model. The image-plot of the cumulative concentrations (Figures 2a and 2c) suggests that only a small number of people were likely to have had significant exposures. The image-plot of the logit-transformation of the cumulative concentrations (Figures 2b) shows a wide area of very low concentration to the northwest of the major cloud.

Given the extremely low odor threshold of pentene (2 ppb), one of the components in chemical cloud, it seems likely that this was the primary source of the unpleasant odor reported by persons exposed to the chemical cloud even at the location far from the major cloud (Figures 2d). Figures 2b and 2d suggest the LPS model gives biased estimates due to lack of residents in the most contaminated area (refer Figure 1).

6 Conclusion

Both deterministic models and self-reported smell intensity can be used to generate estimates of individual exposure. These estimates correspond to the true exposure of interest together with some error component, but in

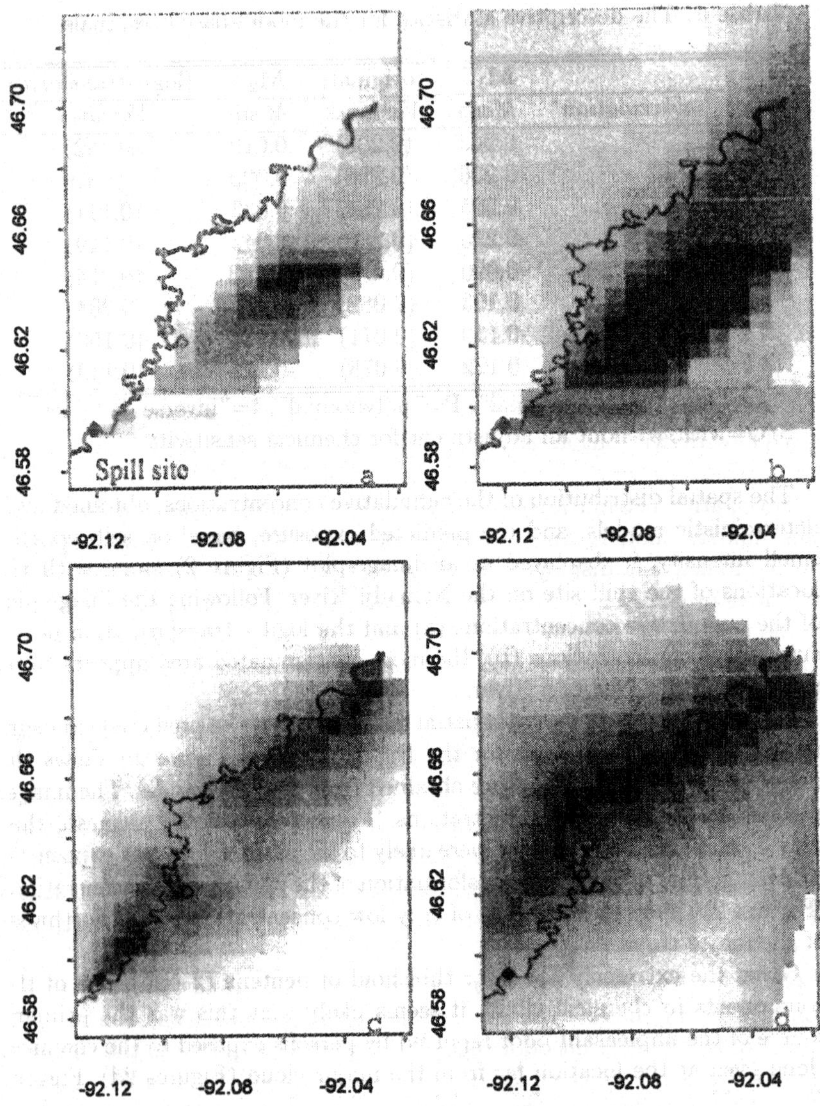

Figure 2. The image of the chemical cloud, based on: (a)- the cumulative concentrations in original scale; (b)- the logit-transformation of the concentrations; (c)- the predicted exposure level, obtained using the self-reported smell intensity, from BIS-model and LPS model (d). The solid diamond indicates the location of the spill site on the Nemadji River.

each case, the sources of error are fundamentally different. The inaccuracies in estimates of exposure from deterministic models result from the simplifying assumptions required by the model and the failure of the model to accurately describe individual microenvironments. Reported smell intensity is affected by reporting biases and by variability in individual sensitivity to odor. Therefore, the overlap between these two estimates should provide information that is relatively free from the two types of error. In other words, the similarity between exposure estimates based on self-reported smell intensity and those derived from deterministic simulation should reflect the underlying spatial stochastic processes corresponding to the true exposure.

The analysis of the data from the spill in Superior suggests that the choice of modeling procedure depends on the specific application of the exposure estimates. Frequently, in the case of a chemical spill, the distribution of individual exposures is highly skewed. If the exposures represented by the tail of the distribution are potentially important, a logit-transformation of cumulative concentration obtained from the deterministic model was found to be best. It was also found that the cumulative logit link predictors agreed well with the logit transformation of the deterministic model. If, on the other hand, we wish to distinguish between exposed and unexposed people, the logit models with binary response will tend to minimize the impact of error on the exposure estimates.The logit models for binary response agreed well with the deterministic model.

Future studies will focus on improving the accuracy and precision of exposure estimates from both types of data. The combination of exposure estimates with various degrees of adjustment for bias can promote better understanding of the association between a chemical spill and health effects. Selected exposure estimates will be used at the next stage in the analysis of the environmental and health effects of the chemical spill as a predictor for the risk of the respiratory diseases and asthma development.

7 References

[1] Agresti, A. (1990) *Categorical Data Analysis.* Wiley: New York.

[2] Akima, H. (1978). A Method of Bivariate Interpolation and Smooth Surface Fitting for Irregularly Distributed Data Points. *ACM Transactions on Mathematical Software* **4**, 148-164.

[3] Chambers, JM and Hastie, TJ. (1993) Statistical Models In S. London: Chapman and Hall.

[4] Cleveland, WS. (1979). Robust Locally Weighed Regression And Smoothing Scatterplots. *Journal of the American Statistical Association* **74**, 829-836.

[5] Dunn, JE. (1996). Interlaboratory Calibration of Measures of Human

Sensitivity to Gaseous Pollutants. Proc. Spruce III Conference - Statistical Aspects of Pollution: Assessment and Control, December, 1995: 21.

[6] EPA: *Users Guide For The Industrial Source Complex Dispersion Models* (Revised), Document EPA-454/B-95-003a, July 1995.

[7] Hastie, TJ and Tibshirani, RJ. (1990). *Generalized Additive Models.* London: Chapman and Hall.

[8] MapINFO Corporation (1996). *MapINFO Professional*, Version 4.02, Troy.

[9] Mccullagh, P and Nelder, JA. (1989). *Generalized Linear Models.* London: Chapman and Hall.

[10] Morris, RD, Naumova, EN, Zhang, C and Chubin, HS. (1996). Human Health Effect Study of a Spill of Aromatis Distillates in Superior, Wisconsin. Technical Report for the Agency for Toxic Substances and Disease Registry.

[11] Statistical Sciences (1995). *Statistical Analysis in S-Plus*, Version 3.3, Seattle: Statsci, Division of Mathsoft, Inc.

[12] Thomas, GB and Finney, RL. (1990). *Calculus and Analytic Geometry.* (7th edition). Massachusetts: Addison-Wesley.

[13] Venables, WN and Ripley, BD. (1994). *Modern Applied Statistics with S-Plus.* New York: Springer-Verlag.

Flexible Response Surface Methods via Spatial Regression and EBLUPS

M. O'Connell*
Becton Dickinson Research Center
United States

R. Wolfinger
SAS Institute
United States

ABSTRACT Spatial regression models provide a complementary alternative to polynomial response surface methods in the context of process optimization. The models enable estimation of design variable effects and, via EBLUPS, smooth data-faithful approximations to the unknown response function over the design space. The covariance structure of the particular spatial models drives the predicted response surfaces and both isotropic and geometrically anisotropic forms are considered. Estimation of covariance parameters is achieved via maximum likelihood or restricted maximum likelihood. A feature of the method is the visually appealing graphical summaries that are produced. These allow rapid identification of process windows on the design space for which the response(s) achieves target performance. The models perform well in association with spatial designs such as the maximin and minimax designs. The EVOP approach is also possible and in this context the models provide a representation of the response over the entire series of designs. An example involving the optimization of assay components in a DNA amplification procedure provides illustration.

Key words and phrases: Spatial regression; Kriging; Process optimization; Mixed models; Response surface methods.

1 Introduction

Response surface methodology (RSM) is a collection of statistical and mathematical techniques useful for developing, improving and optimizing processes (Myers and Montgomery, 1995). Three central ideas are (i) ap-

*We thank W. Keating of Becton Dickinson Microbiology Systems for the data, P. Haaland of Becton Dickinson Research Center for helpful comments on the manuscript and R. Stogner of SAS Institute for help with SAS SPECTRAVIEW. Corresponding author: Michael O'Connell, BDRC, PO Box 12016, RTP NC 27709.

proximating the response surface, (ii) assessing the effects of process variables on the response(s) and (iii) identifying settings of the process variables that provide an optimum value of the response(s) in some sense. Response surface methods typically rely on polynomial models for construction of response surfaces (Box and Draper 1987, Myers and Montgomery, 1995). This characterization is unappealing primarily due to the inflexible, global nature of the fit.

An alternative spatial regression approach, that provides smooth, data-driven approximations to the unknown response function, is described. This approach allows assessment of individual design variable effects and gives realistic predictions of the unknown response over the entire design space. The predicted response surfaces are driven by the covariance structures of the spatial models. Several structures, isotropic and anisotropic, are considered. Estimation of covariance parameters is achieved via maximum likelihood and residual maximum likelihood. An attractive feature of the approach is the visually appealing graphical summaries that are produced. These allow rapid and intuitive identification of process windows on the design space for which the response achieves target performance.

The spatial regression approach can be used with any number of designs including standard response surface method designs such as the central composite second-order polynomial optimal designs (Myers and Montgomery, 1995). Other spatial designs, such as the uniform coverage and maximum spread designs available in SAS PROC OPTEX (SAS Institute Inc., 1995) and the packing designs available in Gosset (Hardin and Sloane, 1994), provide a particularly suitable design complement. An additional feature of the approach is the ability to fit the spatial models equally well for combined data obtained from series of designs on the same space of design variables.

2 Spatial Regression Models: Estimation and Prediction

The spatial regression models considered are similar to the models underlying a geostatistical (universal) kriging analysis. However, in a typical kriging analysis, experimental units lie in 2-dimensional space rather than the multidimensional space studied in process optimization applications. The spatial regression models are written as

$$y_i = X\beta + Z(\boldsymbol{x}_i) + \epsilon_i$$

where y_i is an observed response at the ith combination of design variables $\boldsymbol{x}_i \in \Re^d$, $i = 1, \ldots, n$, X is a mean model matrix, β is a vector of (mean model) coefficients, $Z(\boldsymbol{x}_i)$ is a d-dimensional, second-order stationary stochastic process with $E(Z(\boldsymbol{x}_i)) = 0$ and $\mathrm{Var}(Z(\boldsymbol{x}_i)) = \sigma_Z^2$, and ϵ denotes additive measurement error with $E(\epsilon) = 0$, $\text{Cov}(\epsilon) = \sigma^2 I$. Note that since attention is restricted to stationary stochastic processes

$$\text{Cov}(Z(\boldsymbol{x}_i), Z(\boldsymbol{x}_j)) \equiv C(\boldsymbol{x}_i, \boldsymbol{x}_j; \theta) = C(\boldsymbol{h}; \theta)$$

for $\boldsymbol{h} = \boldsymbol{x}_i - \boldsymbol{x}_j$.

Zimmerman and Harville (1991) discuss a similar spatial regression model, without measurement error, in detail for d=2 in the context of agricultural field experiments and refer to it as a (two-dimensional) random field linear model. For process optimization d is typically in the range d=3-7 design variables.

We consider three forms for the covariance function, an isotropic exponential form and two geometrically anisotropic forms. The exponential covariance function (EXP) is

$$C(\boldsymbol{h}; \theta) \equiv C(r; \theta) = \theta_1 \exp(-\theta_2 r) \tag{1}$$

where $r = (\boldsymbol{h}'\boldsymbol{h})^{1/2}$ for $\boldsymbol{h} = \boldsymbol{s} - \boldsymbol{t}$. Note that if $C(\boldsymbol{h}, \theta)$ depends on $\boldsymbol{h}$ only through its norm $r = (\boldsymbol{h}'\boldsymbol{h})^{1/2}$, then $Z(\boldsymbol{x})$ and $C(\boldsymbol{h}; \theta)$ are referred to herein as an isotropic stochastic process and an isotropic covariance structure.

The anisotropic power covariance function (POWA) is

$$C(\boldsymbol{h}; \theta) = \theta_0 \prod_{k=1}^{d} \theta_k^{h_k} = \theta_0 C^*(\boldsymbol{h}; \theta^*) \tag{2}$$

and the anisotropic exponential covariance function (EXPA) is

$$C(\boldsymbol{h}; \theta, p) = \theta_0 \prod_{k=1}^{d} \exp(-\theta_k {h_k}^{p_k}) = \theta_0 C^*(\boldsymbol{h}; \theta^*, p) \tag{3}$$

where $h_k = \mid s_k - t_k \mid$ is a measure of distance in the kth design variable dimension, $k = 1, ..., d$. The latter model was given by Sacks et al. (1989) who resticted the power parameter p_k to the interval $0 < p_k \leq 2$. In the implementation herein, p_k is considered as both unconstrained and fixed at $p_k = 2\, \forall k$. Note that if $p_k = 1\, \forall k$ this model reduces to a reparameterization of model(2).

For all the spatial regression models given above the variance of Y is conveniently written as $V = \sigma^2(I + \alpha C^*) \equiv \sigma^2 W$ for $\alpha = \sigma_Z^2/\sigma^2 = \theta_0/\sigma^2$. The additive measurement error σ^2 is analogous to a nugget effect in the spatial statistics literature.

Given V, the maximum likelihood estimate (MLE) of β is the GLS estimate

$$\hat{\beta} = (X^T W^{-1} X)^{-1} X^T W^{-1} Y$$

and the MLE of σ^2 is

$$\hat{\sigma}^2 = (1/n)Y^T P_W Y$$

for $P_W = W^{-1} - W^{-1}X(X^T W^{-1}X)^{-1}X^T W^{-1}$. The stochastic process covariance parameters are estimated by maximizing a profile log likelihood

$$l^*(\theta^*, \alpha \mid y) = -\frac{1}{2}\log \mid W \mid -\frac{n}{2}\log(Y^T P_W Y)$$

or profile residual log likelihood

$$l_R^*(\theta^*, \alpha \mid y) = -\frac{1}{2}\log \mid W \mid -\frac{1}{2}\log \mid X^T W^{-1} X \mid -\frac{n-p}{2}\log(Y^T P_W Y)$$

where p is the number of parameters in the mean model.

For the numerical maximization of l^* or l_R^* a ridge-stabilized Newton-Raphson algorithm with MIVQUE(0) starting values performs very well in practice. The algorithm requires the computation of the first and second derivatives with respect to the parameters in θ^* and α. Wolfinger, Tobias, and Sall (1994) provide general analytical expressions and computational details.

Estimation of the response surface is of central importance to the analysis. As is the case with kriging, the response surface is constructed via the best linear unbiased predictor (BLUP). Given V, the BLUP for prediction at a new point $\boldsymbol{g}$ is

$$\hat{y}(\boldsymbol{g}) = \boldsymbol{g}^T\hat{\beta} + c^T(\boldsymbol{g},\boldsymbol{x})V^{-1}(y - X\hat{\beta})$$

where $c(\boldsymbol{g},\boldsymbol{x})$ is the vector of covariances between the Z's at the new point $\boldsymbol{g}$ and the design points $\boldsymbol{x}_i$, $i = 1,\ldots,n$. For example, in the model of Sacks et al. (1989),

$$c(\boldsymbol{g},\boldsymbol{x}_i) = \theta_0 \prod_k \exp(-\theta_k h_{ik}^{p_k})$$

where $h_{ik} = \mid g_k - x_{ik} \mid$. The variance of the predicted response surface (e.g. Harville, 1990) is as follows:

$$\begin{aligned}\mathrm{Var}[\hat{y}(\boldsymbol{g}) - y(\boldsymbol{g})] &= \sigma^2 + \sigma_Z^2 - c^T(\boldsymbol{x},\boldsymbol{g})V^{-1}c(\boldsymbol{x},\boldsymbol{g}) + \\ &[\boldsymbol{g}^T - c^T(\boldsymbol{x},\boldsymbol{g})V^{-1}X](X^T V^{-1}X)^{-1}[\boldsymbol{g} - X^T V^{-1}c(\boldsymbol{x},\boldsymbol{g})]\end{aligned}$$

In practice V is usually unknown, so the empirical BLUP (EBLUP) and its estimated prediction error are obtained by substituting ML or REML estimates of the covariance parameters ($\hat{V}$) into the previous expressions. Even though the estimated prediction error has a slight downward bias (see Cressie 1991, pp. 297-299), this deficiency can often be overcome by using t instead of Gaussian distributions for inference.

Construction of the (predicted) response surface and the prediction standard error surface is accomplished by setting up a grid of combinations of the design variables. For example, to construct a 2 dimensional surface showing the combined effect of two design variables one might set up a $20\times20 = 400$ point grid matrix G. The (predicted) response surface is then

$$\hat{y}(G) = G\hat{\beta} + C(G, X)\hat{V}^{-1}(y - X\hat{\beta})$$

where $C(G, X)$ is the $400\times n$ matrix of covariances between the grid and the design.

3 Example: A Diagnostic Assay Based on DNA Amplification

A DNA amplification procedure, strand displacement amplification (SDA), has been developed at Becton Dickinson Research Center and forms the basis for instrumented diagnostic assay identification of bacterial pathogens (Walker at al. 1992). SDA involves probe capture of target DNA sequences, polymerase extension, enzyme recognition, and strand displacement via further polymerase extension. The displaced strand is then available for subsequent probe capture so that exponential production of the target DNA sequence may be achieved under certain conditions. The response of interest, the amount of target production, is proportional to the amount of target present in the sample and is measured in relative light units (RLU) produced with a sandwich assay. The optimal conditions for amplification involve suitable quantities and concentrations of enzyme co-solvents (e.g. DMSO) and substances required for efficient polymerase extension (e.g. KPO_4 and MgOAc). The study described herein involves a sequence of five response surface experiments in three design variables: DMSO, KPO_4 and MgOAc, with the measured responses representing signal strengths in RLU for a particular target denoted as tDNA1. A total of 64 experimental runs were completed. RLU responses were calibrated by experiment and analyzed as log(RLU) using the spatial regression methods described above.

The three spatial regression models were fit to the RLU response data and the results are summarized in Table 1. Zero-order (intercept only), first-order (intercept plus linear terms in the design variables) and second-order (intercept plus linear, quadratic and interaction terms in the design variables) models were fit as mean models along with each covariance model. All models are fit using scaled design points, $(x_{ik} - \min_i(x_{ik}))/\text{range}_i(x_{ik})$ for each of the k dimensions.

Estimation is performed by maximizing the log likelihood objective l^* given above. The MLEs are obtained using SAS PROC MIXED (SAS Institute Inc., 1996). The EBLUP calculations as performed for this example are available in PROC MIXED, Release 6.12. SAS code for model fitting and visualization is available from the authors.

TABLE 1. Summary of fit for isotropic and geometrically anisotropic covariance models

model	mean params	covar params	total params	AIC	BIC	$-2l^*$
		Intercept-Only Mean Models				
EXP	1	3	4	-145.5	-149.8	283.0
POWA	1	5	6	-144.2	-150.6	276.3
EXPA2	1	5	6	-141.5	-148.0	271.0
EXPA	1	8	9	-144.0	-153.7	270.0
		Second-order Mean Models				
EXP	10	3	13	-140.6	-154.6	255.1
POWA	10	5	15	-139.3	-155.5	248.5
EXPA2	10	5	15	-139.1	-155.3	248.1
EXPA	10	8	18	-141.4	-160.8	246.8

Notes: Models fit are: EXP: exponential, Model (1.1); POWA: anisotropic power, Model (1.2); EXPA: anisotropic exponential, Model (1.3) with upper limits on power parameters p_k of 2.5; EXPA2: anisotropic exponential, Model (1.3) with fixed $p_k = 2 \quad \forall k$. Mean params, covar params, total params refer to number of parameters in the mean model, covariance model and total, respectively. Model evaluation criteria: AIC $= l^* - p$ and BIC $= l^* - 0.5p \log n$, where p is the total number of parameters and $n = 64$ is the sample size.

Table 1 provides a comparison of the models fit via Akaike's Information Criterion (AIC), Schwarz's Bayesian Information Criterion (BIC), and minus twice the value of the log likelihood. AIC and BIC are in larger-is-better form. The decomposition into large scale and small scale variation as specified in the spatial regression models is not unique. Estimated main effects, interactions and quadratic effects from second order models provide useful information on relative sizes of the effects of the design variables. However an intercept-only model is preferable for construction of the response surface. Cressie (1991, pp. 162-163) gives some discussion of this issue.

Of the intercept-only mean models the anisotropic covariance model EXPA2 (model (3) with all θ_k's fixed at 2) gives the best fit in terms of both AIC and BIC. The EXPA2 covariance model also performs well among the second-order mean models. The t-values for the second-order effects are displayed via a Pareto plot in Figure 1. This indicates that the assay is particularly sensitive to MgOAc and that combinations of MgOAc

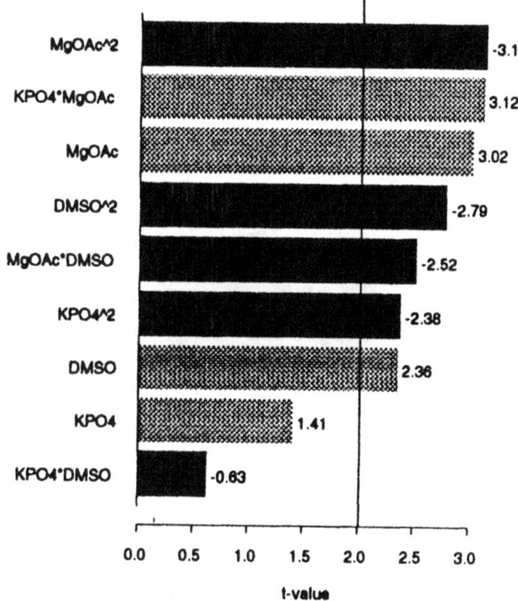

FIGURE 1. Pareto Plot of t-values associated with (large scale) design variable effects as estimated from a second-order mean model with EXPA2 (anisotropic exponential with fixed $p_k = 2, \;\; k = 1,2$) covariance structure. The vertical line is at the 5% critical value of a t_{54} distibution.

concentration with KPO4 and DMSO concentrations are of critical importance.

Due to the format of this proceedings paper response surfaces are not shown. The reader is referred to O'Connell and Wolfinger (1997) for visualization methods and displays. Instead, an isosurface and point cloud of grid points with the largest estimated RLU responses is shown in Figure 2. The isosurface is constructed at a log(RLU) value of 8.7, which is 85% of the optimum value of 10.2. The isosurface and point cloud reveal areas of the design space at which near optimum conditions can be obtained. This includes a region at higher DMSO which is not readily seen from the response surfaces.

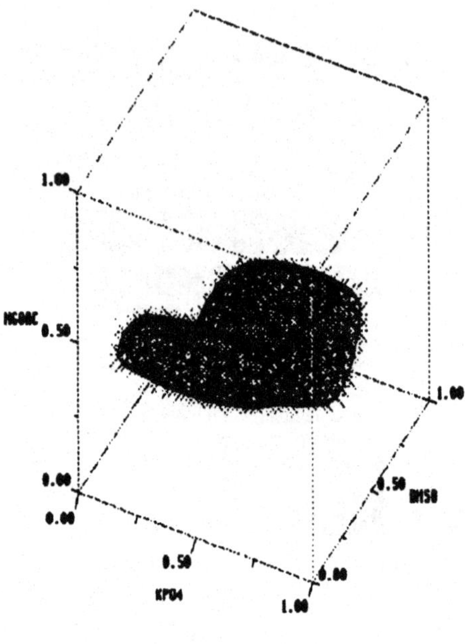

FIGURE 2. Point cloud and isosurface of the grid points with the largest predicted RLU response for the model with EXPA2 covariance and intercept-only mean. The isosurface is constructed at an RLU value of 8.7 which is 85\% of the optimum value of 10.2 and shown as a wire frame.

4 Design Issues

The DNA amplification assay data analyzed above was generated from a sequence of five response surface designs. These included fractional factorial and central composite designs. The spatial regression methods seem to work well in analyzing data from such combined experiments. Other designs that make no attempt to incorporate model based information, and are optimal only in terms of some distance-based criteria, also work well in combination with the spatial models described above (O'Connell et al. 1995). These designs may be chosen as a subset of a candidate point cloud of possible experimental conditions in $\Re^d$ that either 'covers' (U-optimality) or is broadly 'spread' (S-optimality) over the point cloud. These designs may be generated using SAS PROC OPTEX (SAS Institute Inc., 1995). Hardin and Sloane (1994) provide packing designs for which design points are chosen to minimize the reciprocal of the minimum distance between design points. Their software, Gosset, allows these designs to be generated over useful regions in the design space such as hypercubes and hyperspheres.

5 Discussion

Spatial regression models provide a useful characterization of response surfaces in the context of process optimization and we recommend their use in response surface method applications. In particular, an intercept-only mean model, used in combination with an anisotropic covariance structure, provides a flexible and informative response surface. Also, large scale effects of design variables may be quantified using a second-order mean model thus allowing assessment of their relative importance.

The flexible response surface resulting from the fit to the DNA amplification data enables insight into the relationship between the design variables and the measured response. For example, a process window is readily identified from the two-dimensional projections by shading regions above a given contour. Further, sensitivity or robustness information on the design variables is available from the response surfaces. The approach is also suited to analysis of multiple responses such as the mean and standard deviation in which case overlaying of contour slices may identify a process window which satisfies targets on both mean and variance.

The spatial regression models are very similar to thin plate spline smoothers. Connections between these models are discussed in O'Connell and Wolfinger (1997). Thin plate spline models may be fit using the software library FUNFITS (Nychka et al., 1996) which is available from StatLib.

While the application presented involves characterization of data from a sequence of experiments, use of a single design over an unknown design space, may provide a more efficient search strategy. Such designs may be chosen by optimizing a distance-based criterion to pack or cover the design space and analyzed by the same spatial regression models presented above.

6 References

[1] Box, G.E.P. and Draper, N.R. (1987). *Empirical Model Building and Response Surfaces.* Wiley: New York.

[2] Cressie, N.A.C. (1991). *Statistics for Spatial Data.* Wiley: New York.

[3] Hardin, R.H. and Sloane, N.J.A. (1994). *Operating manual for Gosset: A general purpose program for constructing experimental designs.*AT&T Bell Laboratories, Murray Hill, NJ.

[4] Harville, D.A. (1990). BLUP (Best Linear Unbiased Prediction), and Beyond. *Advances in Statistical Methods for Genetic Improvement of Livestock*, (D. Gianola and K. Hammond, eds.). pp. 239-276. Springer-Verlag: New York.

[5] Myers, R.H. and Montgomery, D.C. (1995). *Response Surface Methodology* Wiley: New York.

[6] Nychka, D., Bailey, B., Ellner, S., Haaland, P. and O'Connell, M. (1996). FUNFITS Data Analysis and Statistical Tools for Estimating Functions. Institute of Statistics Mimeo Series. North Carolina State University, Raleigh, NC.

[7] O'Connell, M., P. Haaland, S. Hardy and D. Nychka (1995). Nonparametric Regression, Kriging and Process Optimization. in *Statistical Modeling, Lecture Notes in Statistics* Volume 104. (G.U.H. Seeber, B.J. Francis, R. Hatzinger and G. Steckel-Berger, eds.). Springer-Verlag: New York.

[8] O'Connell, M. and Wolfinger, R. (1997). Spatial Regression, Response Surfaces and Process Optimization. *J. Comp. and Graph. Stat.* in press.

[9] Sacks, J., Welch, W.J., Mitchell, T.J. and Wynn, H.P. (1989). Design and Analysis of Computer Experiments. *Statistical Science* 4, 409-435.

[10] SAS Institute Inc. (1995). *SAS QC Software: Usage and Reference, Version 6, First Edition, Volume 1.* Cary NC: SAS Institute, Inc.

[11] SAS Institute Inc. (1996). *SAS/STAT Software: Changes and Enhancements through Release 6.11* SAS Institute Inc., Cary, NC.

[12] Walker, G.T., M.S. Fraiser, J.L. Schram, M.C. Little, J.G. Nadeau, D.P. Malinowski (1992). Strand Displacement Amplification - an Isothermal, *in vitro* DNA Amplification Technique. *Nucleic Acids Research* **20**, 1691-6.

[13] Wolfinger, R.D., Tobias, R.D., and Sall, J. (1994). Computing Gaussian Likelihoods and their Derivatives for General Linear Mixed Models. *SIAM Journal on Scientific Computing* **15**(6), 1294-1310.

[14] Zimmerman, D.L. and Harville, D.A. (1991). A Random Field Approach to the Analysis of Field-Plot Experiments and Other Spatial Experiments. *Biometrics* **47**, 223-239.

Robust Semivariogram Estimation in the Presence of Influential Spatial Data Values

Richard F. Gunst and Molly I. Hartfield*
Southern Methodist University
United States

1 Introduction

Semivariogram modeling is central to the prediction of point values and areal averages of geostatistical random fields. Additionally, estimates of semivariogram model parameters themselves are of intrinsic interest because of the information they provide about spatial dependence across a region. The fitting of semivariogram models is in turn critically dependent on the shape of sample semivariogram plots. Basu et al. (1995) document that the presence of influential spatial data values can seriously distort sample semivariogram plots and can affect both the choice of semivariogram models and the estimation of model parameters. Moreover, they found that the application of some of the more popular robust methods to data files containing influential data does not always satisfactorily accommodate these influential observations. In this paper, we discuss several robust estimators of semivariogram values that aid in the identification and accommodation of influential spatial data values and that can be used with very large data sets where it is sometimes prohibitive to interactively investigate the presence of influential observations.

2 Effects of Influential Observations

We begin with the usual definition of semivariogram values, under assumptions of isotropy and second-order stationarity (see, for example, Cressie,

*Address for correspondence: Department of Statistical Science, Southern Methodist University, P.O. Box 750332, Dallas, TX 75275-0332, U.S.A.

1991). Let $\gamma(d) = var\{z(s_i) - z(s_j)\}/2$, where $z(s)$ denotes a spatial variate measured at location s and $d = \|s_i - s_j\|$ is the separation distance between the spatial locations. Semivariogram values quantify the spatial covariance structure of the spatial random variables at prescribed distances d and are used to fit models of spatial dependence.

The classical (sample) method-of-moments estimator (Matheron, 1962) is

$$\hat{\gamma}(d) = \sum_{N(d)} \{z(s_i) - z(s_j)\}^2 / 2N_d, \tag{1}$$

where $N(d)$ denotes the set of all pairs of locations binned together at (nominal) separation distance d and N_d is the number of such pairs of locations. Cressie and Hawkins (1980) introduced a robust estimator of semivariogram values that is less susceptible to influential data values than the sample estimator (1):

$$\hat{\gamma}_{CH}(d) = \frac{\left\{\sum_{N(d)} |z(s_i) - z(s_j)|^{1/2} / N_d\right\}^4}{2(0.457 + 0.494/N_d)}. \tag{2}$$

The research discussed in this paper was motivated by many spatial data analyses in which it was observed that a small proportion of data values had a disproportionate affect on both of these semivariogram estimators.

Figure 1 shows estimated directional semivariogram values calculated using the robust estimator (2) for soil nitrate concentrations. See Gunst and Hartfield (1996) for more details about the data and the calculations. The semivariogram values represented by the solid lines were calculated using all the available nitrate values while those indicated by the dashed lines were calculated from a reduced data set in which the 8 largest nitrate values were removed. Notice that the spatial variability as indicated by the solid lines is not isotropic and that there is no apparent sill, while the spatial variability as indicated by the dashed lines appears to be isotropic white noise with a common sill. This implies that the apparent anisotropy and lack of a sill are entirely attributable to the 8 largest nitrate values. We do not recommend blindly eliminating data; however, this example shows what a striking effect a small portion of the data can have on a semivariogram plot.

Anisotropy and lack of a sill are only two of the disturbing features that can be induced in semivariogram plots by influential data values. Figures 2 and 3 are plots of both sample and robust semivariogram estimators for two data sets that were analyzed in Basu et al. (1995). Figure 2 is a semivariogram plot for November 1990 European temperature anomalies (temperature differences from an average temperature over a stated time period). There is an apparent linear trend in the plot, several sharp spikes, and no sill. These effects can be traced to influential data values, notably a very large anomaly for Copenhagen.

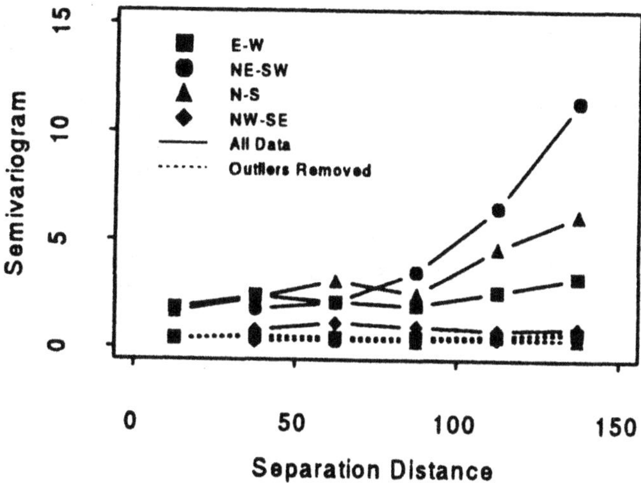

FIGURE 1. Directional semivariogram estimates for soil nitrate concentrations at 36 to 48 inches. Estimates calculated using the robust estimator.

Figure 3 is a semivariogram plot for soil nitrate concentrations from the same field as those in the first plot but from a different depth. This picture includes a mound shape in the center of the plot, termed an *excitation crest* in Basu et al. (1995), which is disturbing because it suggests that the spatial dependence between nitrate concentrations initially decreases with distance between locations but then unexpectedly increases with distance between locations. As in the previous examples, the excitation crest is largely due to the presence and location of an influential concentration. Excitation crests have also been found in a number of other data sets, including semivariogram plots of temperature anomalies for station locations in latitude bands around the globe.

Gunst and Hartfield (1996) derive influence functions for the classical and robust semivariogram estimators (1) and (2). Figure 4 shows theoretical semivariograms calculated from the influence functions. A spatial random field was assumed, the parameters of which were estimated from the nitrate data used in Figure 3. The horizontal line at 40 represents the theoretical value of the sample or robust semivariogram estimator if the random field were a white-noise process and there were no influential data values. The other lines in the plot represent sample and robust semivariogram estimates assuming the presence of one aberrant data value of the same size and location as that found in the actual data. The excitation crests in each of these theoretical semivariograms are evident, as is the lesser effect of the influential data value on the robust semivariogram values than on the sample semivariogram values.

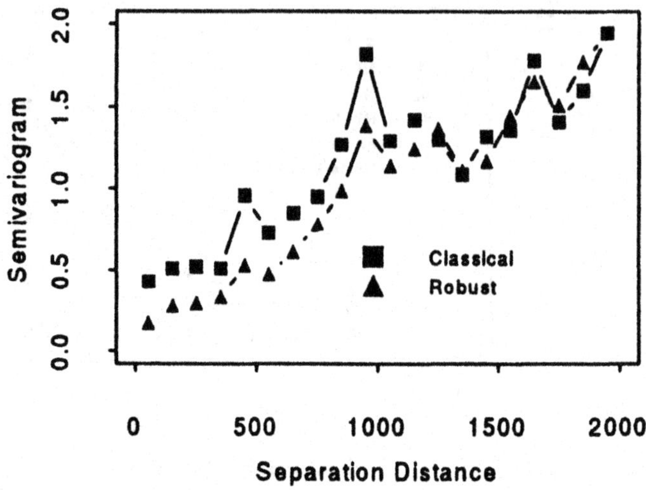

FIGURE 2. Semivariogram estimates for November 1990 European temperature anomalies.

3 Alternative Robust Estimators

Prior to discussing possible alternative robust estimators, it is important to recognize difficulties that arise as a result of the necessary data reuse in the estimation of semivariogram values. The fact that each observation is used many times in semivariogram estimation can exacerbate the effects of unusual data values on semivariogram estimates. For example, in a given bin, it is possible that the percentage of differences which include an influential data value will greatly exceed the percentage of influential data values in the data set. A particular bin may contain a large percentage of differences which include influential data, while many fewer or none of the differences in neighboring bins contain such influential points, leading to spikes in the semivariogram plot. Depending on the proportions of pairs in a bin that involve influential data, the excitation crests discussed previously also can be a result of data reuse. Robust estimators which accommodate such difficulties are needed. Many robust estimators operate on differences in bins with many influential data in the same way as they operate on differences in bins with few or no influential data values, thereby tending to overestimate spatial variability in some bins and underestimate it in others. Both (1) and (2) are such estimators.

The examples and issues discussed above provide motivation for the evaluation of alternative robust estimators. The following alternatives are typical of those evaluated in this study and include those found to be most effective.

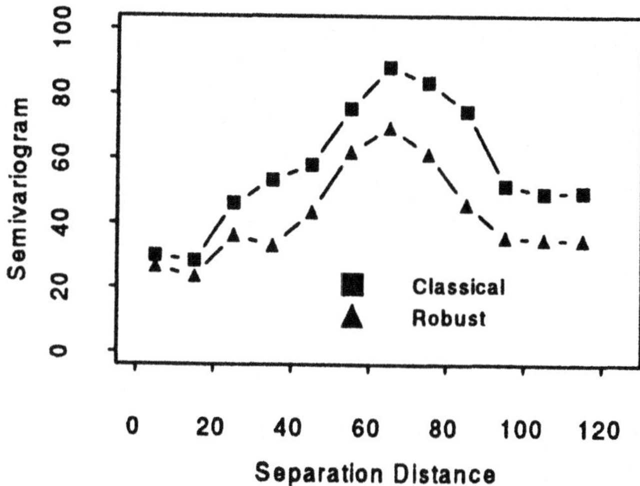

FIGURE 3. Semivariogram estimates for soil nitrate concentrations at 0 to 6 inches.

3.1 Trimming Fixed Percentages

Two trimming estimators were considered: trimming a fixed percentage of raw data values in the data set or trimming a fixed percentage of differences in each bin, and then applying the sample semivariogram estimator (1) to the remaining raw data or differences, respectively. However, because of data reuse issues raised above, such trimming estimators tend to be problematic. In the discussion below, we include, for comparison purposes only, one trimming estimator that trims 5% of the largest raw data values.

3.2 Robust M-Estimator for Location

An alternative to trimming is a robust M-estimator of location. Similar to the approach taken by Cressie and Hawkins (1980), the M-estimates used in our work are calculated separately for each bin. Let N_d denote the number of pairs of locations binned a nominal separation distance d apart. Let M_d denote the median of the square-root differences in the bin and S_d the corresponding median absolute deviation: $M_d = med\{|z(s_i) - z(s_j)|^{1/2}\}$, $S_d = med\{||z(s_i) - z(s_j)|^{1/2} - M_d|\}/0.6745$.

A one-step robust M-estimator of location was calculated as:

$$\hat{\gamma}_M(d) = \frac{\left\{M_d + S_d \frac{\sum \psi(y_{ij})}{\sum \dot{\psi}(y_{ij})}\right\}^4}{2(0.457 + 0.494/N_d)},$$

where $y_{ij} = [\{|z(s_i) - z(s_j)|\}^{1/2} - M_d]/S_d$, and $\dot{\psi}$ is the derivative of Tukey's

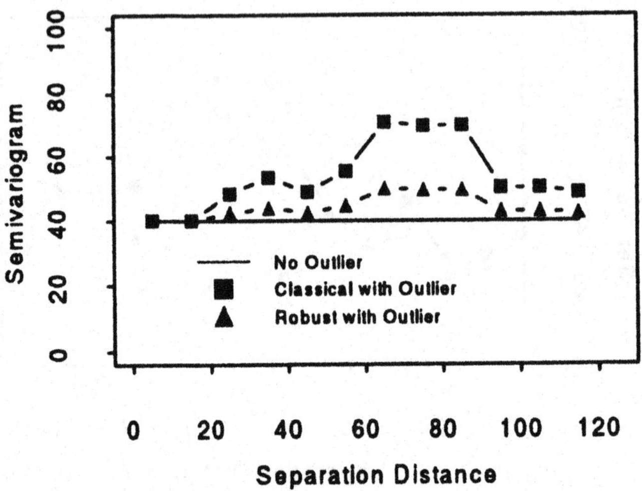

FIGURE 4. Theoretical semivariogram values for soil nitrate concentration at 0 to 6 inches, calculated using influence functions.

biweight ψ (Hampel et al. 1986, Staudte and Sheather 1990):

$$\psi(t) = \begin{cases} t(4^2 - t^2)^2 & |t| \geq 4 \\ 0 & |t| > 4 \end{cases}$$

3.3 *Preliminary Test Estimators*

Two of the robust estimators considered are based on preliminary tests to determine whether any raw data values in the data set or any differences in a given bin are highly influential. For the raw data values, the preliminary test is a robust version of a t-test. Raw data values were judged to be highly influential and were deleted if $|t_i| > 3$, where

$$t_i = \frac{z(s_i) - M}{S}, \tag{3}$$

$M = median\{z(s_i)\}$, and $S = median\{|z(s_i) - M|\}/0.6745$. Differences in each bin were tested for their influence using (3) with obvious modifications. Following the preliminary test on raw data or on differences, remaining data values or differences are used with the sample semivariogram estimator (1) to calculate semivariogram values in the usual way.

4 Simulation Results and Data Analysis

To assess the relative merits of the semivariogram estimators, a wide variety of simulations and analyses of actual data were conducted. The simulations

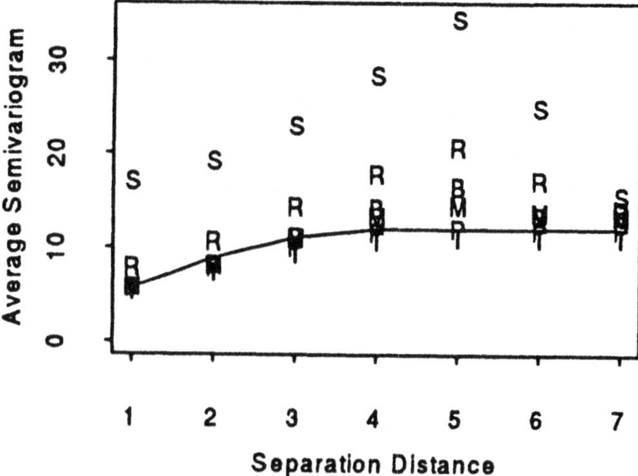

FIGURE 5. Average semivariogram estimates versus lag. 200 simulated realizations, each with outlying data value of 25.

consisted of generating random field data, with spatial correlations induced by specifying semivariogram models. Influential data were then added with stipulated probabilities so that the random field was a known mixture of a specified random field process and influential data values. Consistent results were obtained over a wide range of models, model parameters, sample sizes and mixture proportions on both transects and two-dimensional grids.

Figures 5-7 show the results from a simulation of 200 realizations from an ordinary kriging model $z(s) = \mu + e(s)$ with mean $\mu = 0$ and spatially correlated errors $e(s)$ generated by a spherical semivariogram model

$$\gamma(d) = \begin{cases} \theta_1 + \theta_2\{1.5(d/\theta_3) - 0.5(d/\theta_3)^3\} & d \leq 4 \\ \theta_1 + \theta_2 & d > 4 \end{cases}$$

with nugget $\theta_1 = 2$, sill $\theta_1 + \theta_2 = 12$, and range $\theta_3 = 4$. Each realization consisted of data from a 10x10 grid. At the center of the grid, an influential observation of magnitude $\delta_m = 25$ was inserted in place of the randomly generated data value. The calculated semivariogram values averaged over the 200 realizations are shown in Figure 5 and are indicated by the following symbols: sample (S), Cressie-Hawkins robust (R), M-Estimator (M), sample estimate following 5% trimming of raw data values (T), sample estimate following a preliminary test on the raw data values (P), and sample estimate following a preliminary test on the binned differences (B). The solid curve is the theoretical semivariogram. The variability among the 200 realizations at each lag are shown in Figure 6. Figure 7 shows the results from a simulation identical to that described above, except no aberrant observation was added.

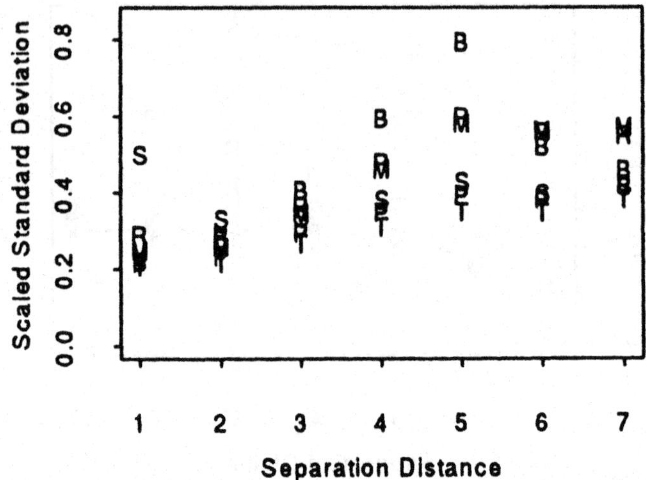

FIGURE 6. Variance of semivariogram estimates versus lag. 200 simulated realizations, each with outlying data value of 25.

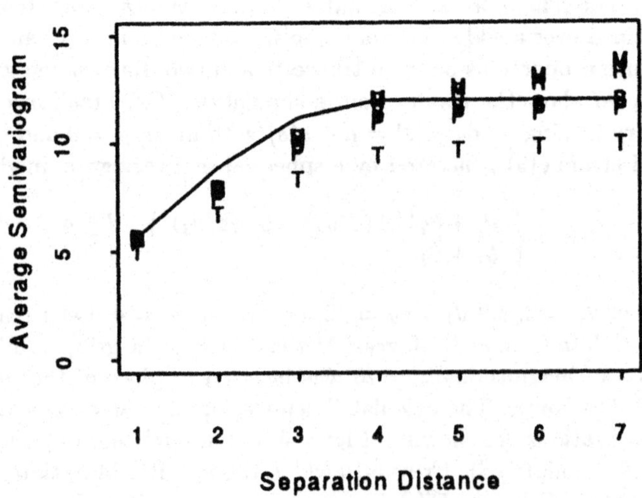

FIGURE 7. Average semivariogram estimates versus lag. 200 simulated realizations, with no outliers.

The results displayed in Figures 5-7 are typical of the simulation results. The sample semivariogram estimator S was the most sensitive to aberrant data, while the trimmed estimator T consistently underestimated the true value of the semivariogram, and was particularly biased when no aberrant data were present. The Cressie-Hawkins robust estimator R was less sensitive to aberrant data values than the sample semivariogram, but tended to be more affected than the M-estimator and preliminary test estimators P and B. The M-estimator and the preliminary-test estimators were much closer over a wide range of models to the theoretical semivariogram than other estimators. Each provided excellent protection against serious bias due to influential observations. Each also was typically among those with the smallest variation. In addition, each provided informative diagnostics for influential observations: the weights $\psi(t)/t$ for the M-estimator and the t values for the preliminary-test estimators. Of the three, the preliminary test estimator P was most often among the estimators with least bias and smallest variation.

These semivariogram estimators also were applied to the data sets discussed in Section 1. Only the results for the European temperature deviations are shown here. The trimmed estimator T will not be discussed because of its poor performance in the simulations. Figure 8 compares semivariogram estimates for the European temperature anomalies. As in the simulations, the M-estimator performs similarly to the Cressie-Hawkins robust estimator. The preliminary test estimator B tracks the sample semivariogram estimator S and is identical to it for many bins. The preliminary test estimator P identifies ($t = 5.9$) and removes Copenhagen, as well as 6 other influential data values that have t values ranging from 3.1 to 4.0. Copenhagen's t value certainly would cause one to investigate it further. The 6 other temperature stations are all clustered nearby one another and may represent a regional temperature difference. The most striking feature of this plot is that only the preliminary test estimator P reaches a sill.

5 Conclusion

The preliminary test estimator P was most effective overall in identifying and accommodating highly influential spatial data values. The M-estimator and the preliminary test estimator B also were generally effective, but occasionally, as in Figure 8, they did not satisfactorily accommodate one or more influential data values. Perhaps the most important conclusions from this work are that robust estimators are preferable to the classical estimator and that estimators such as the preliminary test estimators and the M-estimator are well-suited to large data sets because they efficiently identify highly influential data.

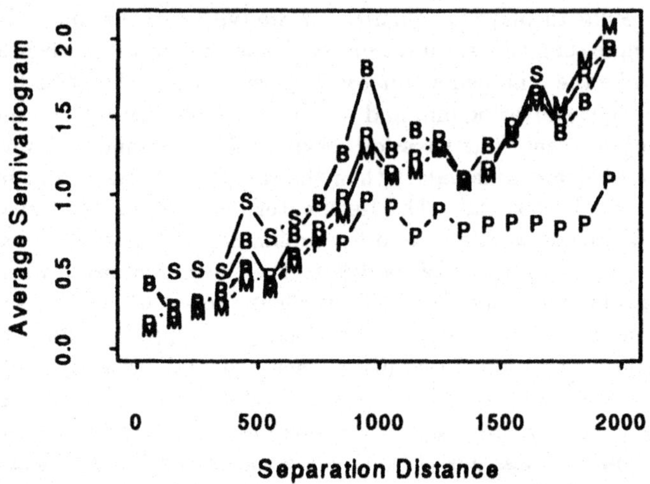

FIGURE 8. Semivariogram estimates for November 1990 European temperature anomalies.

6 References

[1] Basu, S., Gunst, R.F., Guertal, E.A., and Hartfield, M.I. (1995) The effects of influential observations on sample semivariograms. Technical Report SMU/DS/TR 270, Department of Statistical Science, Southern Methodist University, Dallas, TX. Submitted for publication.

[2] Cressie, N. (1991) *Statistics for Spatial Data.* New York: John Wiley and Sons, Inc.

[3] Cressie, N. and Hawkins, D.M. (1980) Robust estimation of the variogram: I. *Mathematical Geology,* 12, 115-125.

[4] Gunst, R.F. and Hartfield, M.I. (1996) Robust semivariogram estimation in the presence of influential data values. Technical Report SMU/DS/TR 286, Department of Statistical Science, Southern Methodist University, Dallas, TX.

[5] Hampel, F.R., Ronchetti, E.M., Rousseeuw, P.J., and Stahel, W.A. (1986) *Robust Statistics.* New York: John Wiley and Sons, Inc.

[6] Matheron, G. (1962) *Traite de Geostatistique Appliquee, Tome I. Memoires du Bureau de Recherches Geologiques et Minieres, No. 14,* Paris: Editions Technip.

[7] Staudte, R.G. and Sheather, S.J. (1990) *Robust Estimation and Testing.*New York: John Wiley and Sons, Inc.

Elephant Seal Movements: Dive Types and Their Sequences *

David R. Brillinger
University of Califonria, Berkeley
United States

Brent S. Stewart
Hubbs-Sea World Research Institute, San Diego
and
University of California, Berkeley
United States

ABSTRACT This paper is concerned with the time-depth curves recorded for northern elephant seals that are migrating. The curves show a succession of dives of varuying depths, durations and types. A mixture model is employed to estimate the various curves present. An advantage of this procedure over the ones that have been employed, is that it is automatic. Further, a categorical-valued series is developed for the sequence of dives. It is examined for evidence of serial dependence for both dives of one type and amongst dives of different types.

Key words and phrases: Categorical-valued time series, dive patterns, elephant seals, foraging behavior, longitudinal data, mixture model.

1 Introduction

Studies of the foraging behavior of a variety of marine vertebrates (e.g., seals, sea lions, penguins, sea birds, sea turtles) have been conducted in recent years using micro-processor controlled event recorders to document diving patterns. The data generated from these recorders are time series

---

*The work of DRB supported by the Office of Naval Research Grant N00014-94-1-0042 and the National Science Foundation Grant DMS-9625774. Elephant seal dive data were collected in previous studies with partial support of a contract to BSS from the Space and Missile Command, U.S. Department of the Air Force.

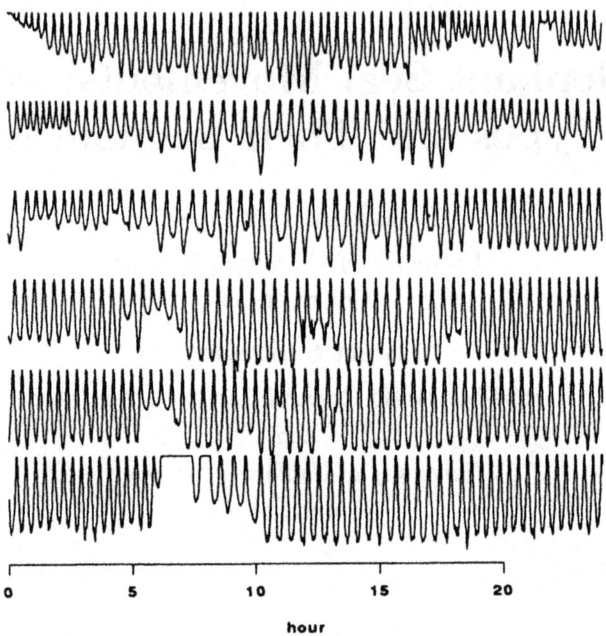

FIGURE 1. Six days diving for one seal. The curves from top to bottom represent the seal's depth as a function of hour for six successive days. Depth was measured every 30s.

of depth measurements made at regular intervals (5s to 60s) over days to months. These data are often displayed graphically as two-dimensional plots of depth versus time. Consequently the two-dimensional shapes of dives, which lack spatial components (i.e.latitude and longitude), have been described and used to separate them into discrete categories of similar shapes, sometimes according to maximum depths reached and durations of dives. For the most part, the dives have been classified into a small number of shape categories by visual inspection (eg. [1], [10], [17], [20], [9], [22], [26], [27]).

The function (eg., swimming, hunting, exploring) of various dives have been inferred from their two dimensional shapes. Further, the inferred functions have been incorporated into discussions of animal physiology and energetics. Thus, the ability to classify dives according to shapes based on time and depth interactions has had utility in developing hypotheses about foraging strategies and efficiency in free-ranging aquatic predators.

Using time-depth series collected for foraging northern elephant seals (*Mirounga angustirostris*). We earlier developed, [8], a computer-assisted method to automatically and quickly describe dive shape with an algorithm to fit joined straight line segments employing the BIC criterion to estimate the number of segments. Here we develop an alternate approach.

As in other species studied, the individual dives of northern elephant seals seem to consist of a restricted number of types, possibly indicating different activity and function (see Figures 1 and 2). In addition to basic questions and inferences of function of particularly shaped dives, it is important to assess the patterns of sequences and mix of the various types to explore hypotheses concerning navigation and orientation, sleep, predator avoidance and the influences of geographic location on foraging strategy.

The data studied in the paper may be seen as curves or segments stretched one after the other. Experiments in which the basic data are curves have been studied in various ways, see [2], [3] and the references therein. One technique is principal components, see [15], [24]. Others are presented in [18] and [28]. In particular, longitudinal data analysis and modelling are discussed in the books [13], [19] and [14]. The data of this paper differ from the usual longitudinal data in that there is but one subject (here a seal) and the curves run one after the other. These data are of the character of the response in an evoked response experiment, see [4].

The observations of discrete categories of two-dimensional shapes of types leads to consideration of a mixture model involving particular functional forms occurring with particular probabilities. That having been said, the model considered in this paper is: the data are curves with $Y_j(u)$ referring to the seal's depth u time units after the start of the j-th dive. The variate $Y_j(u)$ has conditional expected value $a_k(u)$, with probability P_k, $k = 1, ...$ indexing the types.

After this model has been fit, one can go on to estimate the type, $\hat{k}$, of a particular dive, and thence obtain a sequence of dive types, $\hat{k}_1$, $\hat{k}_2$, ... This categorical-valued time series can be examined for short and long range temporal dependence for example.

Some details of the data are provided in Section 2. Section 3 indicates the fitting procedure employed to obtain estimates of the various dive types. The results of this fitting are presented in Section 4. The next section refers to the sequence of dive types and presents the results of analyses looking for serial dependence. Section 6 provides discussion, particularly of the problem of identifiability, and summary.

There are three other papers concerned with the data for this particular seal, [5], [6], [7].

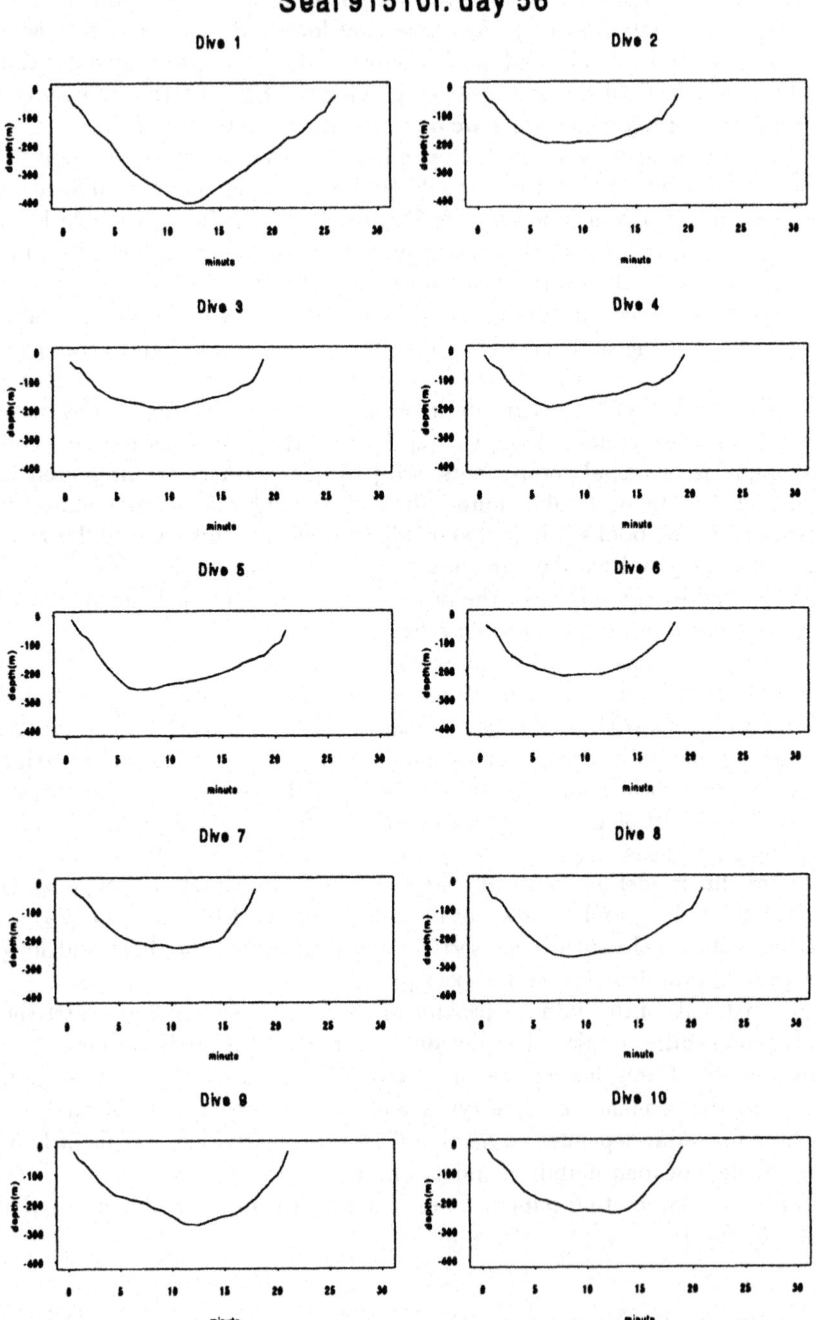

FIGURE 2. The first 10 dives of Day 56.

2 The Data

The data set analyzed in the present work is for a female northern elephant seal (*Mirounga angustirostris*). This species breeds on offshore islands and at a few mainland sites along the coasts of California and Baja California ([30], [32]). Adults are ashore briefly in winter to breed and again in spring (females) or summer (males) to molt but spend the remainder of the year, 8-10 months, at sea foraging. They make two solitary, long-distance migrations each year between islands in southern California and offshore foraging locations in the mid-North Pacific, Gulf of Alaska and along the Aleutian Islands covering 18,000 to 20,000 km (surface movements alone) during the double migrations ([29]). The seals dive continually during these migrations; dives average 20 to 40 minutes long (longest = 2 hours) and 350 to 650 meters deep (deepest = 1560 meters) and are only separated briefly for 2-3 minutes while the seals are at the sea-surface breathing (e.g., [12], [29]). The data studied here are depth measurements made at 30 second intervals throughout the periods at sea (See Figures 1 and 2.) They are recorded by a microprocessor-controlled event-recorder which is harmlessly glued to a seal's hair (e.g.[29], [1], [31]). The instruments are attached at the end of the breeding or molt season and then recovered when the seals next return to shore several months later.

The dives' start times could be read from the time-depth record quite clearly allowing individual dives to be selected, as graphed in Figure 2 for example.

3 Fitting a Mixture of Dive Types

Let $Y_j(u)$ denote the depth at lag u in j-th dive. Suppose there are possible types $a_k(u)$, $k = 1, 2, \ldots$, with k to be selected randomly. One may consider the model:

$$Prob\{K = k\} = P_k \tag{1}$$

$$Y_j(u) = a_K(u) + \epsilon_j(u) \tag{2}$$

for $k = 1, 2, \ldots$ and $j = 1, 2, \ldots$ with $\epsilon(.)$ representing noise. Equations (1), (2) provide a mixture model.

EM algorithms are often a convenient way to obtain maximum likelihood estimates in such models, see [11], [23], [25]. In the case that the noise values, $\epsilon(.)$, are assumed independent with variance $\sigma^2(u)$ at lag u and Gaussian, an EM algorithm for estimating the $a_k(u)$ is implemented by the recursion

$$\hat{a}_k(u) = \sum_j Y_j(u)\, \hat{p}_{jk} \;/\; \sum_j \hat{p}_{jk} \tag{3}$$

$$\hat{\sigma}(u)^2 = \sum_j \sum_k (Y_j(u) - \hat{a}_k(u))^2 \hat{p}_{jk} \,/\, J \tag{4}$$

$$\hat{P}_k = \sum_j \hat{p}_{jk} \,/\, J \tag{5}$$

$$\hat{p}_{jk} = \hat{P}_k \, exp\{-\sum_u (Y_j(u) - \hat{a}_k(u))^2 \,/\, 2\hat{\sigma}(u)^2\} \,/\, C_j \tag{6}$$

where C_j is determined so that $\sum_k \hat{p}_{jk} = 1$. The development of such algorithms is indicated in [25].

4 The Estimated Types

Days 56 to 115 of the migration were studied, accounting for 3629 dives. In employing the EM algorithm, starting values are needed. Here the number of dive types for the analysis was taken to be 9 and the initial curves $\hat{a}_k(.)$ were taken to be the averages of the curves in the 9 cells determined by cross-classifying by duration and depth using the 33 and 67 percentiles as the cut points of those variables. The initial values of the $\hat{P}_k$ were 1/9. Apparent convergence occurred quickly.

Figure 3 provides the results of fitting the mixture model. It is interesting that the curves obtained are all unimodal. The first and second curves each occur about 23 percent of the time. The curves may be distinguished from each other by characteristics such as: duration, maximum depth, symmetry, flatness at maximum depth.

In future work other means of generating initial curves will be investigated. Also the number of dive types might be estimated employing the BIC criterion.

5 Categorical-valued Time Series of Types

Suppose that dive types are well-defined and the actual types are given by k_j, $j = 1, 2, \ldots$. This is a categorical-valued time series. One can ask for example: Is the series k_j white noise and if it is not, how might it be described?

In practice one needs to estimate the k_j. A simple procedure is to determine for which shape, $\hat{a}_k(u)$, the j-th dive, $Y_j(u)$, has the smallest mean-squared error. The corresponding categorical-valued series was constructed. For example the estimated types for the 10 dives of Figure 2 are respectively 8, 5, 5, 5, 5, 5, 5, 5, 5, 5 . This constancy may be seen at the start of the second curve in Figure 1.

Seal 91510: estimated dive shapes

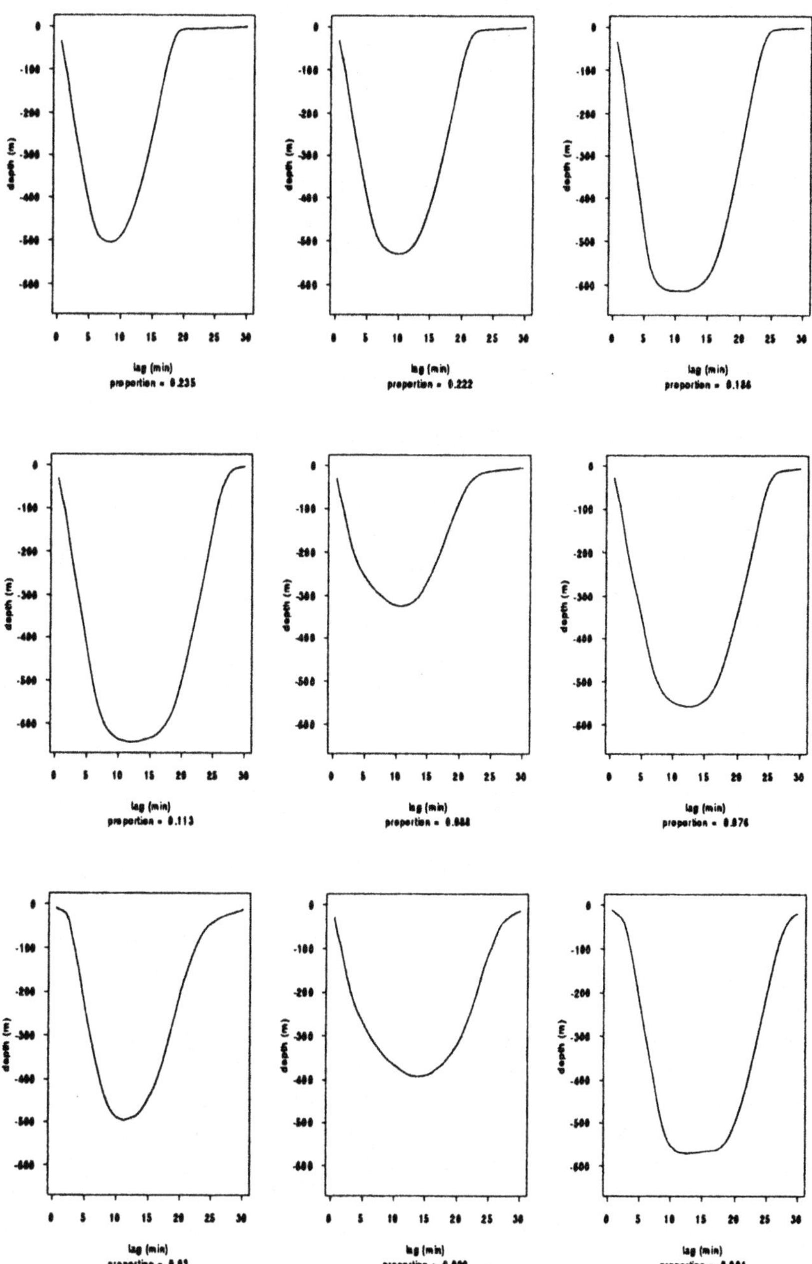

FIGURE 3. The 9 estimated types of dives. They are in the estimated order of prevalence.

For the next analysis, a representation alternate to $\hat{k}_j$ above is useful. Suppose a vector-valued series is constructed whose components are 0-1 valued series corresponding to a particular dive types. In particular set

$$X_{kj} = 1 \quad if\ \hat{k}_j = k$$

and = 0 otherwise for $k = 1, \ldots, 9$ and $j = 1, 2, \ldots$. Then $\mathbf{X}_j$, $j = 1, 2, 3, \ldots$ is a time series indexed by dive number j.

This vector-valued series may now be examined for serial dependence and for interdependence of components. Figure 4 provides estimates of the power spectra, of the 9 components, obtained by averaging 14 periodograms each based on successive stretches of length 256. The vertical arrows indicate the width of approximate 95 percent marginal confidence intervals. When it appears, the high peak on the left corresponds to the seal's regularly diving about 70 times per day. Interestingly series 7 could be white noise, corresponding to that dive type appearing randomly throughout the migration. The other series appear to be far from white noise. For example, the elevated values on the left could correspond to that particular dive type appearing in clusters.

It is of interest to look into the interdependence of the dive types. Because the data have multinomial character, i.e. some dive type has to occur at each time j, the series cannot be completely independent. To alleviate this dependence only the first 8 components of the series will be retained for the next analysis.

A classic test of multivariate dependence is based on comparing the determinant of a sample covariance matrix to the product of the sample variances. A time series extension of this is given in [33]. The likelihood ratio test statistic considered here, of the hypothesis of independence in the stationary time series case, is given by

$$-2n \sum_k \left(\sum_{i=1}^{8} log\ \hat{f}_{ii}(\lambda_k) - log\ \hat{\mathbf{f}}(\lambda_k) \right) \tag{7}$$

where λ_k are the frequencies at which the spectral density matrix, $\mathbf{f}(\lambda)$, is estimated and n is the number of periodograms averaged in forming the spectrum estimates.

These computations were carried out with $n = 28$. Figure 5 provides the individual terms of (7) and the approximate upper 99 per cent marginal null level in the case of independence as a horizontal line. (This last is based on a chi-squared distribution with 8(8-1) = 56 degrees of freedom.) The statistic is above the null level steadily suggesting the presence of some substantial interdependence of the components. The high peak again corresponds to the animal's regularly diving about 70 times per day. The different dive types appear to be particularly tied together at that frequency.

The sampling variability of the $\hat{k}$ has also been ignored in these calculations.

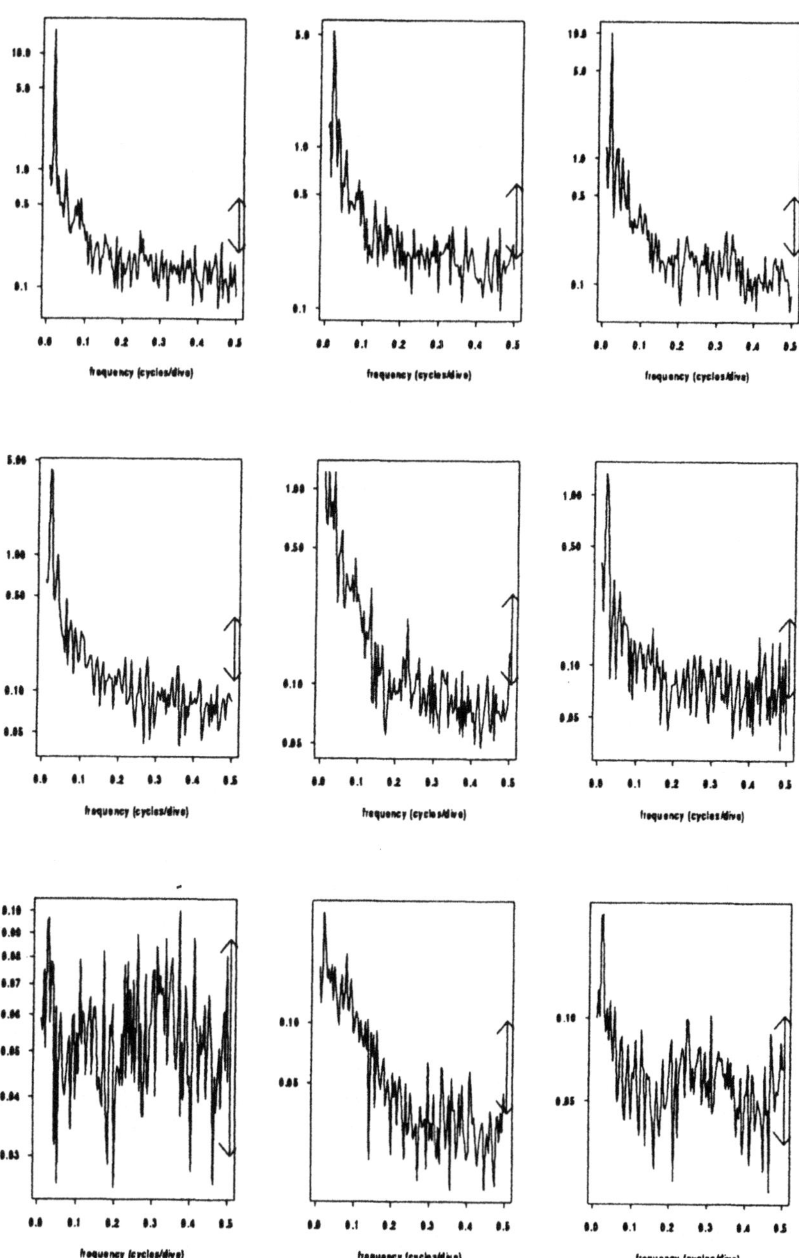

FIGURE 4. Power spectral estimates, for the 0-1 series corresponding to the estimated dive types, obtained by averaging periodograms. The arrows give approximate 95 % confidence bounds.

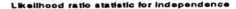

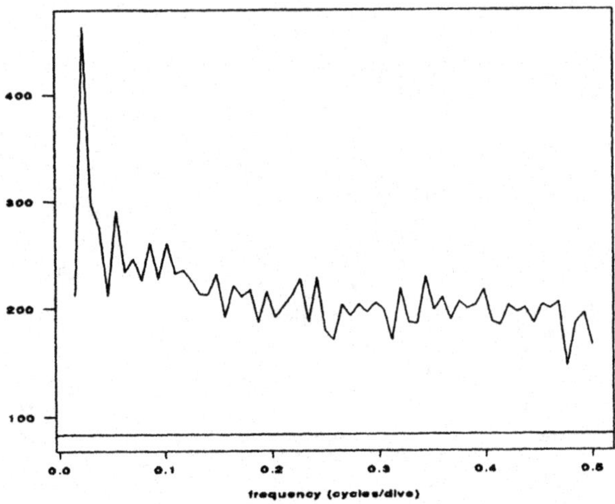

FIGURE 5. Independence test statistic and approximate upper 99 percent null line.

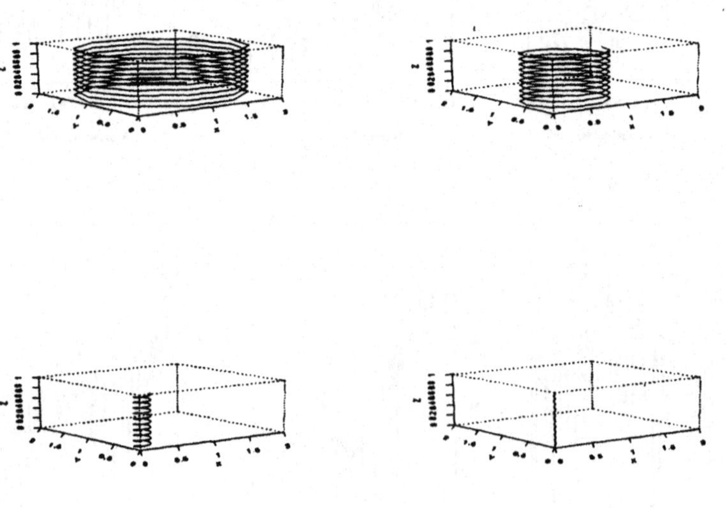

FIGURE 6. Four descents with the same time-depth curve.

Papers concerned with categorical-valued longitudinal data include [21] and [16].

6 Discussion and Summary

There are important difficulties of interpretation of the results of the analyses. Figure 6 shows 4 different possible descent paths of an animal. Each have same time-depth curve, $Y(u) = -\beta u$, yet the paths are very different. The actual descent could in fact be a combination of these. The situation is that conclusions must be drawn carefully. More sophisticated measuring equipment capable of fine scale spatial positioning is required to address this difficulty.

The noise in (2) was taken as statistically independent at the various lags, however it could be modelled as dependent. Then a covariance matrix would be estimated at expression (4) of the EM algorithm.

These preliminary studies indicate that temporal dependence needs to be incorporated into studies of migration to determine whether regularities in behavior imply broad spatio-temporal regularity in the distribution of prey resources or whether oceanographic conditions, season and geographic location influence foraging behavior. Further, additional studies of the spatial components of individual dives are needed to determine how they may confuse or support interpretations of dive form and function based on the necessarily limited shapes that can be categorized from two-dimensional descriptions derived from depth vs. time data series.

7 References

[1] Bengtson, J.L. and Stewart, B.S. (1992). Diving and haulout patterns of crabeater seals in the Weddell Sea, Antartica during March 1986. *Polar Biology* **12,** 635-644.

[2] Brillinger, D. R. (1973). The analysis of time series collected in an experimental design. Pp. 241-256 in *Multivariate Analysis III* Ed. P. R. Krishniah. Academic, New York.

[3] Brillinger, D. R. (1980). Analysis of variance and problems under time series models. Pp. 237-278 in *Handbook of Statistics Vol. 1* Ed. P. R. Krishnaiah. North-Holland, Amsterdam.

[4] Brillinger, D. R. (1981). Some aspects of the analysis of evoked response experiments. Pp. 155-168 in *Statistics and Related Topics* Eds. M. Csorgo, D. A. Dawson, J. N. K. Rao and A. K. Md. E. Saleh. North-Holland, Amsterdam.

[5] Brillinger, D. R. (1997). A particle migrating randomly on a sphere. *J. Theor. Prob.* in press.

[6] Brillinger, D. R. and Stewart, B. S. (1997a). Elephant seal movements: some frequency based studies. *Rev. Bras. Prob. Stat.* in press.

[7] Brillinger, D. R. and Stewart, B. S. (1997b). Elephant seal movements: modelling migration. Submitted.

[8] Brillinger, D. R., Stewart, B. S. and Wong, A. (1995). Computer-assisted, automatic evaluation of two-dimensional profiles (time vs. depth) of time series data for diving marine mammals. Poster at Eleventh Biennial Conference on the Biology of Marine Mammals, Orlando.

[9] Chappell, M. A., Shoemaker, V. H., Janes, D. N., Bucher, T. L., and Maloney, S. K. (1993). Diving behavior during foraging in breeding Adelie penguins. *Ecology* **74**, 1204-1215.

[10] Crocker, D. E. (1994). Swim speed and dive function in a female northern elephant seal. Pp. 328-339 in *Elephant Seals: Population Ecology, Behavior, and Physiology.* Eds. B. J. Le Boeuf and R. M. Laws. University of California Press, Berkeley.

[11] Dempster, A. P., Laird, N. and Rubin, D. H. (1977). Maximum likelihood from incomplete data via the EM algorithm. *J. Roy. Statist. Soc. B* **39**, 1-38.

[12] DeLong, R.L. and Stewart, B.S. (1991). Diving patterns of northern elephant seal bulls. *Marine Mammal Science* **7**, 369-384.

[13] Diggle, P. J., Liang, K-Y. and Zeger, S. L. (1993). *The Analysis of Longitudinal Data.* Oxford Univ. Press, Oxford.

[14] Fahrmeir, L. and Tutz, G. (1994). *Multivariate Statistical Modelling Based on Generalized Linear Models.* Springer-Verlag, New York.

[15] Freeman, W. J. (1980). Measurement of cortical evoked potentials by decomposition of their wave forms. *J. Cybernetics Infor. Sci.* **2**, 44-56.

[16] Gilula, Z. and Haberman, S. J. (1994). Conditional log-linear models for analyzing categorical panel data. *J. Amer. Statist. Assoc.* **89**, 645-656.

[17] Hindell, M. A., Slip, D. J. and Burton, H. R. (1991). The diving behaviour of adult male and female southern elephant seals, *Mirounga leonina* (Pinnipedia; Phocidae). *Australian J. Zoology* **39**, 595-619.

[18] Jones, M. C. and Rice, J. A. (1992). Displaying the important features of a large collection of similar curves. *American Statistician* **46**, 140-145.

[19] Jones, R. H. (1993). *Longitudinal Data With Serial Correlation.* Chapman and Hall, London.

[20] Jonker, F. C. and Bester, M. N. (1994). The diving behaviour of adult southern elephant seal, *Mirounga leonina*, cows from Marion Island. *South African J. Antarctic Research* **24**, 75-93.

[21] Kalbfleisch, J. D. and Lawless, J. F. (1985). The analysis of panel data under a Markov assumption. *J. Amer. Statist. Assoc.* **80**, 863-871.

[22] Kooyman, G. L., Cherel, Y., Le Maho, Y., Croxall, J. P., Thorson, P. H., Ridoux, V. and Kooyman, C. A. (1992). Diving behavior and energetics during foraging cycles in King Penguins. *Ecological Monographs* **62**, 143-163.

[23] Laird, N. (1978). Nonparametric maximum likelihood estimation of a mixing distribution. *J. Amer. Statist. Assoc.* **73**, 805-811.

[24] Rao, C. R. (1958). Some statistical models for comparison of growth curves. *Biometrics* **14**, 1-17.

[25] Redner, R. A. and Walker, H. F. (1984). Mixture densities, maximum likelihood and the EM algorithm. *SIAM Review* **26**, 195-202.

[26] Schreer, J. F. and Testa, J. W. (1995). Statistical classification of diving behavior. *Marine Mammal Science* **11**, 93-96.

[27] Schreer, J. F. and Testa, J. W. (1996). Classification of Wedell seal diving behavior. *Marine Mammal Science* **12**, 227-250.

[28] Segal, M. R. (1994). Representative curves for longitudinal data via regression trees. *J. Comp. Graph. Stat.* **3**, 214-233.

[29] Stewart, B. S. and DeLong, R. L. (1995). Double migrations of the northern elephant seal. *J. Mammalogy* **76**, 196-205.

[30] Stewart, B. S. and Huber, H. R. (1993). *Morounga angustirostris. Mammalian Species* **449**, 1-10.

[31] Stewart, B. S., Leatherwood, S., Yochem, P. K. and Heide-Jorgensen,M. P. (1989). Satellite telemetry of locations and dive durations of a free-ranging harbor seal (*Phoca vitulina richardsi*) in the Southern California Bight. *Marine Mammal Science* **5**, 361-375.

[32] Stewart, B. S., Yochem, P. K., Huber, H. R., DeLong, R. L., Jameson, R. J., Sydeman, W., Allen, S. G. and Le Boeuf, B. J. (1994). History and present Status of the northern elephant seal population. Pp. 29-48 in *Elephant Seals: Population Ecology, Behavior and Physiology* Eds. B. J. Le Boeuf and R. M. Laws. University of California Press, Los Angeles.

[33] Wahba, G. (1968). On the distribution of some statistics useful in the analysis of jointly stationary time series. *Ann. Math. Statist.* **39**, 1849-1862.

Models for Continuous Stationary Space-time Processes

Richard H. Jones*
University of Colorado
Health Sciences Center
United States

Yiming Zhang
Research Data Inc.
United States

ABSTRACT Existing statistical methodologies for space-time processes are usually developed for equally spaced data. This paper develops methods for unequally spaced data. Stochastic partial differential equations driven by white noise are used to describe continuous spatial temporal processes. The models considered here are based on the heat or diffusion equation in one or two spatial dimensions and time. Spectral density functions of these processes can be calculated and inverted using Fourier transforms to obtain the corresponding covariance functions. In two spatial dimensions, numerical integrations are necessary for calculating the correlation functions for these models since Hankel transforms without closed form solutions are involved. FORTRAN subroutines are available to calculate these Hankel transforms and covariance functions. Maximum likelihood estimation can be used assuming Gaussian errors. For small data sets (up to several hundred observations) exact maximum likelihood estimates can be calculated directly. For larger data sets, nearest neighbor methods can be used to reduce the computation and obtain approximate likelihoods. Two examples are discussed.

1 Introduction

Whittle (1954) introduced spatial covariance structures based on stochastic partial differential equations. This work was extended by Vecchia (1985, 1988, 1992), Jones (1989) and Jones and Vecchia (1993). Most work on space-time processes has been for lattice data (see for example, Cliff et al.,

*Department of Preventive Medicine and Biometrics, School of Medicine, Box B-119, University of Colorado Health Sciences Center, Denver, CO 80262. (rhj@times.uchsc.edu).

1975; Cliff and Ord, 1975; Martin and Oeppen, 1975; Pfeifer and Deutsch, 1980; Aroian, 1985; and Cressie, 1993). Linear stochastic difference equations are used to describe the discrete space-time processes. However, there are many occurrences of data that are unequally spaced. It is therefore necessary to develop appropriate methods for fitting continuous spatial temporal models to unequally spaced data.

The linear regression models that we consider for unequally spaced spatial temporal data in this study are of the form

$$z(x,y,t)=\sum_{j=0}^{p-1}\beta_j f_j(x,y,t)+\xi(x,y,t),$$

where $f_j(x,y,t)$ are the independent variables that are functions of space and time, and $\beta_0,..,\beta_{p-1}$ are unknown linear regression parameters. $\xi(x,y,t)$ is a homogeneous Gaussian spatial temporal random field with mean zero. If there are n observations in space and time, there is a covariance matrix for these n observations, $\sigma^2\mathbf{V}$, which is assumed to be a function of the spatial distance and time lag. In geostatistics, predictions based on this formulation are known as "universal kriging". The observations may include measurement error and can be expressed as

$$z_i = z(x_i,y_i,t_i)+\eta_i,$$

where η_i's are independent Gaussian observational errors with zero mean and constant variance. Observational error is often referred to as the "nugget effect" in geostatistics. Here, we describe the continuous space-time processes $\xi(x,y,t)$ via linear stochastic partial differential equations with constant coefficients. Some of them are commonly seen in mathematical physics.

Maximum likelihood estimation is used assuming Gaussian errors. The likelihood function of n observations can be written as

$$\ell = n\ln(2\pi\sigma^2)+\ln|\mathbf{V}|+\frac{1}{\sigma^2}(\mathbf{z}-\mathbf{X}\boldsymbol{\beta})'\mathbf{V}^{-1}(\mathbf{z}-\mathbf{X}\boldsymbol{\beta}), \tag{1}$$

where $\mathbf{z}$ is an $n\times 1$ vector of all the observations and $\mathbf{X}$ is an $n\times p$ matrix of the independent variables at the corresponding point in space and time. Nonlinear optimization routines such as subroutine POWELL from *Numerical Recipes* (Press, et al. ,1992, p. 411) combined with a subroutine that calculates the likelihood function for given values of the unknown variance and covariance parameters can be used to obtain maximum likelihood estimates when there are not too many observations (say, less than 1,000 total in space and time). Since the likelihood function is characterized by the covariance structure, and smoothness of the spatial temporal prediction is also directly related to the covariance structure, we focus on the theoretical development of valid spatial temporal covariance structures. Emphasis is given to one and two dimensional space. However, it is not difficult to extend this study to space dimensions higher than two.

2 Separable Space-Time Models

The elementary temporal process is the continuous AR(1) process represented by the following stochastic differential equation (Jones, 1993, p. 57)

$$\left(\frac{d}{dt} + \alpha\right) \xi(t) = \epsilon(t),$$

with spectral density function

$$s(\omega) = \frac{\sigma^2}{\omega^2 + \alpha^2},$$

where $\epsilon(t)$ is continuous time zero mean Gaussian 'white noise' with variance σ^2 per unit time, and ω is angular frequency.

The elementary continuous spatial process for a fixed time point, given no interaction occurs between space and time, is governed by the following Laplace equation (Whittle, 1954)

$$\left(\frac{\partial^2}{\partial x^2} + \frac{\partial^2}{\partial y^2} - \phi^2\right) \xi(x, y) = \epsilon(x, y),$$

with spectral density function

$$s(k_1, k_2) = \frac{\sigma^2}{(k_1^2 + k_2^2 + \phi^2)^2},$$

where $\epsilon(x, y)$ is a zero mean Gaussian 'white noise' field with variance σ^2 per unit area, and k_1 and k_2 are wave numbers in the two spatial directions. The associated correlation functions for the above two independent processes in time and space are $e^{-\alpha t}$ and $\phi r K_1(\phi r)$, respectively, where t is the absolute value of the time difference, r is the separation distance between observation points and K_1 is the modified Bessel function of the second kind, order one.

When a space-time process is generated by these two separate elementary processes in space and time, the resulting correlation function is

$$\Gamma(r, t) = e^{-\alpha t} \phi r K_1(\phi r),$$

which corresponds to a spectral density function

$$s(k_1, k_2, \omega) = \frac{\sigma^2}{(k_1^2 + k_2^2 + \phi^2)^2 (\omega^2 + \alpha^2)}.$$

The process with such a spectral density function may be formally written as

$$\left(\frac{\partial^2}{\partial x^2} + \frac{\partial^2}{\partial y^2} - \phi^2\right) \left(\frac{\partial}{\partial t} + \alpha\right) \xi(x, y, t) = \epsilon(x, y, t).$$

Although it is difficult to visualize a physical mechanism which would lead to such a relation, the generated correlation structure is theoretically valid. This correlation function has been used by Rodriguez-Iturbe and Mejia (1974) in designing rainfall networks.

3 Non-Separable Models

For non-separable space-time processes, the simplest stochastic partial differential equation for a one dimensional process is the parabolic type,

$$\left(\frac{\partial^2}{\partial x^2} - c\frac{\partial}{\partial t} - \phi^2\right)\xi(x,t) = \epsilon(x,t),$$

which is the heat conduction equation or diffusion equation. Heine (1955) derived the correlation function with respect to both space and time for this one dimensional space process when time is involved,

$$\rho(r,t) = \frac{1}{2}\left[e^{-r\phi}\text{Erfc}\left(\frac{2t\phi - cr}{2\sqrt{ct}}\right) + e^{r\phi}\text{Erfc}\left(\frac{2t\phi + cr}{2\sqrt{ct}}\right)\right], \tag{2}$$

where $\text{Erfc}(z) = \frac{2}{\sqrt{\pi}}\int_z^\infty e^{-v^2}dv$ when z$\geq$ 0, and $\text{Erfc}(-z) = 2 - \text{Erfc}(z)$ when z$<$ 0. The correlation between the same space point at different times is

$$\rho(0,t) = \text{Erfc}\left(\phi\sqrt{\frac{t}{c}}\right),$$

while the correlation between two space points at the same time is

$$\rho(r,0) = e^{-\phi r}.$$

For computing purposes, it is convenient to define dimensionless scaled distance and time variables. Using dimensionless variables allows functions to be set to zero for large values of the arguments. In the functions considered here, values of the scaled distance and time variables greater than 20 are considered to be large. Let

$$r^* = \phi r \qquad \text{and} \qquad t^* = \frac{\phi^2}{c}t. \tag{3}$$

Now (2) becomes

$$\rho(r,t) = \frac{1}{2}\left[e^{-r^*}\text{Erfc}\left(t^* - \frac{r^*}{2\sqrt{t^*}}\right) + e^{r^*}\text{Erfc}\left(t^* + \frac{r^*}{2\sqrt{t^*}}\right)\right],$$

and

$$\rho(0,t) = \text{Erfc}\left(\sqrt{t^*}\right) \qquad \text{and} \qquad \rho(r,0) = e^{-r^*}.$$

Whittle (1962) commented that if the space dimension is greater than one, the diffusion mechanism does not smooth ϵ sufficiently and causes the spectrum to die away too slowly at infinity, which leads to an infinite variance. This is a consequence of the extreme irregularity of the input function ϵ, which itself has infinite variance. Whittle (1963) discussed the process defined by the following elliptic type equation

$$\left(\sum_{1}^{n} \frac{\partial^2}{\partial x_i^2} - \phi^2\right)^p \xi(\mathbf{x}) = \epsilon(\mathbf{x}). \tag{4}$$

Handcock and Wallis (1994) have used (4) to model meteorological fields. They refer to the associated covariance functions as the Matérn class.

Now, it is natural to consider the following process

$$\left[\left(\sum_{1}^{n} \frac{\partial^2}{\partial x_i^2} - \phi^2\right)^p - c\frac{\partial}{\partial t}\right] \xi(x_1, ..., x_n, t) = \epsilon(x_1, ..., x_n, t).$$

The corresponding spectral density function in wave-number and frequency space is

$$s(k, \omega) = \frac{\sigma^2}{(k^2 + \phi^2)^{2p} + c^2\omega^2},$$

and the associated covariance function is (Zhang, 1995)

$$\begin{aligned} \Gamma(r,t) &= \frac{r^{-n/2+1}\sigma^2}{(2\pi)^{n/2+1}} \int_0^\infty \int_{-\infty}^\infty \frac{k^{n/2}e^{i\omega t}}{(k^2+\phi^2)^{2p} + c^2\omega^2} J_{n/2-1}(kr)d\omega dk \\ &= \frac{r^{-n/2+1}\sigma^2}{2(2\pi)^{n/2}c} \int_0^\infty \frac{k^{n/2}e^{-(k^2+\phi^2)^p t/c}}{(k^2+\phi^2)^p} J_{n/2-1}(kr)dk. \end{aligned} \tag{5}$$

When $t = 0$,

$$\begin{aligned} \Gamma(r,0) &= \frac{r^{-n/2+1}\sigma^2}{2(2\pi)^{n/2}c} \int_0^\infty \frac{k^{n/2}}{(k^2+\phi^2)^p} J_{n/2-1}(kr)dk \\ &= \frac{\sigma^2 (r/\phi)^{p-n/2} K_{p-n/2}(\phi r)}{2^p c\Gamma(p)(2\pi)^{n/2}}, \end{aligned}$$

which diverges at $r = 0$ if $p \leq n/2$.

When $n = 2$, the covariance function (5) becomes a zero order Hankel transform, and can be calculated using a numerical integration method developed by Anderson (1979, 1982). A zero order Hankel transform of the kernel $f(k)$ is

$$H(r) = \int_0^\infty f(k) J_0(kr)dk,$$

where J_0 is the Bessel function of the first kind of order 0.

When $n = 2$ and $p = 2$, the correlation function (5) is

$$\rho(r,t) = 2\phi^2 \int_0^\infty \frac{ke^{-\frac{(k^2+\phi^2)^2 t}{c}}}{(k^2+\phi^2)^2} J_0(kr)dk,$$

which can be written using the scaled distance and time (3), with a change of the variable of integration so that it, too, is dimensionless, $g = k/\phi$, as

$$\rho(r,t) = 2\int_0^\infty \frac{ge^{-(g^2+1)^2 t^*}}{(g^2+1)^2} J_0(gr^*)dg.$$

The marginal correlation functions are

$$\rho(r,0) = r^* K_1(r^*),$$

which is the familiar elementary correlation function for a two dimensional spatial process, and

$$\rho(0,t) = e^{-t^*} - \sqrt{\pi t^*}\mathrm{Erfc}(\sqrt{t^*}).$$

The parameter p in the above space-time process can also take non-integer values as long as it is greater than $n/2$. When p approaches ∞ the covariance function approaches the Gaussian covariance function which is usually considered to be "too continuous" to be physically realizable (Matérn, 1986). Note that p must be greater than 1 in order for the two dimensional spatial process to have a finite variance.

4 Parameter Estimation

For space time processes, a direct method can be used to calculate the likelihood function if the total number of observations is not too large (several hundred?). Jones and Vecchia (1993) give specific computational details for with fitting spatial regression models along with homogeneous spatial ARMA errors. Parameter estimation for space-time processes is not very different from that for space processes. In fact, having a time ordering is an advantage. If we substitute weighted least squares estimates for the vector $\boldsymbol{\beta}$ and σ^2,

$$\begin{aligned}
\hat{\boldsymbol{\beta}} &= (\mathbf{X}'\mathbf{V}^{-1}\mathbf{X})^{-1}\mathbf{X}'\mathbf{V}^{-1}\mathbf{z}, \\
\hat{\sigma}^2 &= \frac{1}{n}(\mathbf{z} - \mathbf{X}\hat{\boldsymbol{\beta}})'\mathbf{V}^{-1}(\mathbf{z} - \mathbf{X}\hat{\boldsymbol{\beta}}),
\end{aligned}$$

into the -2 ln likelihood function (1), we get

$$\ell = n\ln(2\pi\hat{\sigma}^2) + \ln|\mathbf{V}| + n.$$

This depends only on the parameters in the covariance matrix $\mathbf{V}$. In this problem there are three parameters in the $\mathbf{V}$ matrix, ϕ, c, and a positive quantity added to the diagonal elements of the $\mathbf{V}$ matrix representing the observational error or nugget effect. The $\mathbf{V}$ matrix is actually a correlation matrix except for the inflated diagonal elements. The parameters are constrained to be positive in the nonlinear optimization by using log transformations. Initial guesses are supplied for parameters in $\mathbf{V}$, and the nonlinear optimization routine searches for the values that minimize ℓ. The normal equation method using Cholesky factorization described in Jones and Vecchia (1993) directly applies here. If the total number of observations is too large so that the $\mathbf{V}$ matrix cannot be handled directly, the nearest-neighbor methods described in that paper can be used.

The actual computational procedure for a moderate number of observations is to calculate and store the upper triangular part of the $\mathbf{V}$ matrix augmented by the $\mathbf{X}$ matrix and the vector of observations, $\mathbf{z}$,

$$[\ \mathbf{V} \quad \mathbf{X} \quad \mathbf{z}\ ].$$

The Cholesky factorization, or square root method (Graybill, 1976, page 231) factors $\mathbf{V}$ into the product of an upper triangular matrix premultiplied by its transposed, $\mathbf{V} = \mathbf{T}'\mathbf{T}$. It also modifies the augmented part of the matrix by premultiplying by $(\mathbf{T}')^{-1}$. Let $\mathbf{X}^* = (\mathbf{T}')^{-1}\mathbf{X}$ and $\mathbf{z}^* = (\mathbf{T}')^{-1}\mathbf{z}$. After factorization, the augmented matrix now is

$$[\ \mathbf{T} \quad \mathbf{X}^* \quad \mathbf{z}^*\ ].$$

This operation is carried out in place without requiring additional storage. The determinant term in the likelihood is the sum of squares of the diagonal elements of $\mathbf{T}$. The weighted total sum of squares, $\text{TSS} = \mathbf{z}'\mathbf{V}^{-1}\mathbf{z}$, is $(\mathbf{z}^*)'\mathbf{z}^*$. The weighted normal equations for regression are accumulated,

$$[\ (\mathbf{X}^*)'\mathbf{X}^* \quad (\mathbf{X}^*)'\mathbf{z}^*\ ].$$

This augmented matrix is reduced using the Cholesky factorization, and the sum of squares of the augmented column calculated to give the weighted regression sum of squares. The difference between the weighted total sum of squares and the weighted regression sum of squares is the weighted residual sum of squares, $n\hat{\sigma}^2$. This difference causes the loss of significant digits, so double precision calculations are necessary. Other methods that work directly with the $\mathbf{X}$ matrix rather than forming the normal equations, such as the Householder QR decomposition are more numerically stable (Kitagawa and Gersch, 1996, p. 18).

Before going to the nearest neighbor methods, it is necessary to understand the concept of the Cholesky factorization. Numbering the points in any order, the contribution to the likelihood is calculated from the first point. The second point is predicted from the first point, and, from the residual, the orthogonal contribution to the likelihood is calculated conditional on the first point. Then the third point is predicted using the first two points, etc. This is like a Kalman filter except there is no natural ordering so there is no Markov property, and all the previous points must be used in the predictions. The final likelihood will not depend on the numbering of the points. The nearest neighbor methods do not select the nearest neighbors from all the points, but select them from the previous points. In other words, if the points are numbered from 1 to n, and we are at point k, we select the nearest neighbors from the previous $k-1$ points. This is important to preserve the orthogonality when calculating an approximate likelihood.

For space-time processes, it is natural to order the points with respect to time noting that there may be many observations at a given time, so that the ordering at a given time is arbitrary. This allows, in large data sets, the possibility of setting a maximum time interval when searching backwards for nearest neighbors. This can result in a substantial saving of computer time. There is also the problem of measuring distance in a space time process when space and time have different units. Since the correlation functions we are considering here are monotonically decreasing to zero, we use correlation as a measure of distance. High correlation is small distance, and low correlation is high distance. This requires that the parameters of the process be known approximately since correlation depends on these parameters (ϕ and c). Since nearest neighbors are calculate up front at the beginning of the program and saved, good guesses are necessary for ϕ and c, so when the nonlinear optimization program converges, it is usually necessary to rerun the program with improved estimates of ϕ and c.

5 Applications

The model for two spatial dimensions plus time has been applied to modelling plutonium contamination around Rocky Flats plant in Colorado. Observations are yearly, equally spaced in time, but unequally spaced in space. There are a total of 550 observations over a time period of 23 years. The data exhibit very strong time correlation as well as spatial correlation, but there is no evidence of a time trend.

The second application involves one spatial dimension plus time. The data were obtained courtesy of NASA/JPL Science Working Team, NSCT project at the National Center for Atmospheric Research. Data from a satellite measures the east west component of surface winds over the Pacific Ocean at the equator. The data set consists of 15,555 observations that are unequally spaced in both space and time. Nearest neighbor methods are used to predict the space time field on a grid so that contour maps can be drawn. The results are a significant improvement over interpolation methods since an artifact of a pattern caused by the sampling scheme is reduced.

Acknowledgement

The first author is partially supported by the Geophysical Statistics Project, National Center for Atmospheric Research, Boulder, Colorado, sponsored by the National Science Foundation under grant DMS93-12686. (http://www.cgd.ucar.edu/stats).

6 REFERENCES

[1] Anderson, W. L. (1979), Numerical integration of related Hankel transforms of orders 0 and 1 by adaptive digital filtering, *Geophysics*, 44, 1287–1305.

[2] Anderson, W. L. (1979), Algorithm 588, Collected Algorithms from ACM. *ACM Trans. Math. Software*, **8**, 369–370, and 444–468.

[3] Aroian, L. A. (1985), *Time Series Analysis: Theory and Practice*, Vol. 6, O. D. Anderson, J. K. Ord, and E. A. Robinson, eds. North-Holland, Amsterdam, The Netherlands.

[4] Cliff, A. D., Haggett, P., Ord, J. K., Bassett, K. A. and Davies, R. B. (1975), *Elements of Spatial Structure: A Quantitative Approach*, New York: Cambridge University Press.

[5] Cliff, A. D. and Ord, J. K. (1975), Model building and the analysis of spatial pattern in human geography, *Journal of the Royal Statistical Society, Ser. B,*, **37**, 297–384.

[6] Cressie, N. (1993), *Statistics for Spatial Data*, New York: John Wiley.

[7] Graybill, F. A. (1976), *Theory and Application of the Linear Model*, Duxbury Press, North Scituate, Massachusetts.

[8] Handcock, M. S. and Wallis, J. R. (1994), An approach to statistical spatial-temporal modeling of meteorological fields (with discussion), *Journal of the American Statistical Association*, **89**, 368–378.

[9] Heine, V. (1955), Models for two-dimensional stationary stochastic processes, *Biometrika*, **42**, 170–178.

[10] Jones, R. H. (1989), Fitting a stochastic partial differential equation to aquifer data. *Stochastic Hydrology and Hydraulics*, **3**, 85–96.

[11] Jones, R. H. (1993), *Longitudinal Data with Serial Correlation: A State-space Approach*, London: Chapman & Hall.

[12] Jones, R. H. and Vecchia, A. V. (1993), Fitting continuous ARMA models to unequally spaced spatial data, *Journal of the American Statistical Association*, **88**, 947–954.

[13] Kitagawa, G. and Gersch, W. (1996), *Smoothness Priors Analysis of Time Series*, New York: Springer-Verlag.

[14] Martin, R. L. and Oeppen, J. E. (1975), The identification of regional forecasting models using space-time correlation functions, *Transactions of the Institute of British Geographers*, **66**, 95–118.

[15] Matérn, B. (1986), *Spatial Variation*(2nd ed.), Lecture Notes in Statistics, 36, Berlin: Springer-Verlag.

[16] Pfeifer, P. E. and Deutsch, S. J. (1980), A three-stage iterative procedure for space-time modeling, *Technometrics*, **22**, 35–47.

[17] Press, W. H., Teukolsky, S. A., Vetterling, W. T. and Flannery, B. P. (1992), *Numerical Recipes in FORTRAN: the Art of Scientific computing*, Second Edition, Cambridge University Press.

[18] Rodriguez-Iturbe, I. and Mejia, J. M. (1974), The design of rainfall networks in time and space, *Water Resources Research*, **10**, 713–728.

[19] Vecchia, A. V. (1985), A general class of models for stationary two-dimensional random processes, *Biometrika*, **72**, 281–291.

[20] Vecchia, A. V. (1988), Estimation and model identification for continuous spatial processes, *Journal of the Royal Statistical Society*, Ser. B, **50**, 297–312.

[21] Vecchia, A. V. (1992), A new method of prediction for spatial regression models with correlated errors, *Journal of the Royal Statistical Society*, Ser. B, **54**, 813–830.

[22] Whittle, P. (1954), On stationary processes in the plane, *Biometrika*, **41**, 434–449.

[23] Whittle, P. (1962), Topographic correlation, power-law covariance functions, and diffusion, *Biometrika*, **49**, 305–314.

[24] Whittle, P. (1963), Stochastic processes in several dimensions, *Bulletin of the International Statistical Institute*, **40**, 974–985.

[25] Zhang, Y. (1995), Autoregressive models for continuous space-time processes. Ph.D. dissertation, Department of Preventive Medicine and Biometrics, University of Colorado Health Sciences Center, Denver.

A Comparison of Two Spatio-temporal Semivariograms with Use in Agriculture

Annette Kjær Ersbøll*

The Royal Veterinary and Agricultural University
Denmark

ABSTRACT In a space-time process with a limited number of measurements separable spatio-temporal semivariograms can be difficult to estimate due to high correlations between the parameters. A parsimonious semivariogram model with common nugget effect and common partial sill for the combined spatio-temporal process is proposed. Parameter estimations in the separable and the parsimonious models are compared for an agricultural example.

Keywords and phrases: Separable semivariogram, parsimonious semivariogram, agriculture, long-term field trial.

1 Introduction

Ersbøll [4] and Kristensen and Ersbøll [6] have previously suggested an approach to spatial experimental design of field trials. They illustrated that accounting for the spatial structure during the design of new field trials can have a large influence on the residual variance in the new trial.

If the suggested approach is to be of any value in planning new experiments, the spatial correlation structure should be expected to be rather similar across years for the same field. It is therefore of interest to estimate the spatio-temporal semivariogram for long-term field trials in order to validate the temporal and spatial correlation structure. Different problems

---

*Annette Kjær Ersbøll, Research Associate Professor, PhD, The Royal Veterinary and Agricultural University, Department of Mathematics and Physics, Thorvaldsensvej 40, DK-1871 Frederiksberg C, Denmark. Phone: +45 35 28 23 41, Fax: +45 35 28 23 50, Email: ae@dina.kvl.dk

are encountered during this procedure, first the definition of a valid semivariogram model and second estimation of the semivariogram parameters with only a limited number of measurements at our disposal. A parsimonious semivariogram model is proposed with a common nugget effect and common partial sill for the combined spatio-temporal process.

Agricultural experiments often contain spatial correlation due to the experimental layout with a number of neighbouring plots. Furthermore, repeated sampling in field trials seems to become more common. Therefore, there seems to be a need for models which describe the combined process of variation in both space and time. However, traditional field trials are often characterized by a limited number of experimental units, which calls for parsimonious models. A spatio-temporal semivariogram might be used to estimate the variance-covariance matrix for a spatio-temporal analysis of variance where the spatial and temporal correlations are taken into account. Another utilization is estimation (or prediction) using spatio-temporal kriging.

2 Methods

Let $Z(\boldsymbol{x},t)$ be a random function and let $Z(\boldsymbol{x}_i,t_j)$ be the random variable, with position $\boldsymbol{x}_i$ at time t_j

$$Z(\boldsymbol{x},t) = \{Z(\boldsymbol{x}_i,t_j), \forall \boldsymbol{x}_i \in D, t_j \in T\}$$

where $D \subset R^d$ and T={1,2,... }.

Let the random function $Z(\boldsymbol{x},t)$ be given as

$$Z(\boldsymbol{x},t) = \mu(\boldsymbol{x},t) + \varepsilon(\boldsymbol{x},t)$$

where $\mu(\boldsymbol{x},t)$ is the mean and $\varepsilon(\boldsymbol{x},t)$ is a (zero mean) stochastic process.

The random function $Z(\boldsymbol{x},t)$ is assumed to be second order stationary.

Given the realization $z(\boldsymbol{x}_i,t_j)$, $i = 1,\ldots,n_x$ and $j = 1,\ldots,n_t$ where n_x is the number of experimental units (e.g. plots) and n_t is the number of repeated measurements, the empirical semivariogram can be estimated.

The spatio-temporal semivariogram is estimated including both correlations in space and time and combinations of these. An empirical semivariogram is estimated using the robust semivariogram estimator suggested by Cressie and Hawkins [2]

$$\hat{\gamma}(\boldsymbol{h},\tau) = \frac{\left(\frac{1}{N(\boldsymbol{h},\tau)}\sum_{i=1}^{N(\boldsymbol{h})}\sum_{j=1}^{N(\tau)}\sqrt{|\, z(\boldsymbol{x}_i+\boldsymbol{h},t_j+\tau) - z(\boldsymbol{x}_i,\tau_j)\,|}\right)^4}{2\left(0.457 + \frac{0.494}{N(\boldsymbol{h},\tau)}\right)}$$

where $N(\boldsymbol{h})$ and $N(t)$ are the number of pairs of observations separated by spatial distance $\boldsymbol{h}$ and temporal distance τ, respectively. The total number of pairs separated by spatial distance $\boldsymbol{h}$ and temporal distance τ equals $N(\boldsymbol{h}, \tau)$.

A model can be fitted to the empirical spatio-temporal semivariogram. A number of proposals have been given for spatio-temporal semivariogram models. Posa [7] has given a model which assumes a range of influence independent of the time. Rouhani and Hall [10] and Bilonick [1] suggested to introduce the time as an additional dimension and rely on a geometric or a zonal anisotropy. Another possibility is to use a separable semivariogram model [9, 2]. The separable model is a valid model which combines the spatial and temporal correlation under an hypothesis of second order stationarity.

With second order stationarity the separable spatio-temporal covariogram and semivariogram are defined as

$$C(\boldsymbol{h}, \tau) = C_h(\boldsymbol{h})C_\tau(\tau) \quad \text{and} \quad \gamma(\boldsymbol{h}, \tau) = C(\boldsymbol{0}, 0) - C(\boldsymbol{h}, \tau)$$

where $C_h(\boldsymbol{h})$ and $C_\tau(\tau)$ are the spatial and temporal covariogram, respectively.

The separable model can be written as

$$\gamma(\boldsymbol{h}, \tau) = C_h(\boldsymbol{0})\gamma_\tau(\tau) + C_\tau(0)\gamma_h(\boldsymbol{h}) - \gamma_h(\boldsymbol{h})\gamma_\tau(\tau) \tag{1}$$

where γ_h and γ_τ are the spatial and temporal semivariograms, respectively. The separable spatio-temporal semivariogram has a nugget effect and a partial sill for both space and time and also a range of influence for both space and time, giving a total of six parameters, as can be seen in

$$\gamma(h, \tau) = \begin{cases} 0 & (h, \tau) = (0, 0) \\ C_{h0}C_{\tau0} + C_hC_{\tau0} + (C_{h0}C_\tau + C_hC_\tau)\delta(\tau) & h = 0,\ \tau > 0 \\ C_{h0}C_{\tau0} + C_{h0}C_\tau + (C_hC_{\tau0} + C_hC_\tau)\delta(h) & h > 0,\ \tau = 0 \\ C_{h0}C_{\tau0} + C_hC_{\tau0} + C_{h0}C_\tau & \\ \quad + C_hC_\tau[\delta(h) + \delta(\tau) - \delta(h)\delta(\tau)] & h > 0, \tau > 0 \end{cases}$$

where $\delta(h)$ and $\delta(\tau)$ are valid semivariogram models (e.g. exponential or spherical) with no nugget effect and sill equals one for space and time, respectively. C_{h0} and $C_{\tau0}$ are the nugget effects for space and time and C_h and C_τ are partial sills for space and time, respectively. A discontinuity is seen in the semivariogram model when either the spatial distance or the temporal distance equals zero.

A proposal for a valid parsimonious semivariogram model is

$$\gamma(h, \tau) = \begin{cases} 0 & (h, \tau) = (0, 0) \\ C_0 + C[\delta(h) + \delta(\tau) - \delta(h)\delta(\tau)] & (h, \tau) \neq (0, 0) \end{cases} \tag{2}$$

where $\delta(h)$ and $\delta(\tau)$ are valid semivariogram models (e.g. exponential or spherical) with no nugget effect and sill equals one for space and time, respectively. Here C_0 and C are nugget effect and partial sill for the combined process.

With an exponential model for both space and time the model (2) is

$$\gamma(h,\tau) = \begin{cases} 0 & (h,\tau) = (0,0) \\ C_0 + C[1 - \exp(-\frac{h}{a} - \frac{\tau}{\alpha})] & (h,\tau) \neq (0,0) \end{cases}$$

where a and α are the ranges of influence in space and time, respectively. (For exponential models the practical range of influence is three times as large.)

This spatio-temporal semivariogram model has a limited number of model parameters to be estimated with common nugget effect and common partial sill. In comparison the separable model (1) has individual nugget effects and partial sills for space and time. These four parameters are highly correlated, which is also seen in the following example.

The parameters in the spatio-temporal semivariograms have been estimated using the weighted least squares method [2] by minimizing

$$\sum_{i=1}^{k}\sum_{j=1}^{l} N(h_i,\tau_j)\left\{\frac{\hat{\gamma}(h_i,\tau_j)}{\gamma(h_i,\tau_j)} - 1\right\}^2$$

where k and l are the lags in space and time and $\hat{\gamma}$ and γ are the empirical semivariogram and the semivariogram model, respectively.

3 Data

A Danish 14 year long-term field experiment (1973-86) with continuous spring barley is used as an example. During the 14 years of experimentation the experimental treatments were: reduced soil tillage and Italian ryegrass as catch crop. A strip-plot design with four blocks has been used with six levels of reduced soil tillage (combinations of stubble cultivating, ploughing, seed bed preparation and Italian ryegrass) and three levels of nitrogen fertilizer. The same experimental design and layout was used every year. The average yield for each of the 18 treatment combinations is seen in Figure 1. For further details cf. Rasmussen [8].

Treatment effects have been estimated for each year using a spatial estimation procedure [4]. The treatment effects are eliminated and only the residuals are used in the following spatio-temporal analyses.

4 Results

A histogram is given in Figure 2 for the residuals in the long-term field trial where treatment effects are eliminated.

The empirical spatio-temporal semivariogram is seen in Figure 3. A three years periodic effect is seen in the empirical semivariogram which could also be seen in Figure 1.

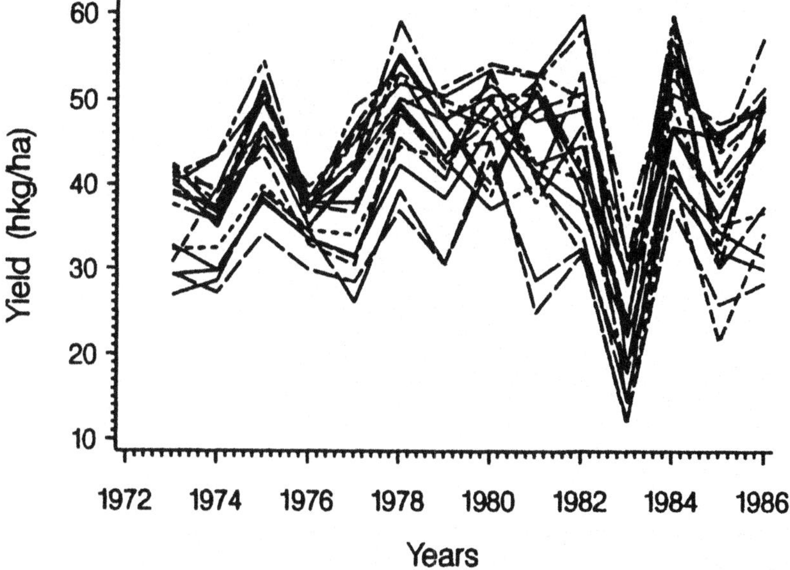

FIGURE 1. Average yield per year for each of the 18 treatment combinations.

In order to remove the periodicity the residuals have been standardized to zero mean and standard error one. The empirical spatio-temporal semivariogram for the standardized residuals is seen in Figure 4. A separable semivariogram model has been fitted to the empirical semivariogram for the standardized residuals with an exponential model for both space and time. The fitted model is seen in Figure 5. The estimated model parameters are given in Table 1 and the correlations between the model parameters are seen in Table 2. The adjusted R^2 is 0.94. Convergence of the model fit was very difficult to obtain. It is seen that the (asymptotic) standard errors for the nugget effects and partial sills are huge, which is also reflected in the large confidence intervals. Furthermore, Table 2 shows that the nugget effects and partial sills are highly correlated.

The parsimonious spatio-temporal semivariogram model has been fitted using an exponential model for both space and time. The fitted model is seen in Figure 6. The estimated model parameters are given in Table 3 and the correlations between the estimated semivariogram parameters are seen in Table 4. The adjusted R^2 is 0.96. The correlations are seen to be resonable for the parsimonious model.

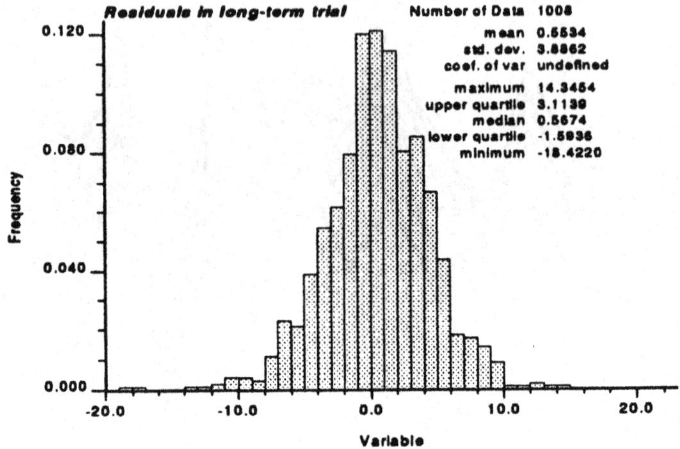

FIGURE 2. Histogram for the residuals in the long-term field trial, where treatment effects have been estimated and eliminated.

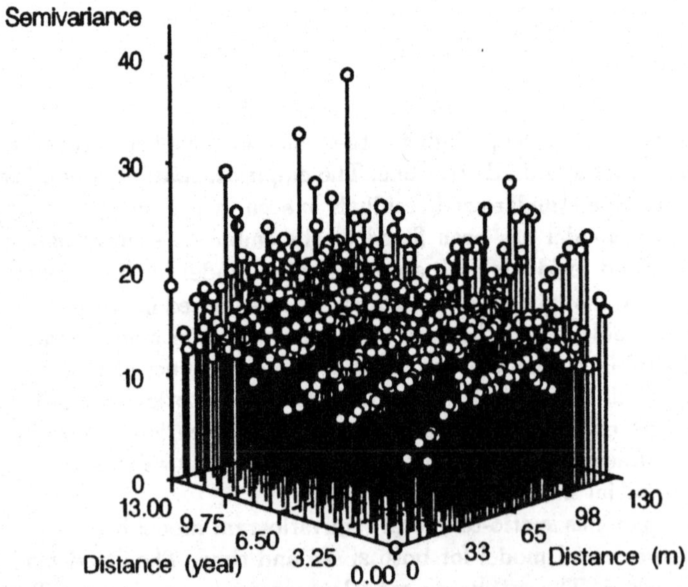

FIGURE 3. The empirical spatio-temporal semivariogram for the residuals.

TABLE 1. Parameter estimates for the separable spatio-temporal model with an exponential model for space and time.

Parameter	Estimate	Asymptotic standard error	95% confidence limits lower	upper
a	50.4	11.3	28.2	72.7
α	19.3	5.3	8.9	29.7
C_{h0}	0.875	7.43	-13.71	15.46
C_h	0.727	6.20	-11.45	12.91
$C_{\tau 0}$	0.329	3.05	-5.66	6.32
C_τ	0.316	2.95	-5.47	6.10

TABLE 2. Correlation matrix for the parameters in the separable spatio-temporal model with an exponential model for space and time.

Correlation matrix	a	α	C_{h0}	C_h	$C_{\tau 0}$	C_τ
a	1	0.754	0.149	0.159	-0.106	-0.099
α	0.754	1	0.320	0.339	-0.266	-0.259
C_{h0}	0.149	0.320	1	0.999	-0.998	-0.998
C_h	0.159	0.339	0.999	1	-0.997	-0.996
$C_{\tau 0}$	-0.106	-0.266	-0.998	-0.997	1	0.999
C_τ	-0.099	-0.259	-0.998	-0.996	0.999	1

TABLE 3. Parameter estimates for the parsimonious spatio-temporal model with an exponential model for space and time.

Parameter	Estimate	Asymptotic standard error	95% confidence limits lower	upper
a	32.9	4.02	25.0	40.8
α	33.6	10.7	12.6	54.5
C_0	0.672	0.023	0.627	0.716
C	0.364	0.021	0.324	0.405

TABLE 4. Correlation matrix for the parameters in the parsimonious spatio-temporal model with an exponential model for space and time.

Correlation matrix	a	α	C_0	C
a	1	0.255	0.625	-0.141
α	0.255	1	0.687	-0.586
C_0	0.625	0.687	1	-0.835
C	-0.141	-0.586	-0.835	1

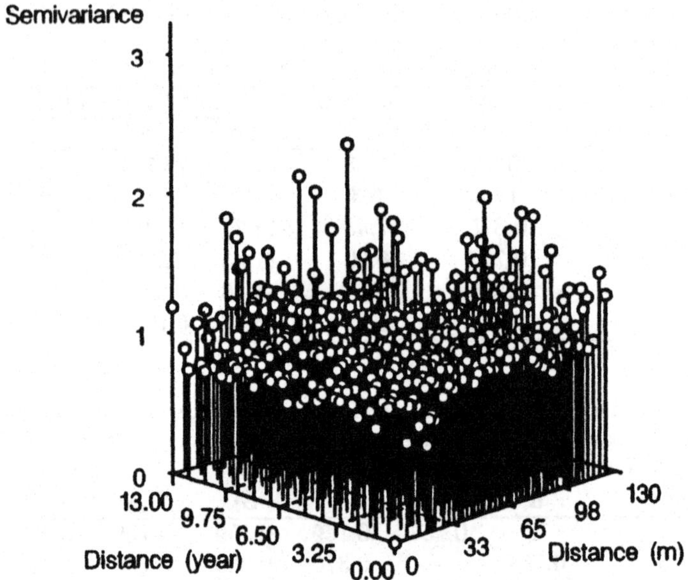

FIGURE 4. The empirical spatio-temporal semivariogram for the standardized residuals.

5 Discussion and Conclusion

In recent years there has been a number of papers using the separable semivariogram models, e.g. Haas [5] and de Cesare et al. [3]. In the long-term field trial described in the present paper the separable semivariogram model has highly correlated parameter estimates with large standard errors. Using the alternative parsimonious semivariogram model the parameters are estimated with smaller standard errors and no extreme correlations between the parameter estimates are seen. However, the separable semivariogram model estimates separate nugget effect and partial sill for space and time, which in some cases might be of interest, even though the parameter estimates are highly correlated.

The correlation between measurements in time is seen to be strong. For the parsimonious model the practical range of influence is estimated at ap-

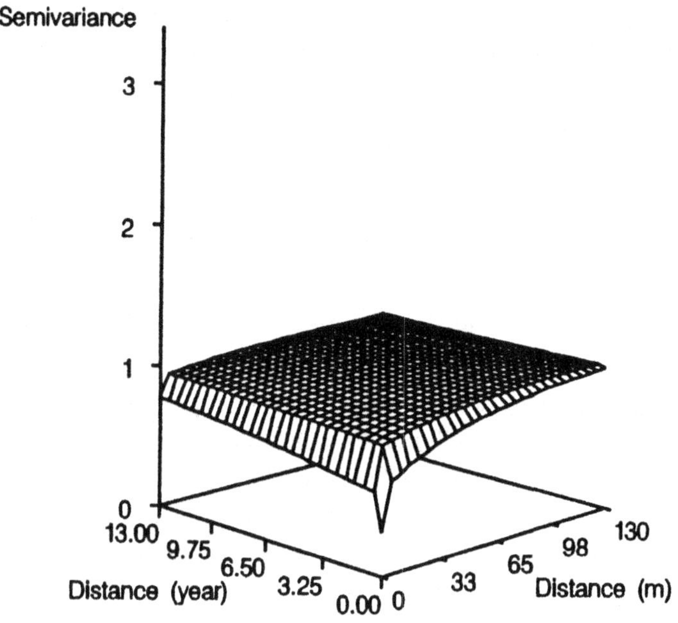

FIGURE 5. A model fitted to the separable spatio-temporal semivariogram with an exponential model in space and time.

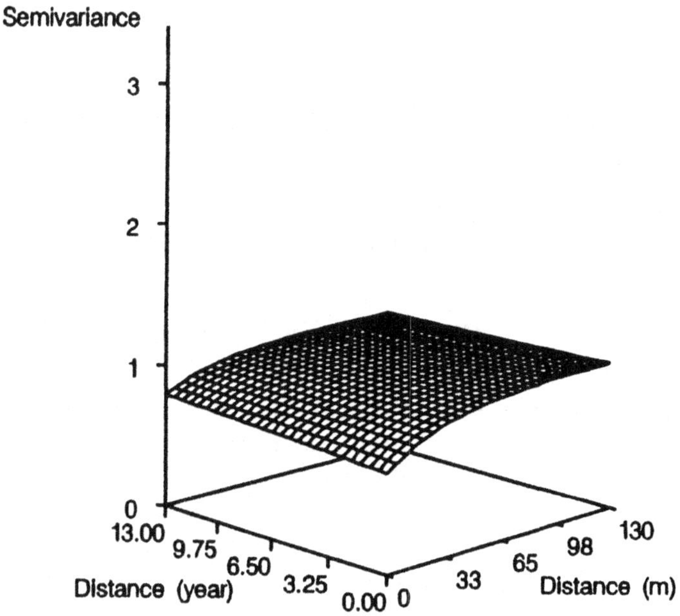

FIGURE 6. A model fitted to the parsimonious spatio-temporal semivariogram with an exponential model in space and time.

proximately 100 years ($\approx 3 \times 33.6$ years). In relation to spatial experimental design, this means that there is a long memory between yield measurements in the field.

6 References

[1] Bilonick, R.A. (1985). The Space-Time Distribution of Sulfate Deposition in the Northeastern United States, *Atmospheric Environment*, **19**, 1829-1845.

[2] Cressie, N. (1991). *Statistics for Spatial Data.* John Wiley & Sons, New York.

[3] de Cesare, L., Myers, D.E., Posa, D. (Accepted for publication). Spatial-Temporal Modelling of SO_2 in Milan District. E.Baafi (ed.), *Geostatistics*, Kluwer Academic Publishers.

[4] Ersbøll, A.K. (Accepted for publication). Estimation of the Spatial Variation in Designed Field Trials. E.Baafi (ed.), *Geostatistics*, Kluwer Academic Publishers.

[5] Haas, T.H. (1995). Local Prediction of a Spatio-Temporal Process with an Application to Wet Sulfate Deposition. *Journal of the American Statistical Association*, **90**, 1189-1199.

[6] Kristensen, K. and Ersbøll, A.K. (1992). The Use of Geostatistical Methods in Planning Variety Trials, *Biuletyn Oceny Odmian*, **24-25**, 139-157.

[7] Posa, D. (1993). A Simple Description of Spatio-Temporal Processes, *Computational Statistics & Data Analysis*, **15**, 425-437.

[8] Rasmussen, K.J. (1991). Reduced Soil Tillage and Italian Ryegrass as Catch Crop. I. Growing Conditions, Yields, Crop Analyses and Weeds, *Tidsskrift for Planteavl*, **95**, 119-138.

[9] Rogriuez-Iturbe, I., Mejia, J.M. (1974). The Design of Rainfall Networks in Time and Space, *Water Resources Research*, **10**, 713-728.

[10] Rouhani, S., Hall, T.J. (1989). Space-Time Kriging of Groundwater Data. M.Armstrong (ed.), *Geostatistics*, Kluwer Academic Publishers.

Structuring Correlation Within Hierarchical Spatio-temporal Models for Disease Rates

Lance A. Waller, Bradley P. Carlin, and Hong Xia *

University of Minnesota

United States

ABSTRACT Hierarchical Bayes models stabilize observed disease rates in low-population areas while maintaining geographic resolution, thereby providing a more accurate map of disease risk. We use a generalized linear mixed model framework to account for covariate effects, and to allow for random effects due to unstructured heterogeneity, spatial correlations, temporal trends, and spatio-temporal interactions. The resulting models are highly parametric and require careful implementation of Markov chain Monte Carlo algorithms. We explore advantages and disadvantages of various parametric correlation models within the hierarchical framework. We compare correlation structures with respect to identifiability, ease of implementation, and interpretation of parameters. We illustrate the method using annual county-specific lung cancer mortality in Ohio counties from 1968 to 1988. The results indicate a changing spatial structure in lung cancer rates over time. Different correlation structures incorporate this feature in different ways.

Key words and phrases: Identifiability, Markov chain Monte Carlo, Metropolis algorithm, model selection.

---

*Lance A. Waller is Assistant Professor, Bradley P. Carlin is Associate Professor, and Hong Xia is graduate student and research assistant, Division of Biostatistics, School of Public Health, University of Minnesota, Box 303 Mayo Memorial Building, Minneapolis, MN 55455. This research was supported in part by National Institute of Allergy and Infectious Diseases FIRST Award 1-R29-AI33466 (BPC and HX), and National Institute of Environmental Health Sciences grant R01 1-R01-ES07750 (LAW and BPC). The views are those of the authors and are not necessarily those of NIH or NIEHS. The authors thank Dr. Owen Devine for the Ohio dataset, and frequent helpful advice.

1 Introduction

The presence of spatial or longitudinal correlation in linear or generalized linear models requires a partitioning of random variation in a convenient and meaningful way. This partitioning is not unique and, as a result, many parameterizations have been proposed. For longitudinal data, the random effects models of Laird and Ware (1982) prove useful where longitudinal correlations are induced by individual-level random effects occurring in a population. An alternate partitioning of covariance, detailed in Diggle, Liang and Zeger (1994, Section 5.2), includes random effects but primarily defines serial longitudinal correlations through a variogram, thus providing a conceptual link to spatial models. For geostatistical models, Cressie (1993, Section 3.1) outlines a partitioning of error into large-scale variation (mean structure), smooth small-scale variation (modeled by a variogram), microscale variation, and measurement error.

A related issue is the assignment of trends in the data to mean effects (perhaps due to covariates) or to covariance effects. In geostatistics, where prediction is the primary concern, there has been some discussion of the need for detrending data (e.g. in universal kriging). In many epidemiologic applications, estimation of covariate effects is of primary interest, and one often regards residual spatial and longitudinal correlations as effects of unobserved (and perhaps unobservable) covariates.

In this paper, we concentrate on hierarchical Bayesian models of disease risk. We outline different partitions of variation into main effects, random effects, and associated correlation-inducing prior distributions. We compare different formulations using a simulation-based model comparison approach for county-specific lung cancer mortality in Ohio from 1968-1988.

2 Motivation: Lung cancer mortality in Ohio

We begin by considering data originally analyzed by Devine (1992, Chapter 4). Let y_{ijkt} denote the number of lung cancer deaths in county i during year t for gender j and race k in the state of Ohio, and n_{ijkt} the corresponding exposed population count (Centers for Disease Control, 1988). The data include $J = 2$ genders (male and female) and $K = 2$ races (white and nonwhite) for each of the $I = 88$ Ohio counties over the $T = 21$ year time period 1968–1988 inclusive, yielding a total of 7392 observations.

The study area and outcome are of interest because of the United States Department of Energy Fernald Materials Processing Center. This facility recycles depleted uranium fuel from U.S. Department of Energy and Department of Defense nuclear facilities. The Fernald plant is located approximately 25 miles northwest of the city of Cincinnati. The recycling process creates radioactive uranium dust, some of which may have been released during peak production from 1951 to the early 1960's. Inhalation is the primary route of the putative exposure, and lung cancer is the most prevalent form of cancer potentially associated with exposure to uranium. We use reported mortality rates for the years 1968-1988 to allow an appropriate (ten- to twenty-year) temporal lag between the putative exposure and disease development.

3 Hierarchical modeling of disease rates

A major complication in the analysis of crude rates of rare outcomes from small areas is the inherent instability of rate estimates based on small numbers of people at risk. Often the highest observed rates occur in regions with very few deaths and few persons at risk. Clayton and Kaldor (1987) define an empirical Bayes approach to "shrink" regional estimates toward a global mean rate thereby gaining precision while maintaining geographic resolution. In the past decade, many other authors also proposed Bayesian or empirical Bayes estimates of regional rates. Clayton and Bernardinelli (1992) provide a thorough review of the area.

We briefly outline the approach below. Suppose the study area is partitioned into I nonoverlapping regions. Let Y_i denote the (random) number of incident deaths, and let n_i denote the number of individuals residing in region i, $i = 1, \ldots, I$. Clayton and Kaldor (1987) propose the following model

$$Y_i \mid \psi_i \overset{ind}{\sim} \text{Poisson}\left(E_i\, e^{\psi_i}\right) , \tag{1}$$

where E_i denotes the expected number of deaths in region i under a constant baseline disease rate, and ψ_i denotes the (unobserved) log relative risk of disease for individuals residing in region i, $i = 1, \ldots, I$. One includes covariate effects (often of direct interest in epidemiologic studies) by defining $\psi_i = \mathbf{z}_i'\boldsymbol{\beta}$, where $\mathbf{z}_i$ denotes a vector of covariate values for region i, and $\boldsymbol{\beta}$ the vector of associated parameters. Often the E_i's are assumed to be known, either *externally* standardized from national rates, or *internally* standardized from the observed disease rate for the entire study area, namely, $E_i = n_i \left(\sum_{i=1}^{I} y_i / \sum_{i=1}^{I} n_i\right)$.

Clayton and Kaldor (1987) suggest a likelihood for $Y_i|\psi_i$, $i = 1, \ldots, I$, comprised of independent Poisson distributions. Spatial correlation is induced through a prior distribution on the ψ_i's. The *conditionally autoregressive* (CAR) prior is a common choice, based on a set of neighbors, denoted ∂_i, for each region i, $i = 1, \ldots, I$. Neighbors are often defined by region contiguity, but could be defined based on a function of distance between regions. Conditionally, the CAR prior can be expressed as

$$\psi_i \mid \psi_{j \neq i} \sim N\left(\bar{\psi}_i, \frac{1}{\lambda m_i}\right),$$

where $\bar{\psi}_i = \sum_{j \in \partial_i} \psi_j / m_i$, and m_i denotes the number of neighbors of region i. Note the conditional variance of $\psi_i | \psi_{j \neq i}$ is inversely proportional to the number of neighbors for region i. The CAR prior is a member of the more general family of pairwise difference priors outlined in Besag et al. (1995).

Stabilized rate maps are based on the posterior distributions of the log relative risks, $p(\psi_i | Y_i)$. Typically, one creates a choropleth map using a set of colors or greyscales to represent ranges of rates.

Besag, York, and Mollié (1991) provide a fully hierarchical Bayesian formulation of the Clayton and Kaldor (1987) approach by considering two random effects for each region. That is, they consider the model

$$\psi_i = \mathbf{z}_i' \beta + \theta_i + \phi_i,$$

where $\theta_i \stackrel{ind}{\sim} N(0, 1/\tau)$, and the ϕ_i's follow a CAR prior with parameter λ, i.e. $\phi_i | \phi_{j \neq i} \sim N\left(\bar{\phi}_i, 1/\lambda m_i\right)$. The hyperparameters τ and λ are given vague but proper priors. The random effect θ_i models excess heterogeneity and serves to shrink rate estimates toward a global mean. The second random effect, ϕ_i, models spatial clustering and serves to shrink estimates toward a local mean of neighboring observations.

Waller et al. (1997) extend the Besag, York, and Mollié (1991) framework to allow for spatio-temporal effects. The random effects are specific to regions within each time period (e.g. year) with the spatial structure allowed to evolve over time. The resulting model is

$$\psi_i = \mathbf{z}_i' \beta + \delta_t + \theta_{it} + \phi_{it}, \tag{2}$$

where $\theta_{it} \stackrel{ind}{\sim} N(0, 1/\tau_t)$ and the ϕ_{it}'s follow a CAR prior with parameter λ_t, for each t. The model allows a time trend through parameters δ_t, $t = 1, \ldots, T$. The authors assign a vague prior to δ_t allowing the data to reveal time trends.

Model (2) offers many possibilities for structuring temporal, spatial, and spatio-temporal correlations. Correlations may be ignored entirely if $\theta_{it} = \phi_{it} = 0$ for $i = 1, \ldots, I$, and $t = 1, \ldots, T$, and δ_s is independent of δ_t for $s \neq t$. We extend the analysis of Waller et al. (1997) by considering longitudinal correlations induced through a time-series structure for δ_t, e.g., an AR(1) prior

$$\delta_t | \delta_{t-1} \sim N\left(\gamma_t + \rho(\delta_{t-1} - \gamma_{t-1}), \sigma_\delta^2\right), \tag{3}$$

with vague priors for hyperparameters γ_t, ρ, and σ_δ^2. The Ohio lung cancer data exhibit a fairly linear increase over time, so we simplify (3) by replacing γ_t with $\gamma_0 + \gamma_1 t$ in the example below. One obtains spatial correlation independent of the longitudinal correlation through region-specific random effects (fixed across time), θ_i and $\phi_i, i = 1, \ldots, I$. Model (2) offers a nested structure for spatio-temporal correlations, i.e. pairs of random effects model spatial correlations within each time period; correlations are within space for each time period.

The variety of possibilities raises a salient point in fitting parametric models of the mean *and* correlation structure: certain data features may appear within models in several different ways. For instance, lung cancer rates are generally increasing during the 20th century. For the Ohio data, such a trend is very apparent, with the state-wide rate increasing from 30.7 to 60.5 deaths per 100,000 people per year from 1968 to 1988. We expect such a feature to appear in the δ_t terms for model (2). However, this effect may be confounded if the model also includes an intercept (e.g. $z_1 = 1$), or if the prior for the spatial effects ϕ_{it} is not centered (say at 0) for each t, since one could add a constant to each ϕ_{it}, and subtract it from each δ_t without affecting the likelihood times prior, hence the posterior. The earlier analysis appearing in Waller et al. (1997) focused on nested spatio-temporal effects, and did not identify separate longitudinal trends in the data. In the analysis below, centering the ϕ_{it}'s (i.e. adding the constraint $\sum_i \phi_{it} = 0$ for all t) provides a useful tool for maintaining identifiability and requiring some anticipated effects to manifest themselves in the appropriate parameters. For example, disallowing an overall intercept, such a constraint forces overall time trends to appear in δ_t for $t = 1, \ldots, T$, as desired.

4 Model choice

With many possibilities for parameterizing spatio-temporal correlations within model (2), the choice of the "best" model is nontrivial. We consider two components to this choice, the first an overall measure of model "fit", and the second an interpretation of effects described by the model.

Bayesian model choice diagnostics are an active area of statistical research. However, for model (2), many of the customary procedures are not applicable. For example, Bayes factors are undefined with flat priors on $\boldsymbol{\beta}$ (and perhaps the δ_t), or with improper CAR priors for the spatial effects. A cross-validatory selection approach (Gelfand, Dey and Chang, 1992) is unavailable, again due to random effects identified only by the prior. Penalized likelihood criteria, where gains in likelihood are offset by penalties for excess parameters, seem attractive, but asymptotic results are based on the sample size increasing relative to the number of parameters (Carlin and Louis, 1996, p. 48). In our case, model dimension increases with sample size, and additional parameters appear with each additional region.

To handle such nonregular models, Gelfand and Ghosh (1995) and Waller et al. (1997) consider a penalized criteria based on predictive space. Consider $\mathbf{y}_{new}$ a replicate of the observed data vector $\mathbf{y}_{obs}$. Let $d(\mathbf{y}_{new}, \mathbf{y}_{obs})$ denote a function quantifying the discrepancy between predicted and observed data. For the generalized linear mixed models considered here, the deviance is a natural choice for the discrepancy function. Given models $M_j, j = 1, \ldots, J$, we select the model that minimizes the expected predictive deviance (EPD),

$$E[d(\mathbf{y}_{new}, \mathbf{y}_{obs})|\mathbf{y}_{obs}, M_j] . \tag{4}$$

The EPD may be recast as

$$\begin{aligned} E[d(\mathbf{y}_{new}, \mathbf{y}_{obs}) \mid \mathbf{y}_{obs}, M_i] = d(E[&\mathbf{y}_{new}|\mathbf{y}_{obs}, M_i], \mathbf{y}_{obs}) \\ &+ \{E[d(\mathbf{y}_{new}, \mathbf{y}_{obs}) \mid \mathbf{y}_{obs}, M_i] \\ &\quad - d(E[\mathbf{y}_{new}|\mathbf{y}_{obs}, M_i], \mathbf{y}_{obs}) \} . \end{aligned} \tag{5}$$

This result partitions EPD into

$$EPD = LRS + PEN, \tag{6}$$

where LRS is essentially a likelihood ratio statistic with the MLE for $\boldsymbol{\psi}$ replaced by $E(\mathbf{y}_{new}|\mathbf{y}_{old}, M_i)$, while PEN is a weighted predictive variability penalty (analogous to the usual penalty for increased model dimension). Smaller EPD values indicate a better model. Computation of (5) requires calculation of predictive expectations, routinely obtained as Monte Carlo integrations under the computational approach outlined in Waller et al. (1997).

5 Space-time modeling of Ohio lung cancer rates

We begin by specifying the available covariates

$$\mathbf{z}_{jk}\boldsymbol{\beta} = s_j\alpha + r_k\beta + s_j r_k \xi \ , \tag{7}$$

where $s_j = 0$ for men, 1 for women, and $r_k = 0$ for white, 1 for non-white. Letting $\boldsymbol{\theta}^{(t)} = (\theta_{1t}, \ldots, \theta_{It})'$, $\boldsymbol{\phi}^{(t)} = (\phi_{1t}, \ldots, \phi_{It})'$, and denoting the I-dimensional identity matrix by $\mathbf{I}$, we adopt the prior structure

$$\boldsymbol{\theta}^{(t)} \mid \tau_t \overset{ind}{\sim} N\left(\mathbf{0} \, , \, \frac{1}{\tau_t}\mathbf{I}\right) \quad \text{and} \quad \boldsymbol{\phi}^{(t)} \mid \lambda_t \overset{ind}{\sim} CAR(\lambda_t) \ , \ t = 1, \ldots, T \ , \tag{8}$$

so that heterogeneity and clustering may vary over time. Note that we assume gender and race do not interact with time or location.

To complete the model specification, we require prior distributions for α, β, ξ, the τ_t, and the λ_t. Since α, β and ξ will be identified by the likelihood, we may employ flat priors for these three parameters. Next, we employ conjugate, conditionally i.i.d. $Gamma(a, b)$ and $Gamma(c, d)$ priors for τ_t and λ_t, respectively. Since only the sum of θ_{it} and ϕ_{it} is identified by the likelihood, proper priors are required to facilitate implementation of an MCMC algorithm in this setting. Waller et al. (1997) suggest the values $a = 1, b = 100$ for the prior on τ, and $c = 1, d = 7$ (i.e., prior mean and standard deviation equal to 7) for the prior on λ. These priors are still quite vague, and are consistent with the advice of Bernardinelli, Clayton and Montomoli (1995), whose study of prior sensitivity for such models suggests heterogeneity parameters have prior standard deviation roughly 7/10 that assigned to clustering parameters when local associations are based on adjacencies. This ratio yields $\lambda \approx \tau/(2\bar{m})$, where $\bar{m}$ is the average number of counties adjacent to a randomly selected county (approximately six for the Ohio data), thereby linking parameters λ and τ, adjusting for the number of neighboring regions.

For each model, we ran 5 parallel, initially overdispersed MCMC chains for 500 iterations, a task which took roughly 20 minutes on a Sparc 10 workstation. We used univariate Gibbs updating steps for parameters with available full conditional distributions, and univariate Metropolis steps for the remaining parameters. Graphical monitoring of the chains for a representative subset of the parameters, along with sample autocorrelations and Gelman and Rubin (1992) diagnostics, indicated an acceptable degree of convergence by around the 100th iteration. Using the final 400 iterations from all 5 chains, we obtained posterior medians and 95% credible sets for all parameters.

Table 1 shows model choice diagnostics for several possible models. The diagnostic values are based on Monte Carlo integration from the MCMC samples, and are therefore subject to Monte Carlo variation. The first four models appear in Waller et al. (1997). Model (a) includes heterogeneity and clustering parameters nested within time. These parameters are not centered around 0, and so the overall increase in disease rates across time appears as a linear trend in the posterior means of ϕ_{it} for each t. Models (b) and (c) illustrate that model (a) tends to overfit the data, and offer considerable improvement in EPD score. Model (d) separates spatial (constant ϕ_i's across time) correlations and a temporal trend (δ_t), but provides poorer fit than models (a)-(c). Waller et al. (1997) prefer model (c) over model (b) based on the posterior distributions of hyperparameters. The posterior distributions of τ_t for model (b) display a very slight increase over time, resulting in fairly consistent excess heterogeneity across time. Model (c) exhibits the linear increase in lung cancer rates through the posterior means of ϕ_{it} for fixed t. Simultaneously, increasing posterior means of λ_t indicate decreasing variance of ϕ_{it} from its spatially neighboring values, resulting in increasing spatial clustering of rates over time. Model (c) provides insight to data trends not apparent from model (b). Given the near equivalence of EPD values, model (c) is preferred.

Many other modeling possibilities remain and we offer two such models here. In both, we center the ϕ_{it}'s around zero for each t. As mentioned in Section 3, this requires any temporal trend to appear in the δ_t terms. For model (e) we use a vague prior for each δ_t, and for model (f) we use equation (3) to define temporal autocorrelation in the model, where we assume a

Model $\psi_{it} =$	Prior for temporal effect	LRS	PEN	EPD
(a) $\mathbf{z}'_{jk}\beta + \theta_{it} + \phi_{it}$	None	5374.87	5806.07	11180.94
(b) $\mathbf{z}'_{jk}\beta + \theta_{it}$	None	4941.32	6017.06	10958.39
(c) $\mathbf{z}'_{jk}\beta + \phi_{it}$	None	5180.25	5808.73	10988.98
(d) $\mathbf{z}'_{jk}\beta + \delta_t + \phi_i$	Uniform	7274.70	5725.19	12999.89
(e) $\mathbf{z}'_{jk}\beta + \delta_t + \phi_{it}$	Uniform	5176.76	5807.48	10984.24
(f) $\mathbf{z}'_{jk}\beta + \delta_t + \phi_{it}$	AR(1)	5182.44	5808.81	10991.25

TABLE 1. Likelihood ratio statistics (LRS), predictive variability penalties (PEN), and overall expected predicted deviance (EPD) scores, spatio-temporal Ohio lung cancer models.

linear model for the main temporal effect, $\gamma_t = \gamma_0 + \gamma_1 t$. Considering the Monte Carlo variation associated with their calculation, the EPD values indicate near equivalent fit for models (b), (c), (e), and (f). Therefore, we explore parameter estimates and graphical assessments of fit for particular years to distinguish between these models.

Models (e) and (f) are attractive since time trends are isolated from the spatial parameters. Model (f) utilizes the near-linearity of lung cancer rates over time, and includes temporal autocorrelation (in addition to the temporally-evolving spatial correlations). The posterior median value of ρ is 0.29, with 95% credible set (-0.28,0.76), indicating modest temporal autocorrelation in the data.

Figure 1 plots (as dots) the posterior median values of δ_t from model (f). The values indicate the near-linear increase state-wide in the logarithm of lung cancer rates, a feature buried in the posterior distributions of the ϕ_{it}'s in model (c). The solid line in Figure 1 illustrates the linear trend defined by the posterior median values of γ_0 and γ_1. Final adjustments to the linear trend due to the autocorrelation parameter, ρ, are shown in the dotted line. The autocorrelation adjustment mirrors the pattern of consecutive positive and negative residuals from the linear trend. Model (f) is more parsimonious than model (e), containing 4 parameters ($\gamma_0, \gamma_1, \rho, \sigma_\delta^2$), rather than 21 ($\delta_1, \ldots, \delta_{21}$) to describe the temporal trend. This feature, coupled with the accommodation of the modest autoregressive trend and near-equivalent EPD scores, offers a substantive reason to prefer model (f) over model (e).

6 Conclusions

The family of hierarchical spatio-temporal models offers great flexibility for data analysis, but requires careful implementation and interpretation. Our analysis of lung cancer in Ohio illustrates that numerical constraints

FIGURE 1. Posterior median values of δ_t from model (f).

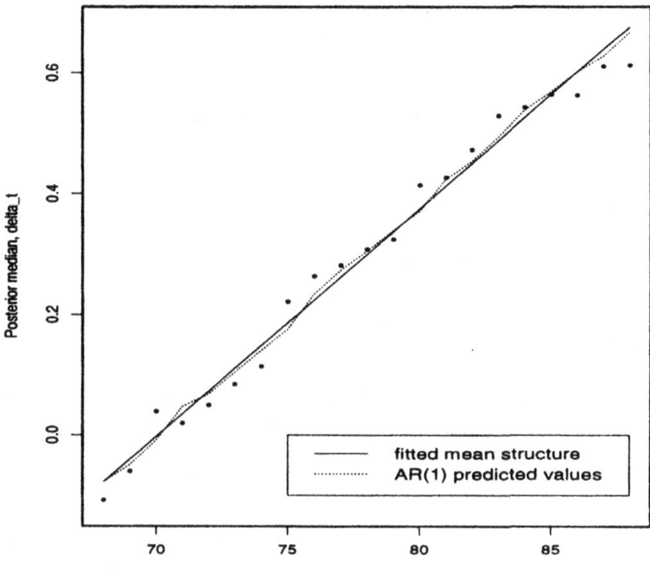

provide a useful tool for guiding data patterns toward appropriate parameters. The expected predictive deviance model choice diagnostics allow us to avoid overfitting models but do not differentiate between some parameterizations of covariance. We find that model (f) offers additional insight into the data and provides a similar fit to earlier models considered by Waller et al. (1997). Model (f) describes an evolving spatial pattern among county-specific lung cancer rates accompanyed by modest temporal correlations.

Many other models in the same general framework are possible. The CAR prior limits spatial correlations to adjacent regions, possibly reasonable for counties, but questionable for smaller areas such as census tracts. More reasonable models in these cases would incorporate weights relating different strengths of spatial correlations to different distances, perhaps through a variogram as in Cressie and Chan (1989).

Finally, the CAR structure offers possibilities for more complex spatio-temporal modeling. For instance, one could define three-dimensional neighborhood structures across space *and* time, where regional rates correlate with current and past spatially neighboring values. Since the magnitude of association would likely differ between space and time, we might employ two CAR priors, $\phi^{(t)} \overset{ind}{\sim} CAR(\lambda_t)$ and $\delta \sim CAR(\lambda_\delta)$. Such a structure will require careful implementation, but could describe migration effects, or offer insight into dynamic patterns of infectious disease.

7 References

[1] Bernardinelli, L., Clayton, D., and Montomoli, C. (1995). Bayesian estimates of disease maps: how important are priors? *Statistics in Medicine*, **14**, 2411–2431.

[2] Besag, J., Green, P., Higdon, D. and Mengersen, K. (1995). Bayesian computation and stochastic systems (with discussion). *Statistical Science*, **10**, 3–66.

[3] Besag, J., York, J.C., and Mollié, A. (1991). Bayesian image restoration, with two applications in spatial statistics (with discussion). *Annals of the Institute of Statistical Mathematics*, **43**, 1–59.

[4] Carlin, B.P. and Louis, T.A. (1996). *Bayes and Empirical Bayes Methods for Data Analysis*, London: Chapman and Hall.

[5] Centers for Disease Control and Prevention, National Center for Health Statistics (1988). *Public Use Data Tape: Compressed Mortality File, 1968–1985*, Hyattsvile, Maryland: U.S. Department of Health and Human Services.

[6] Clayton, D.G. and Bernardinelli, L. (1992). Bayesian methods for mapping disease risk. In *Geographical and Environmental Epidemiology: Methods for Small-Area Studies*. P. Elliott, J. Cuzick, D. English, and R. Stern, eds., Oxford: University Press.

[7] Clayton, D.G. and Kaldor, J. (1987). Empirical Bayes estimates of age-standardized relative risks for use in disease mapping. *Biometrics*, **43**, 671–681.

[8] Cressie, N.A.C. (1993). *Statistics for Spatial Data*, 2nd ed., New York: Wiley.

[9] Cressie, N. and Chan, N.H. (1989). Spatial modeling of regional variables. *Journal of the American Statistical Association*, **84**, 393–401.

[10] Devine, O.J. (1992), *Empirical Bayes and Constrained Empirical Bayes Methods for Estimating Incidence Rates in Spatially Aligned Areas*, unpublished Ph.D. dissertation, Division of Biostatistics, Emory University.

[11] Diggle, P.J., Liang, K.-Y., and Zeger, S.L. (1994) *Analysis of Longitudinal Data*. Oxford: Clarendon Press.

[12] Gelfand, A.E., Dey, D.K., and Chang, H. (1992), Model determination using predictive distributions with implementation via sampling-based methods (with discussion). in *Bayesian Statistics 4*, J.M. Bernardo, J.O. Berger, A.P. Dawid and A.F.M. Smith, eds., Oxford: Oxford University Press, pp. 147–167.

[13] Gelfand, A.E., and Ghosh, S.K. (1995). Model choice: a minimum posterior predictive loss approach. University of Connecticut Department of Statistics Technical Report 95-28.

[14] Gelman, A. and Rubin, D.B. (1992). Inference from iterative simulation using multiple sequences. (with discussion), *Statistical Science*, **7**, 457–511.

[15] Laird, N.M. and Ware, J.H. (1982). Random-effects models for longitudinal data. *Biometrics*, **38**, 963-974.

[16] Waller, L.A., Carlin, B.P., Xia, H., and Gelfand, A.E. (1997, to appear) Hierarchical spatio-temporal mapping of disease rates. *Journal of the American Statistical Association.*

Generalized Linear Mixed Measurement Error Models

Raymond J. Carroll, Xihong Lin and Naisyin Wang *
Texas A&M University
United States

ABSTRACT We consider generalized linear mixed models (GLMM) in a sampling design consisting of clusters and then units within clusters, when one of the predictors is measured with additive, normal error. We first review some basic ideas and recent results on the structure of such Generalized Linear Mixed Measurement Error Models (GLMMeM), Then we consider a specific example, fit fully parametrically via a Bayesian analysis using the Gibbs sampler with essentially noninformative priors.

Keywords and phrases Gibbs sampling; measurement error; mixed models; random effects; SIMEX; simulation-extrapolation.

1 Introduction

Correlated data are frequently observed in longitudinal studies, clinical trials, familial studies, etc. Generalized linear mixed models (GLMMs) have become increasingly popular for analyzing such correlated and overdispersed data, see Breslow & Clayton (1993) for examples. A variety of methods for fitting such models have been proposed, including Monte–Carlo EM (McCulloch, 1994), Laplace approximations (Liu and Pierce, 1993; Breslow and Lin, 1995); Penalized Quasilikelihood (PQL) (Schall, 1991; Breslow and Clayton, 1993); corrected penalized quasilikelihood (CPQL) (Lin and Breslow, 1996); and Bayesian procedures including EM–type algorithms (Stiratelli, Laird and Ware, 1984) and the Gibbs sampler (Zeger and Karim, 1991).

---

*The research of Carroll and Wang was supported by a grant from the National Cancer Institute (CA–57030). We thank Roberto G. Gutierrez for many helpful conversations. Corresponding author: Raymond J. Carroll, Department of Statistics, Texas A&M University, College Station, TX 77843-3143.

A common problem in analyzing correlated data is the presence of the covariate measurement error. The problem of measurement error with independent observations has a vast literature in linear models (Fuller, 1987) and a growing literature in generalized linear models and other nonlinear models (Carroll, Ruppert and Stefanski, 1995). Generally, the literature distinguished between functional modeling, in which nothing is assumed about the unobserved predictors, and structural modeling, in which specific assumptions are made about the distributional structure of these unobserved predictors.

In this paper, we study a class of models proposed by Carroll, Gutierrez, Lin and Wang (1996, hereafter denoted by CGLW), the generalized linear mixed measurement error models (GLMMeMs), which model the correlation and the measurement error simultaneously. CGLW study the bias induced by ignoring measurement error, and propose functional methods for estimation in this context, in particular the SIMEX method of Cook & Stefanski (1994). They also derive functional score tests for variance components, generalizing work of Lin (1997) in the no–error problem. Lin, Wang and Carroll (1996, hereafter denoted by LWG) study structural models fit by likelihood methods, comparing full maximum likelihood and approximate (LaPlace) likelihood estimators. We first review the results of CGLW on the bias induced by ignoring measurement error in a specific case where sampling is done in clusters with repeated observations within each cluster. We also describe the estimation approaches they used. Finally, we study in detail a specific example, using a fully parametric model fit via Bayesian Gibbs sampling with essentially noninformative priors, comparing the results to those obtained by CGLW and LWC.

2 The Generalized Linear Mixed Measurement Error Model

In this section, we review the model and the results of CGLW. We will use boldface for vectors and matrices.

2.1 The General Model

Suppose that the data are obtained from m independent clusters with outcome variable Y_{ij}, unobserved true covariate $\mathbf{X}_{ij}$ ($p_1 \times 1$), observed $\mathbf{X}_{ij}$-related covariate $\mathbf{W}_{ij}$, and other observed covariates $\mathbf{Z}_{ij}$ ($p_2 \times 1$) and $\mathbf{B}_{ij}$ ($q \times 1$) associated the fixed and random effects, respectively, where $i = 1, \cdots, m$ identifies the cluster and $j = 1, \ldots, n_i$ identifies subjects within clusters. Given the covariates $\mathbf{X}_{ij}$, $\mathbf{Z}_{ij}$, $\mathbf{B}_{ij}$, and an unobserved $q \times 1$ random effect vector $\mathbf{b}_i$, the observations Y_{ij} in the ith cluster are assumed to be independent with means $\mu_{ij,x}^{\mathbf{b}_i}$ and variance $\phi a_{ij}^{-1} v(\mu_{ij,x}^{\mathbf{b}_i})$, where ϕ is a scale parameter, a_{ij} is a prior weight, and $v(\cdot)$ is a variance function. The generalized linear mixed model (GLMM) of $\mathbf{Y}$ given $\mathbf{X}$ is constructed by assuming that the conditional mean $\mu_{ij,x}^{\mathbf{b}_i}$ is related to $\mathbf{X}_{ij}$, $\mathbf{Z}_{ij}$ and $\mathbf{b}_i$ through a generalized linear model

$$g(\mu_{ij,x}^{\mathbf{b}_i}) = \beta_0 + \mathbf{X}_{ij}^T\boldsymbol{\beta}_x + \mathbf{Z}_{ij}^T\boldsymbol{\beta}_z + \mathbf{B}_{ij}^T\mathbf{b}_i, \tag{1}$$

where $g(\cdot)$ is a monotonic differentiable link function and the $\mathbf{b}_i$ are independent and identically distributed normal random vectors with mean zero and covariance matrix $\mathbf{D}(\boldsymbol{\theta})$, where $\boldsymbol{\theta}$ is an $l \times 1$ vector of variance components. The integrated quasi-likelihood of the $\mathbf{Y}_i$ given the $(\mathbf{X}_i, \mathbf{Z}_i)$ in the ith cluster is thus

$$\begin{aligned} &L_i(\mathbf{Y}_i|\mathbf{X}_i, \mathbf{Z}_i\boldsymbol{\beta}_x, \boldsymbol{\beta}_z, \boldsymbol{\theta}) \qquad (2) \\ &\propto |\mathbf{D}|^{-1/2} \int \exp\left\{ \sum_{j=1}^{n_i} \ell_{ij}(Y_{ij}|\mathbf{X}_{ij}, \mathbf{Z}_{ij}, \mathbf{b}_i) - \frac{1}{2}\mathbf{b}_i^T\mathbf{D}^{-1}\mathbf{b}_i \right\} d\mathbf{b}_i, \end{aligned}$$

where $\mathbf{Y}_i = (Y_{i1}, \ldots, Y_{in_i})^T$, $\mathbf{X}_i = (\mathbf{X}_{i1}^T, \ldots, \mathbf{X}_{in_i}^T)^T$, $\mathbf{Z}_i$ is defined similarly and

$$\ell_{ij}(Y_{ij}|\mathbf{X}_{ij}, \mathbf{Z}_{ij}, \mathbf{b}_i) = \int_{Y_{ij}}^{\mu_{ij}^{\mathbf{b}_i}} \frac{a_i(Y_{ij} - u)}{\phi v(u)} du \tag{3}$$

denotes the conditional log quasilikelihood of Y_{ij} given $\mathbf{b}_i$.

The model is completed by assuming that the measurement error is additive, so that

$$\mathbf{W}_{ij} = \mathbf{X}_{ij} + \mathbf{U}_{ij}, \tag{4}$$

where the $\mathbf{U}_{ij}$ are independent and normally distributed with mean zero and covariance matrix $\boldsymbol{\Sigma}_{uu}$. When $\mathbf{W}$ and $\mathbf{X}$ are scalar, we will write the measurement variance $\boldsymbol{\Sigma}_{uu}$ simply as σ_u^2. Assuming that the U's are independent of the X's, the Z's and the Y's, the joint quasilikelihood in the ith cluster is

$$L_i(\mathbf{Y}_i, \mathbf{W}_i, \mathbf{Z}_i) = \int L_i(\mathbf{Y}_i|\mathbf{X}_i, \mathbf{Z}_i)L_i(\mathbf{W}_i|\mathbf{X}_i)L_i(\mathbf{X}_i|\mathbf{Z}_i)d\mathbf{X}_i, \tag{5}$$

where $L_i(\mathbf{X}_i|\mathrm{ß})$ is the likelihood function of $\mathbf{X}_i$ given $\mathbf{Z}_i$ (so far unspecified).

The additive model (4) is not a requirement. Carroll, et al. (1995, pages 16–17) note that the only real requirement is nondifferential measurement error, i.e., that $\mathbf{W}_i$ is conditionally independent of $\mathbf{Y}_i$ given $(\mathbf{Z}_i, \mathbf{X}_i)$. Thus, multiplicative models or models where the errors depend on covariates are possible. In addition, we have assumed that the errors are independent even within a cluster. This is not required, see Wang, et al. (1996) for an example.

2.2 Models for the Unobservables

As indicated in (5), a full likelihood analysis requires that one specify a distribution for $\mathbf{X}_i$ given $\mathbf{Z}_i$. Here we consider the case that the X_{ij} are scalar random variables. Then CGLW and LWC suggest modeling the X's within a cluster to follow a linear–GLMM. Specifically, given random effects $\mathbf{e}_i$, the unobserved (and hence latent) $\mathbf{X}_i$ within a cluster are independent with conditional mean

$$\gamma_0 + \mathbf{Z}_i \boldsymbol{\gamma}_z + \mathbf{C}_i \mathbf{e}_i \tag{6}$$

and conditional variance $\sigma_x^2 \mathbf{I}$. The simplest model for the random effects here is $\mathbf{C}_{ij}^T \mathbf{e}_i = \mathbf{1} e_i$, where $\mathbf{1}$ is a vector of ones and e_i is a scalar normal random variable with mean zero and variance $\sigma_{x\mu}^2$. For this simple model, the terms $\mathbf{X}_{ij}$ have mean $\gamma_0 + \mathbf{Z}_{ij}^T \boldsymbol{\gamma}_z$, variance $\sigma_x^2 + \sigma_{x\mu}^2$ and common covariance $\sigma_{x\mu}^2$.

It is worthwhile at this point to note once again the difference between functional and structural modeling. In the structural model under consideration here, we have made two critical assumptions: (a) that $\mathbf{X}_i$ follows a linear GLMM with a random intercept; and (b) that the random variable in this linear GLMM are normally distributed. By way of contrast, the functional approach taken by CGLW makes neither assumption. The functional approach thus has the advantage of model robustness, while the structural approach may lead to more precise inferences if the assumed model really holds.

2.3 Biases for Large Number of Clusters

CGLW obtain expressions for the bias in maximum likelihood parameter estimates due to ignoring measurement error when there are no covariates $\mathbf{Z}$ measured exactly, and when the GLMM has a random cluster-level intercept with variance θ. They study what the call the *homogeneous* case in which $\mathbf{e}_i = 0$ in (6) as well as in the general case, which they call *heterogeneous*. In their work, the number of clusters $m \to \infty$ while the number of observations n within a cluster remains fixed.

Their results are fairly complete in the homogeneous case, and can be summarized briefly as follows:

- In the normal, probit, logistic and Poisson GLMM model, the bias in estimating $\boldsymbol{\beta}_x$ is the same as in the ordinary regression model (clusters of size 1), see Carroll, et al. (1995) for details.
- Likelihood estimates are consistent for the random effect θ in the linear model, but attenuated in the probit and logistic models, with the asymptotic bias essentially independent of the cluster size.

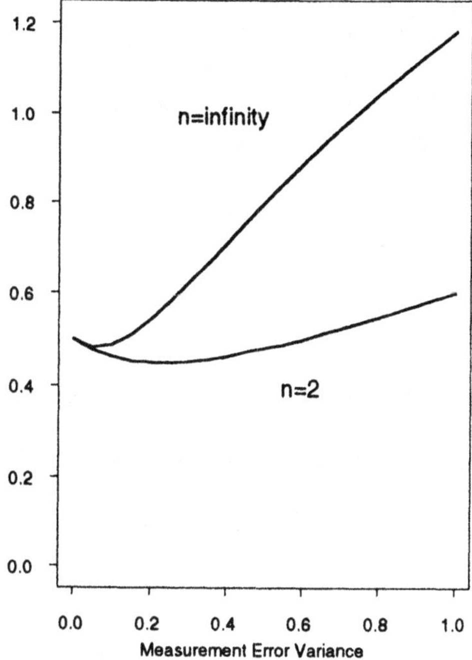

FIGURE 1. The asymptotic (as the number of clusters increases) limit of the maximum likelihood estimate for the variance component θ in a logistic–GLMM as a function of the measurement error variance σ_u^2. Here n refers to the number of observations per cluster. This is logistic regression with $\beta_0 = -2$, $\beta_x = 2$, $\theta = 0.5$, $\sigma_x^2 = 1$ and $\sigma_{x\mu}^2 = 1.5$.

- Likelihood estimates overestimate the random effect θ in the Poisson model, with the biases decreasing as the cluster size increases.

In the more realistic heterogeneous model, CGLW find that the bias in the parameter estimates may depend strongly on the number n of observations within each cluster. In many realistic cases, ignoring measurement error causes attenuation in estimating β_x, with the bias increasing as the cluster size increases. Similarly, the effect of measurement error is typically to overestimate the variance component θ, with the bias in this estimate often being most severe for a large number of observations within a cluster. CGLW display one specific example of logistic regression where there is almost no bias for estimating the variance component when the cluster size is $n = 2$ whereas the maximum likelihood estimate is biased by a factor greater than 2 when the cluster size n is large. This occurs in the case of no $\mathbf{Z}$ in a logistic–GLMM, with variance component $\theta = 0.5$ and $\beta_0 = -2$, $\beta_x = 2, \sigma_x^2 = 1$ and $\sigma_{x\mu}^2 = 1.5$. In Figure 1, we display the limit of the maximum likelihood estimate of θ for varying amount of measurement error. Note the strong dependence on the cluster size.

3 An Example

3.1 Background

Many of these ideas can be illustrated by considering data from the Framingham Heart study. CGLW and LWC should be consulted for full details. The particular part of the Framingham study under consideration here consists of a series of exams taken two years apart. The binary indicators Y correspond to the presence ($Y = 1$) or absence ($Y = 0$) of Left Ventricular Hypertrophy (LVH) diagnosed by Electrocardiogram (ECG). Seventy five patients who have coronary heart disease (CHD) developed before or during the study period and who have not received diuretics are included in the study. The primary interest is to study the association between LVH measured over an eight year period and a covariate systolic blood pressure (SBP) (X) after adjusting for other control covariates Z, namely age, smoking status, body mass index and exam number with values 1–4. The SBP measures were transformed to log(SBP-50) as suggested in Carroll, et al (1995) to achieve approximately normality.

The number of clusters (in this case individuals) is $m = 75$. Most individuals have $n = 4$ observations, although some have fewer. The total number of observations is 271.

As noted previously, a parametric structural analysis in the GLMMeM framework consists of three parts.

1. The model for $\mathbf{Y}_i$ given $(\mathbf{X}_i, \mathbf{Z}_i)$ used here is a logistic GLMM with a cluster level random intercept having variance θ. Thus, given mean zero random effects b_i with variance θ, Y_{ij} follows a logistic model with mean $H(b_i + \beta_0 + \beta_x X_{ij} + \mathbf{Z}_{ij}^T \beta_z)$, where $H(\cdot)$ is the logistic distribution function.

2. The model for $\mathbf{X}_i$ given $\mathbf{Z}_i$ is a linear GLMM with a cluster level random intercept having variance $\sigma_{x\mu}^2$. Thus, given mean zero random effects e_i with variance $\sigma_{x\mu}^2$, the X_{ij} are independent and follow a linear model with mean $e_i + \gamma_0 + \mathbf{Z}_{ij}^T \gamma_z)$ and variance σ_x^2.

3. A reasonable model for measurement error is that the errors are independent, so that W_{ij} given X_{ij} is normally distributed with mean X_{ij} and variance σ_u^2.

4. In sum, the parameters are $(\beta_0, \beta_x, \boldsymbol{\beta}_z, \gamma_0, \boldsymbol{\gamma}_z)$ (fixed effects) and $(\theta, \sigma^2_{x\mu}, \sigma^2_x, \sigma^2_u)$ (random effects).

Note that in the functional approach, the assumptions in step 2 are not made. Model robustness is thus achieved, albeit at the possible loss of efficiency.

Under the structural model, within a cluster the W_{ij}'s have mean $\gamma_0 + \mathbf{Z}_{ij}^T\gamma_1$, variance $\sigma^2_x+\sigma^2_u+\sigma^2_{x\mu}$ and covariance $\sigma^2_{x\mu}$. A standard linear–GLMM analysis thus yields estimates of $(\gamma_0, \gamma_1, \sigma^2_{x\mu}, \sigma^2_x+\sigma^2_u)$. CGLW report strong evidence in favor of the heterogeneous model, finding that the residuals from regressing W on Z have approximately 2/3 of their observed variability due to cluster–to–cluster variation, i.e., $\sigma^2_{x\mu} > 0$. In addition, $\gamma_1 \neq 0$, since observed blood pressure W depends on body mass index, a component of Z.

3.2 Identifiability

As noted above, neither σ^2_x nor σ^2_u but only their sum are identified from $(\mathbf{W}, \mathbf{Z})$ observations alone. It can be shown that identifiability holds if one takes into account the logistic–GLMM for $(\mathbf{Y}, \mathbf{W}, \mathbf{Z})$ as well as the assumed normality in the linear–GLMM for $(\mathbf{X}, \mathbf{Z})$. It is however, little comfort from a modeling robustness viewpoint to note that identifiability of the measurement error variance depends so heavily on the model specifications relating $(\mathbf{Y}, \mathbf{X}, \mathbf{Z})$.

We believe that experiments should be designed so that the measurement error variance σ^2_u can be identified from observations on $(\mathbf{W}, \mathbf{Z})$ alone. In this example, such a design would have some replicated SBP's at additional times close to each of the regular exams, so as to capture the daily variation inherent in SBP's. By identifying the error properties via replication independent of the response and any assumed distribution for unobserved covariates, one has a realistic opportunity to check the logistic–GLMM.

Because we want to compare the results to the functional methods of CGLW, for illustrative purposes here we assume that a person's true SBP does not change after taking into account $\mathbf{Z}$, so that all within–person variability is due to measurement error and secular time trends, and hence $\sigma^2_x = 0$, and $X_{ij} = X_{i1}$. This is obviously an oversimplification, but likely to be not too far from the mark.

3.3 Model Fitting

We estimated all the remaining parameters using a Bayesian analysis via Gibbs sampling, using the following steps.

1. We first standardized W and each component of $\mathbf{Z}$ so that they have mean zero and variance 1 in the data.

2. The fixed effect parameters $(\beta_0, \beta_x, \beta_z, \gamma_0, \gamma_z)$ had independent proper but essentially noninformative normal priors with mean zero and standard deviation 10.

3. The random effect parameters $(\theta, \sigma^2_{x\mu} \sigma^2_u)$ had independent but essentially noninformative inverse–gamma priors with shape 0.01 and scale 100.

4. Starting values for $(\gamma_0, \gamma_1, \sigma^2_{x\mu}, \sigma^2_u)$ were obtained from a GLMM regression of W on $\mathbf{Z}$.

5. Starting values for $(\beta_0, \beta_x, \beta_z, \theta)$ were obtained from the SIMEX analysis of CGLW.

6. For those conditionals in the Gibbs sampler which were not completely specified, we used Metropolis–Hastings steps.

7. The sampler was run 10,000 times, with a burn–in period of 2,000 steps.

We describe here only the estimate of θ (the variance component). The CPQL–SIMEX, maximum likelihood and Bayesian posterior median estimates of θ were 1.85, 2.20 and 2.33, respectively. The posterior mode is approximately 2.10 as obtained from a kernel density estimate in Splus with the parameter width=1.0, indicating some shrinkage from the maximum likelihood estimate. The lower value of the SIMEX estimate is probably due to CGLW's choice of CPQL as the basic method of fitting.

This posterior kernel density estimate for θ is plotted in Figure 2. It is as expected somewhat skew, with a posterior standard deviation of 0.96. In contrast, for the CPQL–SIMEX method, CGLW found an estimated standard deviation of 1.52 for their estimate of θ. The decrease in standard deviation for the structural–Bayes estimator most likely has much to do with the structural assumptions we have made.

4 Discussion

There are three essential points that need to be kept in mind when considering a GLMMeM.

- The effect of ignoring measurement error depends on the within cluster sample sizes. Typically, biases are more pronounced when the within–cluster sample sizes are large.
- The simplest likelihood structure involves three GLMM's, one for Y given (X, W), one for W given (X, Z) and one for X given Z. Functional approaches require the first two models, but not the third.

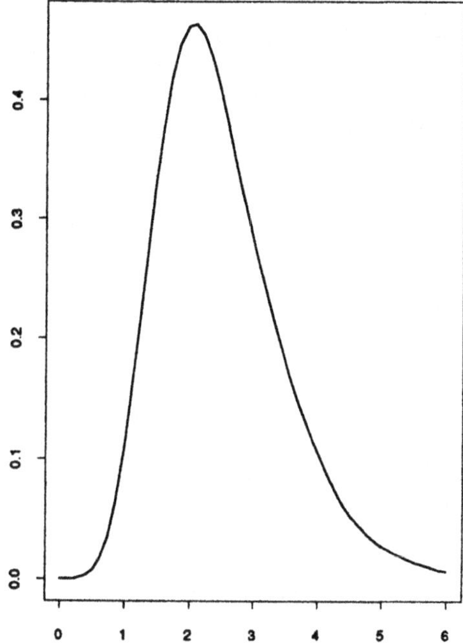

FIGURE 2. Kernel density estimate of the posterior for θ, the variance component in the Framingham data.

- Efficient estimation of all parameters is often compromised by study design. Typically, additional data focusing particularly on the measurement error are required to estimate measurement error structure effectively from the observed covariates only.

5 REFERENCES

[1] Breslow, N. E., and Clayton, D. G. (1993), "Approximate Inference in Generalized Linear Mixed Models," *Journal of the American Statistical Association*, **88**, 9-25.

[2] Breslow, N. E., and Lin, X. (1995), "Bias Correction in Generalized Linear Mixed Models With a Single Component of Dispersion," *Biometrika*, **82**, 81-91.

[3] Carroll, R. J., Küchenhoff, H., Lombard, F., & Stefanski, L. A. (1996). Asymptotics for the SIMEX estimator in structural measurement error

models. *Journal of the American Statistical Association*, **91**, 242–250.

[4] Carroll, R. J., Gutierrez, R. G., Lin, X. and Wang, N. (1996). Bias analysis and SIMEX inference in generalized linear mixed measurement error models. Submitted.

[5] Carroll, R. J., Ruppert, D. and Stefanski, L. A. (1995), *Measurement Error in Nonlinear Models*, Chapman and Hall: London.

[6] Cook, J. & Stefanski, L. A. (1995). A simulation extrapolation method for parametric measurement error models. *Journal of the American Statistical Association*, **89**, 1314–1328.

[7] Fuller, W. A. (1987). *Measurement Error Models.* John Wiley & Sons, New York.

[8] Lin, X. (1997). Variance components testing in generalized linear models with random effects. *Biometrika*, to appear.

[9] Lin, X., and Breslow, N. E. (1996), "Bias Correction in Generalized Linear Mixed Models With Multiple Components of Dispersion," *Journal of the American Statistical Association*, **91**, 1007-1016.

[10] Lin, X., Wang, N. and Carroll, R. J. (1996). Exact and approximate likelihood inference in generalized linear mixed measurement error models. Submitted.

[11] Liu, Q., and Pierce, D. A. (1993), "Heterogeneity in Mantel-Haenzel-type Models," *Biometrika*, **80**, 543-556.

[12] McCulloch, C. E. (1994), "Maximum Likelihood Variance Components Estimation for Binary Data," *Journal of the American Statistical Association*, 89, 330-335.

[13] Schall, R. (1991), "Estimation in Generalized Linear Models With Random Effects," *Biometrika*, **40**, 917-927.

[14] Stiratelli, R., Laird, N., and Ware, J. (1984), "Random Effect Models for Serial Observations With Binary Response," *Biometrics*, **40**, 961-971.

[15] Wang, N., Carroll, R. J. & Liang, K. Y. (1996). Quasilikelihood and variance functions in measurement error models with replicates. *Biometrics*, to appear.

[16] Zeger, S. L., and Karim, M. R. (1991), "Generalized Linear Models With Random Effects: A Gibbs Sampling Approach," *Journal of the American Statistical Association*, **86**, 79-86.

Calculating the Appropriate Information Matrix for Log-linear Models When Data Are Missing at Random

Geert Molenberghs
Limburgs Universitair Centrum
Belgium

Michael G. Kenward *
The University of Kent
United Kingdom

ABSTRACT It is commonly assumed that likelihood based inferences are valid when data are missing at random. In his original work on this topic, Rubin defined precisely the extent to which this statement holds. In particular, the observed but not the expected information matrix can be used for frequentist inference. In the rapidly growing literature on this subject, this fact is not always appreciated. An illustration is given, in the setting of the log-linear model for correlated binary data.

Key words and phrases: dropouts, expected information, likelihood function, missing values, observed information.

1 Introduction

The classification of missing value processes, introduced by Rubin (1976) and Little (1976), is now well established. They define *missing completely at random* (MCAR) to be a process in which the probability of missingness is completely independent of the measurement process. A process is called *missing at random* (MAR) if the probability of missingness is conditionally independent of the unobserved measurements given the observed measurements. The remaining processes are termed *non-ignorable* (NI). Since then, the view has established itself that likelihood methods which

*G. Molenberghs is Assistant Professor, Biostatistics, Limburgs Universitair Centrum, Belgium. M.G. Kenward is a Reader in the Institute of Mathematics and Statistics, The University of Kent, UK

ignore the missing value mechanism are valid under an MAR process, where likelihood is interpreted in a frequentist sense.

Kenward and Molenberghs (1996) provided an exposition of the precise sense in which frequentist methods of inference are justified under MAR processes. They used the classical selection modelling framework, where the joint distribution of measurements and missingness mechanism is factorized into the marginal measurement distribution and the conditional distribution of the non-response mechanism given the measurements.

The log-linear model has an important role in the analysis of correlated binary data (Cox, 1972, Baker, Rosenberger and DerSimonian, 1992). With incomplete binary data, the non-response indicator(s) are naturally incorporated as additional factors in the log-linear model. As a consequence, the resulting likelihood does not typically have the selection modelling factorization. In spite of this, the choice of information matrix is still an issue, which we elucidate.

2 The Sampling Distributions

Let us consider first the general setting. Let the random vector $\boldsymbol{Y}$ correspond to the complete set of measurements on an individual and $\boldsymbol{R}$ the associated missing value indicator. For a particular realization of this pair $(\boldsymbol{y}, \boldsymbol{r})$ the elements of $\boldsymbol{r}$ take the values 1 and 0 indicating respectively whether the corresponding values of $\boldsymbol{y}$ are observed or not. Let $(\boldsymbol{y}_{\text{obs}}, \boldsymbol{y}_{\text{mis}})$ denote the partition of $\boldsymbol{y}$ into the respective sets of observed and missing data.

We want to study the statistical information under MCAR and MAR mechanisms. These mechanisms are defined formally as follows (Little and Rubin, 1987). Under an MCAR mechanism $\mathrm{P}(\boldsymbol{R} = \boldsymbol{r} \mid \boldsymbol{y}) = \mathrm{P}(\boldsymbol{R} = \boldsymbol{r})$ and under an MAR mechanism $\Pr(\boldsymbol{R} = \boldsymbol{r} \mid \boldsymbol{y}) = \Pr(\boldsymbol{R} = \boldsymbol{r} \mid \boldsymbol{y}_{\text{obs}})$. The log-likelihood function usually partitions as follows

$$\ell(\boldsymbol{\theta}, \boldsymbol{\beta}; \boldsymbol{y}_{\text{obs}}, \boldsymbol{r}) = \ell_1(\boldsymbol{\theta}; \boldsymbol{y}_{\text{obs}}) + \ell_2(\boldsymbol{\beta}; \boldsymbol{r}), \tag{1}$$

where $\boldsymbol{\theta}$ and $\boldsymbol{\beta}$ are parameter vectors. This partition of the likelihood has, with important exceptions, been taken to imply that, under an MAR mechanism, likelihood methods based on $\ell_1(\cdot)$ alone are valid for inferences about $\boldsymbol{\theta}$ even when interpreted in the broad frequentist sense. The precise sense in which the different elements of the frequentist likelihood methodology can be regarded as valid in general under the MAR mechanism is the subject of Kenward and Molenberghs (1996).

Under the MAR mechanism $\boldsymbol{r}$ is not an ancillary statistic for $\boldsymbol{\theta}$ in the extended sense of Cox and Hinkley (1974, p. 35) and we are not justified in restricting the sample space from that associated with the pair $(\boldsymbol{Y}, \boldsymbol{R})$. In considering the properties for frequentist procedures we have to define the appropriate sampling distribution to be that determined by this pair. We call this the *unconditional* sampling framework. Clearly, by working within this framework we do need to consider the missing value mechanism. This is to be contrasted with the sampling distribution that would apply if r were fixed by design. We call this the *naive* sampling framework.

Precision of the maximum likelihood estimators is generally derived from the information. For this either the observed information, i_O, can be used where

$$i_O(\theta_j, \theta_k) = -\frac{\partial^2 \ell(\cdot)}{\partial \theta_j \partial \theta_k}$$

or the expected information, i_E, where

$$i_E(\theta_j, \theta_k) = E\{i_O(\theta_j, \theta_k)\}. \tag{2}$$

As pointed out by Little and Rubin (1987, section 8.2.2) and Laird (1988, p. 307) the use of the observed information matrix implicitly assumes the unconditional framework and hence its inverse is valid as an estimate of the asymptotic variance-covariance matrix. In contrast, to calculate the expected information matrix the sampling framework must be made explicit. In other words, the expectation needs to be taken over the unconditional sampling distribution while the use of the naive sampling framework can lead to inconsistencies.

As stated earlier, the log-linear model does not enjoy the classical likelihood factorization (1). The contrast between the unconditional and naive sampling frameworks need to be reconsidered in the light of this. In the next section, this will be done for the simple setting of a bivariate outcome with non-response confined to one component.

3 A Log-Linear Model for Bivariate Binary Data

Suppose that each member of the pair of observations (Y_{i1}, Y_{i2}), from unit i, $i = 1, \ldots n$, is a binary random variable. Let Y_{i1} always be observed and let R_i be a binary random variable indicating whether Y_{i2} is observed ($R_i = 1$) or not ($R_i = 0$). The joint probability mass function for (Y_{i1}, Y_{i2}, R_i) can be represented as a conventional log-linear model:

$$\begin{aligned} p(y_1, y_2, r) &= \frac{1}{D}\exp(\theta_1 y_1 + \theta_2 y_2 + \theta_{12} y_1 y_2 \\ &\quad + \eta r + \eta_1 y_1 r + \eta_2 y_2 r + \eta_{12} y_1 y_2 r), \end{aligned} \tag{3}$$

where D is the normalizing constant. As we are confining attention to an MAR mechanism, which implies conditional independence of R_i and Y_{i2}, given Y_{i1}, model (3) reduces to

$$p(y_1, y_2, r) = \frac{1}{D}\exp(\theta_1 y_1 + \theta_2 y_2 + \theta_{12} y_1 y_2 + \eta r + \eta_1 y_1 r), \tag{4}$$

where

$$D = 1 + e^{\theta_1} + e^{\theta_2} + e^{\theta_1+\theta_2+\theta_{12}} + e^{\eta} + e^{\theta_1+\eta+\eta_1} + e^{\theta_2+\eta} + e^{\theta_1+\theta_2+\theta_{12}+\eta+\eta_1}.$$

For a detailed exploration of the use of this type of log-linear model in missing data settings, see Baker et al (1992).

The log-likelihood for a sample of n units, of which m are observed on both occasions is

$$\begin{aligned} \ell &= \sum_{i=1}^{m} \{\theta_1 y_{i1} + \theta_2 y_{i2} + \theta_{12} y_{i1} y_{i2} + \eta + \eta_1 y_{i1} - \ln D\} \\ &\quad + \sum_{i=m+1}^{n} \{\theta_1 y_{i1} + \ln\left[1 + \exp(\theta_2 + \theta_{12} y_{i1})\right] - \ln D\}. \end{aligned} \quad (5)$$

Our aim is to compare the naive and unconditional information for both main effect parameters θ_1 and θ_2. For θ_1, the score function is

$$S(\theta_1) = \sum_{i=1}^{n} (y_{i1} - p_1),$$

where $p_1 = \mathrm{P}(Y_{i1} = 1)$. It follows immediately that the observed information is equal to $i_O(\theta_1) = np_1(1-p_1)$, and hence that the naive and unconditional information must coincide for θ_1: $i_N(\theta_1) = i_U(\theta_1) = i_O(\theta_1)$. Note that this does not imply that the estimated variances for θ_1 will coincide under both frameworks, because they depend on other elements through the process of matrix inversion.

Turning attention to θ_2, the score function becomes

$$S(\theta_2) = \sum_{i=1}^{m} (y_{i2} - p_2) + \sum_{i=m+1}^{n} (q_i - p_2),$$

where $p_2 = \mathrm{P}(Y_{i2} = 1)$ and

$$q_i = q(y_{i1}) = \frac{e^{\theta_2+\theta_{12} y_{i1}}}{1 + e^{\theta_2+\theta_{12} y_{i1}}}.$$

The observed information is then

$$i_O(\theta_2) = np_2(1-p_2) - \sum_{i=m+1}^{n} q_i(1-q_i). \quad (6)$$

We now make precise what is meant by the naive framework. The naive information is obtained from (6) by taking expectations of $q_i(1-q_i)$ over the marginal distribution of Y_{i1}. This means, marginal over Y_{i2} and the missingness indicator R_i. In contrast to the selection model setting, this marginal distribution still involves the parameters associated with R_i. The expectation equals $p_1 q(1)[1-q(1)] + (1-p_1)q(0)[1-q(0)]$. After some algebra, we get

$$\begin{aligned} i_N(\theta_2) &= np_2(1-p_2) - (n-m) \\ &\times \left[\frac{(1+e^{\eta+\eta_1})}{D} e^{\theta_1} \frac{e^{\theta_2+\theta_{12}}}{1+e^{\theta_2+\theta_{12}}} + \frac{(1+e^{\eta})}{D} \frac{e^{\theta_2}}{1+e^{\theta_2}} \right]. \end{aligned} \quad (7)$$

The unconditional information is derived in two steps. First we obtain the conditional expectation of (6) with respect to $Y \mid R$. This is based on the calculation of

$$\mathrm{P}(Y_{i1}=1|R_i=0)q(1)[1-q(1)] + [1-\mathrm{P}(Y_{i1}=1|R_i=0)]q(0)[1-q(0)].$$

Again, some manipulations lead to

$$i_U(\theta_2) = np_2(1-p_2) - (n-m)\left[\frac{1}{D_1} e^{\theta_1} \frac{e^{\theta_2+\theta_{12}}}{1+e^{\theta_2+\theta_{12}}} + \frac{1}{D_1} \frac{e^{\theta_2}}{1+e^{\theta_2}} \right], \quad (8)$$

where $D_1 = 1 + e^{\theta_1} + e^{\theta_2} + e^{1+\theta_1+\theta_2+\theta_{12}}$. Taking expectations over R_i replaces the factor $(n-m)$ with $n\mathrm{P}(R_i=0) = nD_1/D$. However, when estimating $n\mathrm{P}(R_i=0)$ in practice we would recover $n-m$. Hence, it follows that to study differences between (7) and (8), this factor can be ignored.

It can be shown that, when $\theta_{12}=0$, $i_N(\theta_2)$ and $i_U(\theta_2)$ are equal. In this case, Y_{i2} is independent of both Y_{i1} and R_i and the trivariate outcome splits into two independent groups: (Y_{i1}, R_i) and Y_{i2}. As a consequence, missingness in Y_{i2} is MCAR. Equality also holds (whether or not θ_{12} is zero) when $\eta_1 = 0$, because then $D = (1+e^{\eta})D_1$. In this case, whether or not Y_{i1} and Y_{i2} are correlated, $\eta_1 = 0$ is equivalent to MCAR.

In Table 1, we give a numerical illustration of the fact that naive and unconditional expectations need not be the same when $\theta_{12} \neq 0$ and $\eta_1 \neq 0$. The table contains the ratio $i_N(\theta_2)/i_U(\theta_2)$ for a range of values for θ_{12} and η_1 and with all other model parameters equal to zero. In addition, a small simulation study is conducted. For each of the (θ_{12}, η_1) combinations, 1000 samples of size 500 are generated. The average observed information matrix for each simulation is called i_O. The table shows $i_O(\theta_2)/i_U(\theta_2)$. We clearly see that there is a (small) discrepancy between naive and unconditional information when θ_{12} and η_1 move away from 0. For the most extreme situation ($\theta_{12} = 2$ and $\eta_1 = -2$) the probability of dropout is 0.19 given the first outcome was a success and 0.64 given it was a failure. In contrast, the behaviour of the observed information agrees closely with the (correct) information derived within the unconditional framework.

4 Concluding Remarks

In spite of an early awareness of problems with conventional likelihood-based frequentist inference in the MAR setting, it seems that an apprecia-

TABLE 1. Ratio of naive and unconditional information, and ratio of observed and unconditional information for θ_2, given $\theta_1 = \theta_2 = \eta = 0$, for a range of selected values of θ_{12} and η_1. The observed information is calculated from 500 simulated samples of size 1000.

	η_1				
θ_{12}	-2	-1	0	1	2
			$i_N(\theta_2)/i_U(\theta_2)$		
-2	0.9181	0.9469	1.0000	1.0613	1.0869
-1	0.9618	0.9764	1.0000	1.0205	1.0228
0	1.0000	1.0000	1.0000	1.0000	1.0000
1	0.9411	0.9689	1.0000	1.0144	1.0118
2	0.8486	0.9208	1.0000	1.0349	1.0277
			$i_O(\theta_2)/i_U(\theta_2)$		
-2	1.0043	0.9931	1.0083	0.9847	1.0012
-1	0.9981	1.0109	0.9936	1.0069	1.0016
0	1.0101	0.9968	0.9924	0.9934	1.0028
1	0.9894	1.0102	0.9848	1.0044	1.0021
2	0.9884	1.0012	1.0070	1.0085	0.9976

tion of this has diminished while the number of methods formulated to deal with the MAR situation has risen dramatically. A restatement and exposition of this issue has been given in Kenward and Molenberghs (1996) in the context of selection models. Here, we see that a parallel problem exists in convential log-linear models for correlated binary outcomes with a binary missingness indicator. The different status of the observed information and the conventional expected information (called the naive information in this work) has been clearly shown by contrasting both with the expected information, where the expectation takes the missingness pattern into account (referred to as the unconditional information). We can in practice circumvent the problem with the expected information matrix by using the observed information matrix.

5 References

[1] Baker, S.G., Rosenberger, W.F., Dersimonian, R. (1992). Closed-form estimates for missing counts in two-way contingency tables. *Statistics in Medicine*, 11, 643–657.

[2] Cox, D. R. (1972). The analysis of multivariate binary data. *Applied Statistics*, **21**, 113–120.

[3] Cox, D.R., Hinkley, D.V. (1974). *Theoretical Statistics.* London: Chapman and Hall.

[4] Kenward, M.G., Molenberghs, G. (1996). Likelihood based frequentist inference when data are missing at random. *Submitted for publication.*

[5] Laird, N.M. (1988). Missing data in longitudinal studies. *Statistics in Medicine*, **7**, 305–315.

[6] Little, R.J.A. (1976). Inference about means for incomplete multivariate data. *Biometrika*, **63**, 593–604.

[7] Little, R.J.A., Rubin, D.B. (1987). *Statistical Analysis with Missing Data.* New York: Wiley.

[8] Rubin, D.B. (1976). Inference and missing data. *Biometrika*, **63**, 581–592.

Nonparametric Regression in the Presence of Correlated Errors

J. D. Opsomer *

Iowa State University

United States

ABSTRACT Most automated bandwidth selection methods for nonparametric regression break down in the presence of correlated errors. This problem has been previously studied in the context of kernel regression and the fixed, equidistant design. This article generalizes these results by addressing the problem for local linear regression and allowing for a random design. In this setting, we show that when the errors are correlated, the asymptotically optimal bandwidth for local linear regression depends on the integrated covariance function. A nonparametric plug-in bandwidth estimator that takes this effect into account is proposed. The resulting bandwidth estimator shares many of the same properties in the presence of autocorrelation as traditional plug-in estimators possess when the errors are independent. The extension to the spatial setting is discussed and a simple plug-in bandwidth selection without asymptotic optimality properties is proposed in this case. Two examples are used to demonstrate the proposed bandwidth selection algorithm.

Key words and phrases: Local linear regression, bandwidth selection, spectral density estimation, nitrogen runoff.

1 Introduction

In nonparametric regression, the researcher is typically interested in estimating the mean function $E(Y|X = x) = m(x)$ based on observations $(X_1, Y_1), \ldots, (X_n, Y_n)$, with the X_i either univariate or multivariate. While nonparametric regression allows the researcher to estimate this function without specifying a parametric shape, (s)he still has to select a value for

*The research for this article was partially supported by the Center for Agricultural and Rural Development at Iowa State University. Address: Snedecor Hall, Ames, IA 50014. Email: jopsomer@iastate.edu

the smoothing parameter, often referred to as the *bandwidth*. This introduces an unwanted element of arbitrariness in the estimation procedure, since it is often unclear what the "right" bandwidth choice for a specific data set should be. Several bandwidth selection methods are available, but they typically require that the errors be independently distributed.

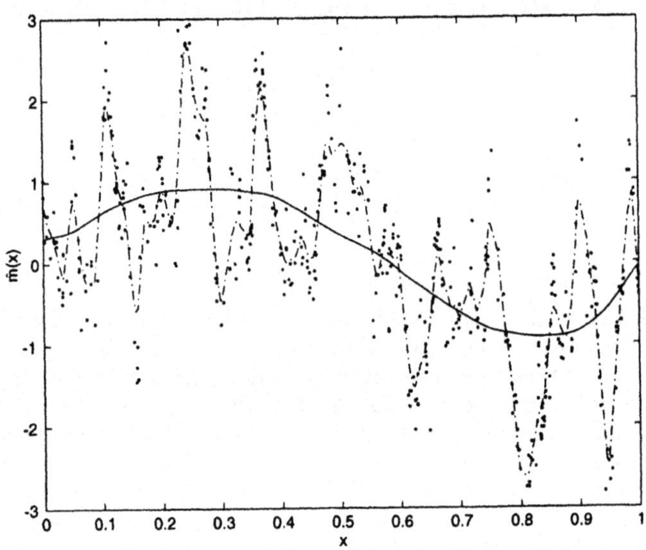

FIGURE 1. Simulated data and estimated mean functions using CV (–·) and CDPI(–).

A simulated example will illustrate the effect of correlation on the bandwidth selection. In Figure 1, data is generated by a simple polynomial trend, and overlaid with errors that follow an AR(1) model. Cross-validation (CV), the most commonly used bandwidth selection method, selects a bandwidth that is far too small and results in an overly "wriggly" estimated mean function in Figure 1. The larger bandwidth selected by the CDPI method developed in this article produces an estimate that is much closer to the true mean function in the data. The reason for the poor performance of cross-validation is easy to understand, since its goal is to minimize the *prediction* error for the dataset, not the *estimation* error. This means that CV attempts to capture all the trend in the data to achieve the best possible function for generating new points from the same random process, resulting in the almost "interpolating" fit seen in Figure 1. Conversely, CDPI allows for short-range structure in the data to be due to correlation and chooses a bandwidth that filters out these short-range effects. Its goal is not optimal prediction but instead optimal estimation (when the errors are independent, the distinction between prediction and estimation vanish, at least in the context of bandwidth selection).

In kernel regression, a number of authors have also shown that correlation leads to the "wrong" choice for the bandwidth parameter, and proposed various methods to remedy the situation (see Opsomer (1995) for an overview of this literature). While providing valuable insights in the problem of nonparametric regression in the presence of correlated errors, all these authors assumed that the observations are available on an equally spaced, fixed grid, and that the covariates are one-dimensional. This is a common setting for time series problems, but many actual datasets are comprised of randomly distributed, multi-dimensional observations that contain correlation. In addition to this somewhat restricted applicability, a methodological drawback of many of these methods is their reliance on kernel regression. Whereas local linear and kernel regression are equivalent in the fixed design case, the latter has been shown to be asymptotically inadmissible in the random design case (Wand and Jones (1995)).

The overview of the current paper follows. In Section 2, we will review the theoretical results of Opsomer (1995) on local linear regression with correlated errors. Section 3 outlines a plug-in bandwidth selection method that accounts for the presence of correlation and can be used for both the random and the fixed designs. Section 4 extends these results to the bivariate case. Examples illustrate the proposed method in Section 5.

2 Mean Squared Error Properties

We consider the following estimation problem: $(X_1, Y_1), \ldots, (X_n, Y_n)$ are a set of random variables in $\mathbb{R}^2$, generated by the process:

$$Y_i = m(X_i) + \varepsilon_i,$$

where m is a smooth function and the ε_i are random variables with $\mathrm{E}(\varepsilon_i) = 0$ and $\mathrm{Cov}(\varepsilon_i, \varepsilon_j) = \sigma^2 \rho_n(X_i - X_j)$ for all $i, j = 1, \ldots, n$, and ρ_n is a symmetric correlation function.

The correlation function ρ_n is an element of a sequence $\{\rho_n\}$ with the following properties for all n:

(P.1) ρ_n is differentiable, $\int n|\rho_n(t-x)|dt = O(1)$ and $\int n\rho_n(t-x)^2 dt = o(1)$ for all x,

(P.2) $\exists\, \xi > 0 : \int |\rho_n(t)| I_{(|t|>\xi h)} dt = o(\int |\rho_n(t)|dt)$,

where h is the bandwidth for the local linear regression. The conditions on the integrals in (P.1) and (P.2) are generalizations of the assumptions for the fixed design (e.g. Altman (1990)), which are necessary to ensure convergence of the estimators.

We introduce some notation. Define $c_n(x) = n\mathrm{E}(\rho_n(X_i - x))$, and let $[a, b]$ represent the support of X_i and f its density function. Let $\boldsymbol{X} =$

$(X_1, \ldots, X_n)^T$ and similarly for $\boldsymbol{Y}$. We use a kernel function K, and write $\mu_r(K) = \int u^r K(u)du$ for any integer $r > 0$ and $R(K) = \int K(u)^2 du$. The local linear estimator of m at a point x is defined as $\hat{m}(x) = \boldsymbol{s}_x^T \boldsymbol{Y}$, with the smoother vector $\boldsymbol{s}_x^T$ defined as

$$\boldsymbol{s}_x^T = \boldsymbol{e}_1^T (\boldsymbol{X}_x^T \boldsymbol{W}_x \boldsymbol{X}_x)^{-1} \boldsymbol{X}_x^T \boldsymbol{W}_x, \tag{1}$$

with $\boldsymbol{e}_1^T = (1, 0)$, $\boldsymbol{W}_x = \frac{1}{h}\text{diag}\{K\left(\frac{X_1 - x}{h}\right), \ldots, K\left(\frac{X_n - x}{h}\right)\}$ and

$$\boldsymbol{X}_x = \begin{bmatrix} 1 & (X_1 - x) \\ \vdots & \vdots \\ 1 & (X_n - x) \end{bmatrix}. \tag{2}$$

The standard technical assumptions on the kernel K, density f and bandwidth h for local linear regression are also required in this case. See Opsomer (1995) for details. We construct an asymptotic approximation to the conditional Mean Average Squared Error (MASE) of $\hat{m}$,

$$MASE(\hat{m}|X) = \frac{1}{n} \sum_{i=1}^{n} \mathrm{E}(\hat{m}(X_i) - m(X_i))^2.$$

Let $R_n = \frac{2n}{b-a} \int_0^{b-a} \rho_n(t)\, dt$ and define $IC_n = \sigma^2(1 + R_n)$, the *Integrated Covariance Function.*

Theorem 2.1 *The conditional Mean Average Squared Error of $\hat{m}$ is approximated by*

$$\begin{aligned} MASE(h|X) &= \left(\frac{\mu_2(K)}{2}\right)^2 h^4\, \mathrm{E}(m''(X_i)^2) + \frac{1}{nh} R(K)(b-a) IC_n \\ &\quad + o_p\left(h^4 + \frac{1}{nh}\right). \end{aligned}$$

In this result, the first term represents the asymptotic squared bias and is unaffected by the presence of correlation, while the second term is the asymptotic variance. Setting $R_n = 0$ yields the results previously derived by others under the assumption of independent errors (see Ruppert and Wand (1994)). An interesting aspect of Theorem 2.1 is that the presence of correlated errors induces an adjustment in the MASE approximations that does *not* depend on the distribution of the observations. It is easy to show that the MASE approximation is therefore valid for both random and fixed designs.

We will refer to the asymptotic MASE approximation in Theorem 2.1 as the Asymptotic MASE, or AMASE. The explicit expression for the bandwidth minimizing the AMASE is given by:

$$h_{AMASE} = \left(\frac{R(K)\,(b-a) IC_n}{n\, \mu_2(K)^2\, \mathrm{E}(m''(X_i)^2)}\right)^{1/5}, \tag{3}$$

so that the optimal rate of h is the same as when the errors are uncorrelated (Ruppert *et al.* (1995)).

3 Plug-In Bandwidth Selection

An estimator of h_{MASE} is found by replacing the unknown quantities in the asymptotic approximation (3) by estimators. This approach is known as *plug-in* bandwidth selection. The choice of estimators to plug into (3) clearly determines the properties of the bandwidth estimator. Following Ruppert *et al.* (1995), we opt for a fully nonparametric method, in which the unknown quantities are themselves estimated by nonparametric estimators. The specific implementation will generalize the *Direct Plug-In* (DPI) method of Ruppert *et al.* (1995) and will be referred to as *Correlation DPI* (CDPI), with the bandwidth estimators denoted by $\hat{h}_{DPI}$ and $\hat{h}_{CDPI}$, respectively. For proposed nonparametric estimates of $\mathrm{E}(m''(X_i)^2)$ and σ^2, see Opsomer (1995). In that article, we also show that

$$\frac{\hat{h}_{CDPI} - h_{MASE}}{h_{MASE}} = O_p(n^{-2/7}),$$

where h_{MASE} is the minimizer of the MASE. This rate is the same as the relative convergence rate for $\hat{h}_{DPI}$ when the errors are uncorrelated. We outline the estimation of IC_n here.

There exists a large literature on estimating the correlation or covariance function for univariate stationary processes, both in the time domain and the frequency domain (see Priestley (1981) for an overview). Since we are only interested in finding an estimate of IC_n for plug-in purposes, the primary objectives in developing an estimator are speed and convenience, rather than accuracy. Frequency domain estimation is therefore particularly attractive in this case, because an estimate of the integrated covariance function can, at least conceptually, be computed in a single step by estimating the spectral density at 0. However, we cannot directly apply existing spectral estimation methods, since they require equally spaced observations. Our approach to circumvent the "problem" of unequally spaced observations is inspired by the recent work by Turlach and Wand (1995) on binning approximations for local polynomial regression.

We contruct a binned dataset with approximately the same correlation structure as the original data, with the number of equally spaced gridpoints equal to $M = O(n)$. Using the notation of Turlach and Wand (1995), let $\delta = (b-a)/M$ and let $g_1 = a + \delta/2 < g_2 < \dots < g_M = b - \delta/2$ be an equally spaced grid over (a, b). We define the binning weights $w_{il} = I_{(|X_i - g_l| < \delta/2)}$ and let $c_l = \sum_{i=1}^n w_{il}$. We replace the original data $(X_i, Y_i), i = 1, \dots, n$ by the binned data $(g_l, z_l), l = 1, \dots, M$, with $z_l = \sum_{i=1}^n w_{il} Y_i / c_l$. Define the variance σ^{*2} and correlation function ρ_n^* for the binned data, and the spectral density of the errors of the binned data as $H^*(\omega) = \frac{\sigma^{*2}}{2\pi^2} \sum_{l=-\infty}^{\infty} \rho_n^*(l) e^{-il\omega}$. Under certain technical assumptions, Opsomer (1995) shows that

$$IC_n = \sigma^2 + \frac{n}{M}(2\pi H^*(0) - \sigma^2) + o(1). \tag{4}$$

We can therefore replace IC_n by the above expression in (3). Unlike in the true equidistant design case, approximation (4) also shows that because of the presence of the adjustment factor n/M, we cannot directly approximate IC_n by $H^*(0)$ but need to estimate both the spectral density at 0 and the variance parameter σ^2.

$H^*(0)$ is estimated by kernel smoothing of the periodogram, a common practice in time-series analysis (Wand and Jones (1995)). Details on the method can be found in Opsomer (1995). The approach is to (1) find a binned "pilot" fit of the mean function by nonparametric regression, (2) perform a Fourier transform of the residuals, and (3) smooth the periodogram by kernel regression with bandwidth parameter ν. The results in Opsomer (1995) provide an expression for the asymptotically optimal choice for ν. They also show that the effect of the pilot fit is asymptotically negligible, so that the periodogram smoothing methods described in standard time-series textbooks such as Priestley (1981) can be applied to the residuals of the pilot fit.

4 Extension to Bivariate Functions

The approach from Sections 2 and 3 can be extended to the spatial setting. Full derivations are in Opsomer (1995). In this case, we consider the random variables $(X_{11}, X_{21}, Y_1), \ldots, (X_{1n}, X_{2n}, Y_n)$ in $\mathbb{R}^3$ and generated by

$$Y_i = m(\boldsymbol{X}_i) + \varepsilon_i$$

where $\boldsymbol{X}_i = (X_{1i}, X_{2i})$, m is again a smooth function and the ε_i are random variables with $\mathrm{E}(\varepsilon_i) = 0$ and $\mathrm{Cov}(\varepsilon_i, \varepsilon_j) = \sigma^2 \rho_n(X_{1i} - X_{1j}, X_{2i} - X_{2j})$ for all $i, j = 1, \ldots, n$. We restrict our attention to tensor product kernels $K(u_1)K(u_2)$, so that the bandwidth parameter is now $\boldsymbol{h} = (h_1, h_2)^T$. As before, $IC_n = \sigma^2(1 + R_n)$, but $R_n = \frac{n}{(b_1-a_1)(b_2-a_2)} \int_{-(\boldsymbol{b}-\boldsymbol{a})}^{\boldsymbol{b}-\boldsymbol{a}} \rho_n(\boldsymbol{t})\, d\boldsymbol{t}$. Finally, let D_k^r represent the rth derivative operator with respect to the kth covariate. Theorem 2.1 can be generalized to:

Theorem 4.1 *The conditional MASE of $\hat{m}$ is*

$$MASE(\boldsymbol{H}|\boldsymbol{X}) = \left(\frac{\mu_2(K)}{2}\right)^2 \sum_{k=1}^{D} \sum_{l=1}^{D} h_k^2 h_l^2\, \mathrm{E}(D_k^2 m(\boldsymbol{X}_i) D_l^2 m(\boldsymbol{X}_i))$$
$$+ \frac{1}{nh_1h_2} R(K)^2 (b_1 - a_1)(b_2 - a_2) IC_n + o_p(h_1^4 + h_2^4 + \frac{1}{nh_1h_2}).$$

This MASE approximation shows that the asymptotically optimal bandwidth choice is $h_k = C_k n^{-1/6}$, a slower rate than that found for the univariate model. This dimensionality effect also has serious implications for the development of a plug-in bandwidth estimator. When the binning and periodogram smoothing approach of Section 3 is extended to the bivariate case, the effect of the pilot fit for the construction of the periodogram is no longer asymptotically negligible. A simpler plug-in without asymptotic optimality properties is therefore developed. Since no bivariate plug-in method is currently available, a generalization of the univariate *Rule of Thumb* (ROT) bandwidth selection method of Ruppert *et al.* (1995) is used and referred to as *Correlation ROT* (CROT).

5 Examples

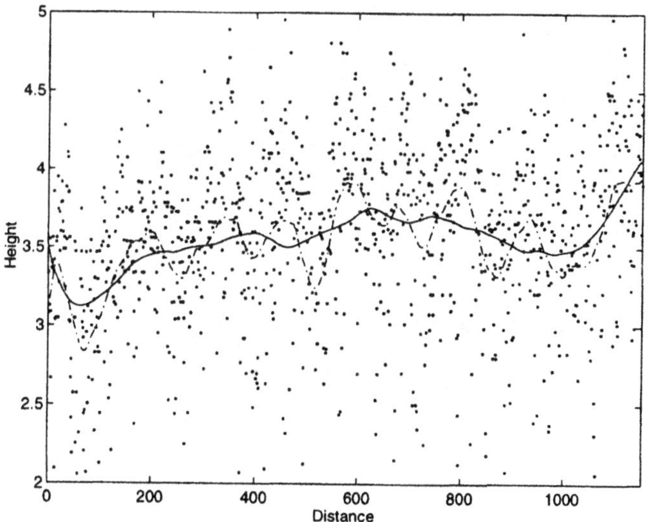

FIGURE 2. DPI (—·) and CDPI (–) fits to the Drum Roller data.

Details on the implementation of the bandwidth selection methods CDPI and CROT, including construction of pilot estimators, are provided in Opsomer (1995). We illustrate its practical behavior for univariate functions with an example previously analyzed by Laslett (1994) and Altman (1994). The data consist of 1,150 equally spaced measurements of height along a drum roller and are further described by Laslett (1994). Both authors note the presence of significant positive autocorrelation. The distance between each two observations was rescaled to be equal to 1. When cross-validation is used for bandwidth selection on these data, the estimated bandwidth $\hat{h}_{CV} = 2.09$ results in a fit that virtually interpolates between the observations, making the resulting fit essentially useless as an estimate of the underlying mean function. Figure 2 only shows the fits using DPI and CDPI, with bandwidth estimates $\hat{h}_{DPI} = 38.98$ and $\hat{h}_{CDPI} = 107.57$, respectively. While DPI performs significantly better than cross-validation in this case, the estimated function is still quite wriggly. CDPI results in the smoothest function. While it is not possible to decide which function represents the true underlying mean function when only one realization of the data-generating process is observed, a smooth function like that generated by CDPI seems the most likely to correspond to what a user of nonparametric regression would consider a "long-range trend," with the periodicities still visible in the DPI fit representing "short-range variability."

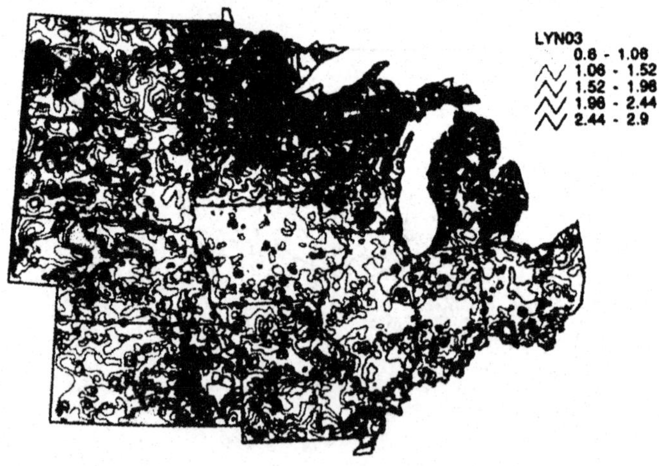

FIGURE 3. Contour plot of the transformed CARD data.

For the bivariate model, we use an spatial dataset generated by Wu *et al.* (1996) at the Center for Agricultural and Rural Development (CARD) at Iowa State University. The dataset is comprised of nitrogen runoff predictions (YN03) at 4,918 locations in the Midwest and Northern Plains of the United States. The predictions were generated by EPIC-WQ, a widely accepted biogeophysical process model developed by U.S. Environmental Protection Agency staff. Nonparametric regression provides a convenient way to perform exploratory data analysis, allowing the CARD researchers to look for spatial trends in the runoff predictions before selecting a particular parametric model. As in many spatial applications, the observations are likely to be correlated, but the exact form of the correlation function is not a priori obvious. In order to reduce the heteroskedasticity of the residuals, we follow Wu *et al.* (1996) and replace YN03 by LYN03 = $\text{YN03}^{1/3.5}$. Figure 3 shows a contour plot of the transformed data.

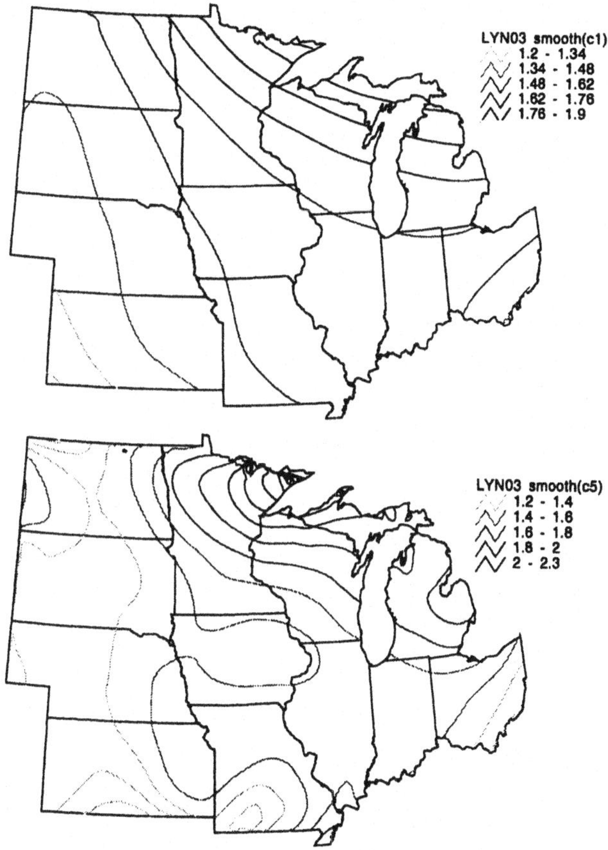

FIGURE 4. Two contour plots of the estimated mean function for the CARD data using different values for the pilot estimates.

Even though CROT avoids the problem of having to select specific values for the bandwidth parameters, it is sensitive to the choice of pilot estimators, so that the process is not completely automatic (this is in marked contrast to CDPI, which is quite insensitive to pilot estimator choice). Nevertheless, by allowing short-range variation to be captured by IC_n instead of the mean function, it is expected that CROT is relatively robust compared to a method that does not allow for correlation in the bandwidth choice. Figure 4 shows the contour maps of predicted values using the smoothest possible pilot estimator (top map), as well as the contour map for a pilot estimator that allows more variability to be captured by the mean function (bottom map). Note that the latter map displays a ridge-shaped pattern in the central and southern regions that is completely absent in the former map. Choosing between these two fits could be done using prior knowledge about the likely distribution of nitrogen runoff in the region of interest. Variograms of the residuals (not shown) from the nonparametric fits indeed indicated the presence of spatial correlation.

6 References

[1] N. S. Altman. Kernel smoothing of data with correlated errors. *Journal of the American Statistical Association*, 85:749–759, 1990.

[2] N.S. Altman. Krige, smooth, both or neither? Technical report, Biometrics Unit, Cornell University, Ithaca, NY, September 1994.

[3] G.M. Laslett. Kriging and splines: an empirical comparison of their predictive performance in some applications. *Journal of the American Statistical Association*, 89:392–409, 1994.

[4] J.-D. Opsomer. Estimating a function by local linear regression when the errors are correlated. Preprint 95–42, Department of Statistics, Iowa State University, 13 December 1995. Submitted to *Journal of the American Statistical Association.*

[5] M. B. Priestley. *Spectral Analysis and Time Series.* Academic Press, London, U.K., 1981.

[6] D. Ruppert and M. P. Wand. Multivariate locally weighted least squares regression. *Annals of Statistics*, 22:1346–1370, 1994.

[7] D. Ruppert, S. J. Sheather, and M. P. Wand. An effective bandwidth selector for local least squares regression. *Journal of the American Statistical Association*, 90:1257–1270, 1995.

[8] B. A. Turlach and M. P. Wand. Fast computation of auxiliary quantities in local polynomial regression. Manuscript, 24 April 1995.

[9] M. P. Wand and M. C. Jones. *Kernel Smoothing.* Chapman and Hall, London, 1995.

[10] J. Wu, P.G. Lakshminarayan, and B.A. Babcock. Impacts of agricultural practices and policies on potential nitrate water pollution in the Midwest and the Northern Plains of the United States. Working Paper 96–WP 148, Center for Agricultural and Rural Development, Iowa State University, February 1996.

Exploratory Modelling of Multiple Non-Stationary Time Series: Latent Process Structure and Decompositions

Raquel Prado and Mike West*

Duke University

United States

ABSTRACT We describe and illustrate Bayesian approaches to modelling and analysis of multiple non-stationary time series. This begins with univariate models for collections of related time series assumedly driven by underlying but unobservable processes, referred to as dynamic latent factor processes. We focus on models in which the factor processes, and hence the observed time series, are modelled by time-varying autoregressions capable of flexibly representing ranges of observed non-stationary characteristics. We highlight concepts and new methods of time series decomposition to infer characteristics of latent components in time series, and relate univariate decomposition analyses to underlying multivariate dynamic factor structure. Our motivating application is in analysis of multiple EEG traces from an ongoing EEG study at Duke. In this study, individuals undergoing ECT therapy generate multiple EEG traces at various scalp locations, and physiological interest lies in identifying dependencies and dissimilarities across series. In addition to the multivariate and non-stationary aspects of the series, this area provides illustration of the new results about decomposition of time series into latent, physically interpretable components; this is illustrated in data analysis of one EEG data set. The paper also discusses current and future research directions.

Key words and phrases: Dynamic latent factor model, Dynamic linear model, Non-stationary time series, Time series decomposition

---

*This research was supported in part by the National Science Foundation under grant DMS-9311071. The EEG data and context arose from discussions with Dr Andrew Krystal, of Duke University Medical Center, with whom continued interactions have been most valuable. Address for correspondence: Institute of Statistics and Decision Sciences, Duke University, Durham, NC 27708–0251 U.S.A. (http://www.stat.duke.edu)

1 Introduction

A wide variety of scientific and socio-economic problems involve study of multiple time series driven by underlying, latent processes characterising the system. In such problems, interest lies in identifying the time evolution and structure of the underlying system, as well as in characterising the univariate series and how they respond to variations in the underlying system. The notion of "exchangeable time series" (e.g., West and Harrison 1997, Section 16.4) has proven useful in some such problems, as have dynamic hierarchical models (e.g., Gamerman and Migon 1993). In other areas, a more direct approach to modelling and inference about the underlying but latent system process is of interest, leading to the notion of *dynamic factor models* that are the focus of this paper. We describe how such models are structured, and elaborate on exploratory univariate time series analyses that provide insight and inferences on underlying latent processes and cross-sectional structure. Our development involves specific, non-stationary time series models for latent processes, based on time-varying, autoregressive component dynamic models. Practical issues of model fitting and computation are briefly noted and illustrated.

One motivating problem arises from a collaboration with Duke psychiatrists studying issues of clinical design and efficacy of various brain seizure treatments, and also concerned with questions of brain function in various neurological conditions. Electroconvulsive therapy (ECT) is a major tool in brain seizure treatment and in fundamental brain research (Weiner and Krystal 1993), and EEG monitoring is the primary method of observation on brain activity during ECT (as in other contexts). ECT induced seizures are monitored by scalp electrodes measuring resulting EEG waveforms at various scalp locations, simultaneously, throughout the seizure episode. Very long EEG time series, of the order of several to a few tens of thousands of recordings, are available for individuals under varying treatment conditions, each with multiple series recorded. The data analysis summarised here comes from one experimentally induced seizure on a single individual under one treatment. We have 18 parallel series from 18 separate EEG "channels" – measured via electrodes at 18 scalp locations, and each generating a record of over 26000 voltage levels at a sampling rate of 256 observations per second. Some data from channel 4 appears in Figure 1 (see also the top time series plot in Figure 2); the general features are typical of the 18 channels, though levels and amplitudes of fluctuations over time do appear quite variable across channel. Of the 26000 plus observations on channel 4, we removed about 2000 at the start and end of the recording interval, and then subsampled the remainder every 6 observations to produce a series of 3600 observations; four sections of 500 consecutive observations from the start, end and two mid-sections of this series appear in Figure 1. Essentially indistinguishable displays are generated from the original data. The EEG time series exhibit a major pattern of quasi-cyclicity with

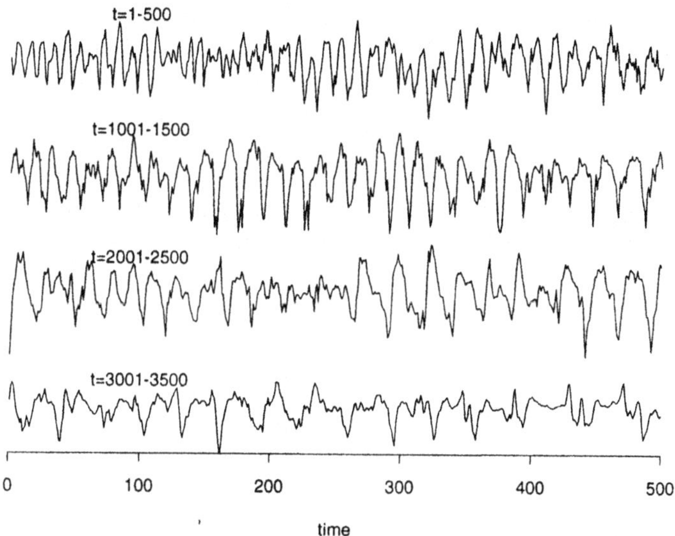

FIGURE 1. Sections of 500 consecutive observations from the recordings of EEG channel 4.

time-varying frequency characteristics, with superimposed high-frequency distortions. The appearance is quite typical of the "slow-wave" activity of epileptiform discharges, with increased amplitudes and wavelengths relative to the common alpha waves, and others, apparent in "normal" EEG traces (Dyro 1989). The frequency of the apparently dominant waveform decays through the course of the seizure, with concurrent time-variation in amplitude and decay characteristics; this represents the initial build up to peak intensity of the seizure, with correspondingly rapid oscillations in EEG levels, followed by gradual dissipation and eventual decline of the fluctuations as the seizure dies out. Modelling these patterns will bear in mind the objective of characterising the seizure through parameters that measure and reflect the level of maturity of the seizure, capturing and quantifying its rate of onset and eventual decay; inferring the beginning, duration and end of actual seizure activity is of critical interest and has proven to be a challenging problem (Weiner and Krystal 1993). Comparing such parameters across channels is of interest in exposing possible differences due to scalp placement of electrodes, and in inferring structure in the driving seizure signal through commonalities across channels. Comparison of inferences about such characterising parameters from EEG records on repeated seizures under differing treatment conditions, and across different individuals, is of further interest, though this is beyond our scope here.

It is apparent from Figure 1 that there is rough stability of the EEG waveform in short periods of perhaps one or two hundred observations, on this time scale. This holds up across channels. Exploratory analysis suggests that, within such short sections, the data appear consistent with a roughly constant AR model of order 10-15, but that the parameters differ as time evolves through the seizure episode. This indicates the global applicability of a time-varying AR model (West and Harrison 1997, Section 9.5). We develop such models below, and explore issues of time series decomposition and multivariate, dynamic factor model structure for the collection of EEG channel series.

2 Non-stationary process models

2.1 *Factor models and time-varying autoregressions*

Suppose a system under study is characterised by a latent process x_t that drives m parallel time series via

$$y_{i,t} = \beta_i x_t + \nu_{i,t} \tag{1}$$

for $i = 1, \ldots, m$ and all t. The β_i are regression parameters, or factor weights, and the $\nu_{i,t}$ assumedly independent noise sequences, here taken as zero-mean normal, $N(\nu_{i,t}|0, s_i)$ for some variances s_i.

Suppose further that the latent x_t series is a time-varying parameter autoregression (TV-AR, as in West and Harrison 1997, Section 9.5). Such models are of particular interest for long series to adapt to time-varying patterns of dependence and non-stationarities; they embody the notion of "local stationarity" but "global" non-stationarity. Specifically, assume that

$$x_t = \sum_{h=1}^{p} \phi_{h,t} x_{t-h} + \epsilon_t \quad \text{and} \quad \phi_{h,t} = \phi_{h,t-1} + \omega_{h,t}, \tag{2}$$

where $\boldsymbol{\phi}_t = (\phi_{1,t}, \ldots, \phi_{p,t})'$ is the time-varying AR parameter vector at time t and $\omega_t = (\omega_{1,t}, \ldots, \omega_{p,t})'$ is the stochastic change in the parameter vector at time t. Further assume that the error terms are independent normal, with distributions $N(\epsilon_t|0, v_t)$ and $N(\boldsymbol{\omega}_t|0, \mathbf{W}_t)$ for some sequence of AR innovation variances v_t, and variance-covariance matrices $\mathbf{W}_t$ controlling variation in $\boldsymbol{\phi}_t$. We refer to (2) as a TV-AR(p) model. This can be written as a dynamic linear model (DLM) in various ways (West and Harrison 1997, Sections 9.4 and 9.5). Variants on this model might include other forms of time-variation for $\boldsymbol{\phi}_t$, beyond this basic random walk, non-normal innovations and evolution errors for outliers and more abrupt changes in structure, and additional DLM components for time-varying trends (West 1995, 1996, 1997a,b,c).

Introduce the "instantaneous" characteristic AR polynomial $\phi_t(u) = 1 - \phi_{1,t}u - \cdots - \phi_{p,t}u^p$ for each t, and the standard back-shift operator B. Then $\phi_t(B)x_t = \epsilon_t$ and (1) implies

$$\phi_t(B)y_{i,t} = \beta_i\epsilon_t + \phi_t(B)\nu_{i,t}. \tag{3}$$

This is a time-varying parameter ARMA(p,p) model, or TV-ARMA(p,p). The TV-AR filter $\phi_t(\cdot)$ is common across series i, just the underlying structure of the latent x_t process. Hence fitting individual TV-ARMA models, or similar, to the $y_{i,t}$ should yield inferences about the AR component that are similar across series, and which may be used to identify structure in the underlying x_t process. This is a key to exploratory modelling to isolate factor structure. A practical strategy is to fit high-order TV-AR models to each of the $y_{i,t}$ series and use these to isolate the dominant TV-AR components, attributing the residual high-frequency components to the MA noise structure. This is a valuable and easily implemented strategy whose success and utility is described below in the EEG context. To be specific, suppose that $p = 4$ and we fit, say, a TV-AR(12) model to $y_{i,t}$, with AR polynomial $\phi_{i,t}(B)$ of order $p = 12$. Then we expect that $\phi_{i,t}(B) \approx \phi_t(B)\theta_{i,t}(B)$ where $\phi_t(\cdot)$ is close to the TV-AR(4) polynomial of the x_t process, and $\theta_{i,t}(B)$ represents a TV-AR(8) component that, when inverted, approximates the TV-MA(4) structure of $\beta_i\epsilon_t + \phi_t(B)\nu_{i,t}$. Our practical experience with a variety of data sets verifies the utility of this approach.

2.2 Decompositions of factor and observation processes

A most useful time series decomposition result is relevant to inference about latent structure and the partitioning of the series x_t into key components. We use this in data analysis below, though space precludes presentation of full details here. The results used generalise West (1997c) to the time-varying case and will be fully reported elsewhere; see also West and Harrison (1997, Section 9.5).

Note that $\phi_t(u) = \prod_{j=1}^{p}(1 - \alpha_{j,t}u)$ where the $\alpha_{j,t}$ are (real or complex) reciprocals of the characteristic roots at time t. Suppose, as is usual, that the roots are distinct, occurring as c pairs of complex conjugates and $r = p - 2c$ real and distinct values. Write the complex roots as $r_{j,t}\exp(\pm i\omega_{j,t})$ for $j = 1, \ldots, c$, noting that the real-valued, non-zero elements $\omega_{j,t}$ correspond to the "instantaneous" frequencies of quasi-cyclical component behaviour in the series at time t, varying over time. Write the real roots as $r_{j,t}$ for $j = 2c+1, \ldots, p$. Based on the development of similar models in DLM theory (West and Harrison 1997, Section 5.4.4), our decomposition result is that x_t may be written as the sum of $c + r$ real processes

$$x_t = \sum_{j=1}^{c} z_{j,t} + \sum_{j=1}^{r} a_{j,t} \tag{4}$$

in which the summands $z_{j,t}$ correspond to the complex roots, and the $a_{j,t}$ to the real roots. The real-valued processes $a_{j,t}$ follow individual, time-varying AR(1) models $a_{j,t} = r_{j,t}a_{j,t-1} + \eta_{j,t}$ for some zero-mean innovations $\eta_{j,t}$, (correlated across component index j). The real-valued $z_{j,t}$ processes follow quasi-periodic, time-varying ARMA(2,1) models, $z_{j,t} = 2r_{j,t}\cos(\omega_{j,t})z_{j,t-1} - r^2_{j,t}z_{j,t-2} + \gamma_{j,t}$ for additional, zero-mean innovations $\gamma_{j,t}$ that are mutually correlated and also correlated with the $\eta_{j,t}$. Based on a specified $\boldsymbol{\phi}_t$ vector and estimated or known values of x_t, extensions of the eigenanalysis results in West (1997c) apply to allow calculation of the defining quantities $r_{j,t}$ and $\omega_{j,t}$, and of the actual values of the latent component processes $a_{j,t}$ and $z_{j,t}$. The time-varying variances of the innovation sequences $\eta_{j,t}$ and $\gamma_{j,t}$ are similarly computed; these are relevant in assessing relative amplitudes of the latent components.

Under the factor model (1) it follows that the latent processes $a_{j,t}$ and $z_{j,t}$ drive the observed series $y_{i,t}$, so that fitting higher-order TV-AR models to the individual $y_{i,t}$ series should yield estimated latent processes that are similar across series (up to multiplicative constant factors β_i). This constructive result is illustrated in decomposition of EEG signals below. We note, in passing, the connections with the AR component models of West (1995, 1996).

2.3 *Multivariate dynamic factor models*

More general dynamic factor models extend (1) to include $k > 1$ latent factor processes and possibly time-varying factor weights. A dynamic, $k-$factor model has the following ingredients: label the $k-$factor processes $x_{j,t}$ for $j = 1,\ldots,k$; let $\beta_{i,j,t}$ be the (possibly time-varying) regression parameter relating $y_{i,t}$ to $x_{j,t}$; write $\mathbf{y}_t = (y_{1,t},\ldots,y_{m,t})'$ and $\boldsymbol{\beta}_{j,t} = (\beta_{1,j,t},\ldots,\beta_{m,j,t})'$ for each j and t. Then the multivariate time series $\{\mathbf{y}_t\}$ is modelled as

$$\mathbf{y}_t = \sum_{j=1}^{k} \boldsymbol{\beta}_{j,t}x_{j,t} + \boldsymbol{\nu}_t \tag{5}$$

over $t = 1,\ldots,n$, where $\boldsymbol{\nu}_t \sim N(\boldsymbol{\nu}_t|\mathbf{0},\mathbf{V})$ are independent noise terms. It will usually be appropriate to assume $\mathbf{V} = \text{diag}(V_1,\ldots,V_n)$ so that the instantaneous dependencies among the $y_{i,t}$ are due entirely to the latent factor processes $x_{j,t}$. Defining the $m \times k$ matrices $\mathbf{B}_t = [\boldsymbol{\beta}_{1,t},\cdots,\boldsymbol{\beta}_{k,t}]$ for each t, (5) can be written as

$$\mathbf{y}_t = \mathbf{B}_t\mathbf{x}_t + \boldsymbol{\nu}_t \tag{6}$$

where $\mathbf{x}_t = (x_{1,t},\ldots,x_{k,t})'$ is the latent factor vector at time t.

A rather general framework models the collection of latent processes $\mathbf{x}_t$ via a DLM. Then (6) results in a highly structured, multivariate DLM for $\mathbf{y}_t$, a fact that has modelling and technical ramifications. One important class of models is that based on lagged latent factors. Suppose that the first factor $x_{1,t} = x_t$ is a TV-AR process as above, and that additional factors are simply lagged values, namely $x_{2,t} = x_{t-1}, \ldots, x_{k,t} = x_{t-k+1}$. In this case, it easily follows that, for each i,

$$\phi_t(B) y_{i,t} = \sum_{j=1}^{k} \beta_{i,j} \epsilon_{t-j+1} + \phi_t(B) \nu_{i,t}, \tag{7}$$

so $y_{i,t}$ is TV-ARMA(p, q) with $q = \max(p, k)$. The comments about fitting higher-order TV-AR models applies here as above.

Typically, applied contexts involve far fewer factor processes than observation series, i.e., k much smaller than m. In the EEG context, for example, we surmise that a small number of underlying factor processes should explain the observed variability across the $m = 18$ channels; two primary, latent though real processes are the invoked seizure waveform and the underlying normal brain activity, respectively. We may need $k > 2$ factor processes if, for example, lagged values of these two major processes are evident in the multi-channel series.

Note that, in the case of constant parameter AR models for the latent $x_{j,t}$ processes, and with constant factor weights $\beta_{i,j,t} = \beta_{i,j}$ for all t, we are in a context close to that of the foundational theory in Peña and Box (1987), which provides useful background material.

3 Some analyses of the EEG data

Following earlier comments, we have undertaken various exploratory analyses of the 18 EEG channels individually using TV-AR(12) models. Inference is based on couching the model in DLM form and then applying standard results, as in West and Harrison (1997, Section 9.5) for example. In particular, we model time-variation in the AR parameters using discount factors, and select model order and discount factors to maximise marginal likelihood functions. Then posterior distributions for the individual TV-AR parameter vector for each series at each time point are computed using standard updating and filtering recursions (West and Harrison 1997, chapter 4); results summarised below are based on posterior means of all TV-AR coefficients. Across the 18 channels, $p = 12$ and a common discount factor of 0.994 are chosen and used in the analyses summarised here. Full details will be reported elsewhere; we note that fitting higher-order models does not materially impact the broad conclusions of interest here.

Across all 18 series, we find that posterior distributions for the TV-AR(12) parameters support moderate degrees of variation through time as the seizure begins, matures and eventually decays. Across series $i = 1, \ldots, 18$ and all time t, TV-AR polynomials exhibit and maintain two key pairs of complex conjugate roots, with moduli and arguments that vary slowly throughout the seizure. The frequencies of these two roots, though time-varying, correspond closely to the known and expected ranges of the seizure slow-wave and the basic alpha rhythm of background brain activity; as a result we identify these four roots as common. In each series at each time point, we now factor the TV-AR polynomial $\phi_{i,t}(B)$ as the product of a TV-AR(4) polynomial with these four roots, and a resulting TV-AR(8) component $\theta_{i,t}(B)$. Inverting each $\theta_{i,t}(B)$ provides an inferred, infinite-order MA representation, and we evaluate the estimated MA coefficients as functions of those of $\theta_{i,t}(B)$. This confirms that, across all channels i and over all time t, only the first three or four coefficients are non-negligible, providing support for the representation (3) and hence for the single factor structure (1) with an underlying TV-AR(4) process (2).

We illustrate the model for a single channel, number $i = 4$. Based on posterior mean estimates of the TV-AR(12) coefficients for this series, we apply the decomposition result of Section 2.2 to isolate estimated latent components. The two dominant pairs of complex-conjugate roots correspond to two quasi-cyclical TV-ARMA(2, 1) components and it happens that these two components dominate the rest in amplitude. We note a basic identification problem: any AR parameter vector generates characteristic roots, and resulting series components, that have no inherent ordering. We surmount this by summarising inferences based on ordering components by estimated amplitude. Various interesting technical and conceptual issues arise due to this inherent identifiability; for example, as amplitude, wavelength and moduli characteristics are time-varying, distinct components may switch positions under any specific ordering. Such issues will be thoroughly explored in a forthcoming article.

Figure 2 displays the first four estimated components of the channel 4 series. Figure 3 is a similar display over a short subseries in the central section of the seizure, more clearly displaying structure in the data and components. The remaining roots contribute components of lower amplitudes than those displayed. Evidently, the first component is dominant, representing the periodic forcing of aggregate transmission of cortical neural networks that drive the slow-wave EEG signal. The second component apparently contributes to the signal, though with a much lower amplitude than the primary wave. Analyses of each of the 18 EEG channels lead to very similar decompositions; channel 4 here is quite typical.

Inferences about the "instantaneous" moduli and frequencies of each of the two dominant components displayed follow directly from inferences on the TV-AR parameter vector. At the posterior mean of the AR vector, at each time point, we obtain estimates of moduli and frequency directly by computing roots of the characteristic polynomial. This is done for each of the 18 series and illustrated in Figures 4 and 5. Figure 4 displays estimates of instantaneous frequency of the dominant seizure waveform over time throughout the seizure episode and for each of the 18 channels.

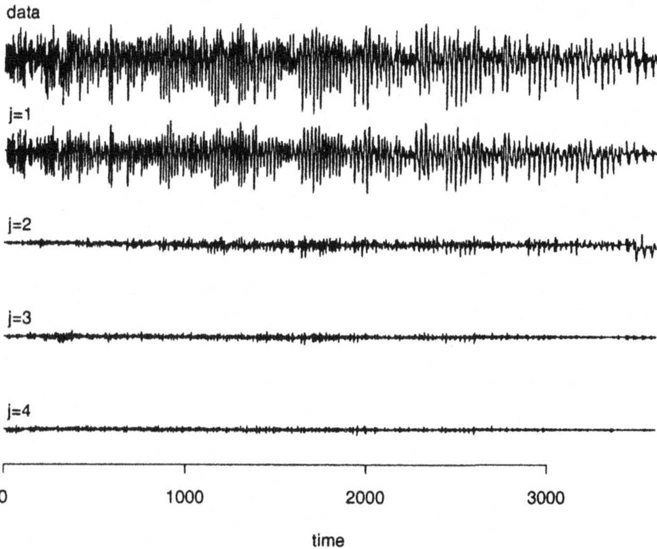

FIGURE 2. First four components of the decomposition of EEG channel 4 signal, evaluated based on posterior mean estimates of the time-varying AR parameter vector.

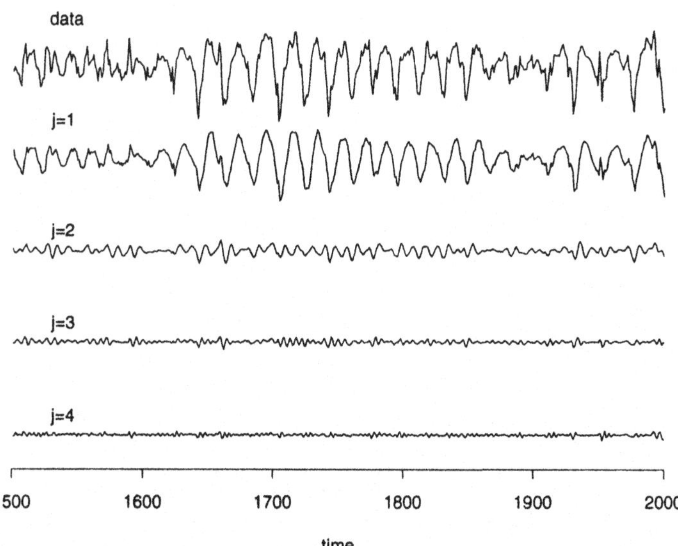

FIGURE 3. First four components of the decomposition of EEG channel 4 signal, as in Figure 2 but restricted to a central section of 500 time points.

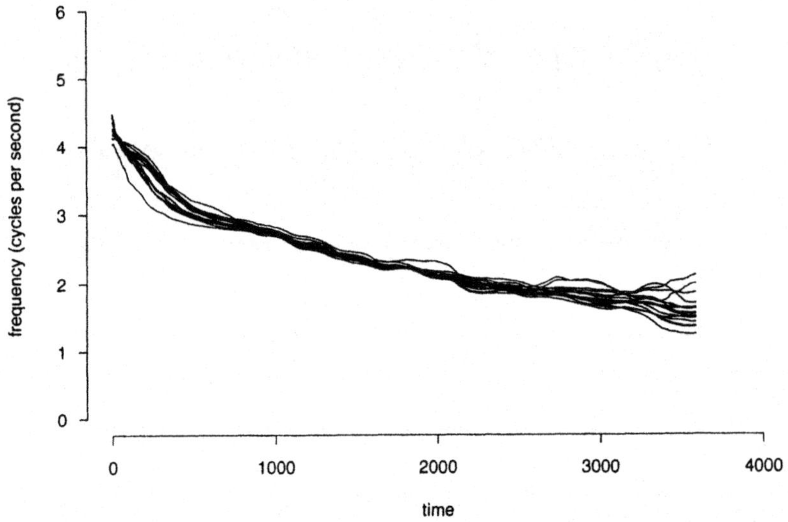

FIGURE 4. Estimated time trajectories of frequencies of the dominant quasi-cyclical components of each of the 18 EEG channels.

We note consistency of the range of frequencies evident here with known and expected ranges of 1-5 cycles per second, gradually decaying as the seizure dies out (Dyro 1989). Figure 5 provides a similar display for estimated moduli of the seizure waveform as a function of time, and for all channels. Similarly, Figure 6 graphs estimated trajectories of amplitudes of the dominant component across channels. Similar figures may be constructed for the second important component, that of the underlying alpha rhythm. The frequency trajectories lie in the 4-9 cycles per second range, consistent with expected ranges of normal brain activity.

The figures indicate that the pattern of time evolution of the dominant seizure waveform is consistent across univariate analyses of the 18 channel series: we see consistency in the decreasing frequency content, in the stable but eventually decaying modulus, and in the form of amplitude trajectories that map the onset, process of maturing and eventual decay of the seizure. Consistency of estimated frequency and amplitude trajectories, and similar consistency of estimated dominant components (not shown), support the notion of an underlying factor model (1) in which the seizure waveform is at least a component of the process x_t. There is similar consistency across channels for the second component corresponding to the background brain activity. Hence we conclude that figures (4-6) give an overall, exploratory description of the nature of the seizure episode, and that an underlying,

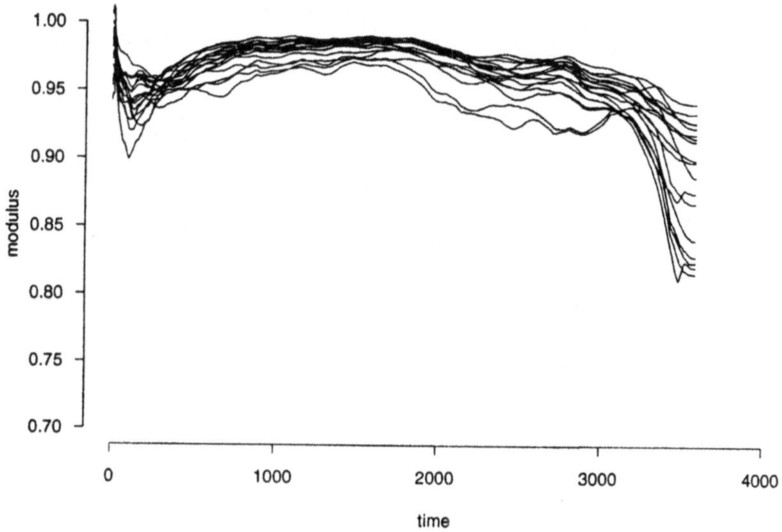

FIGURE 5. Estimated time trajectories of moduli of the dominant quasi-cyclical components of each of the 18 EEG channels.

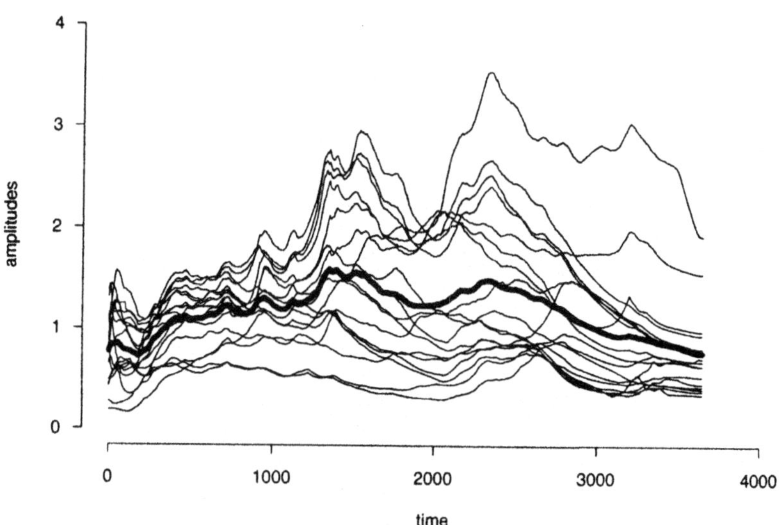

FIGURE 6. Estimated time trajectories of amplitudes of the dominant quasi-cyclical components of each of the 18 EEG channels. The full line through the trajectories represents the average.

latent seizure process contains a seizure signal with frequency, modulus and amplitude characteristics varying as some average of the three sets of trajectories graphed.

The simplest "candidate" factor model, therefore, is a single factor model as in (1) in which the latent driving process x_t is TV-AR(4) with complex root structure generating the decomposition into two quasi-periodic TV-ARMA(2, 1) subseries; these two subseries represent the seizure slow-wave and background alpha rhythm, as identified and described above. Were this appropriate then, as discussed earlier, the TV-AR(12) models for each of the channels would approximately decompose into these two subseries plus low amplitude, higher frequency components; we have seen that this is the case. However, the data exhibit more complex structure. Under this candidate model, (1) implies a simple linear regression of each of the $y_{i,t}$ on the average series $\bar{y}_t = \sum_{i=1}^{18} y_{i,t}/18$, and with each regression having zero-mean and independent errors. This can be directly assessed, and is found to be wanting; residual time series from such simple linear models evidence residual quasi-periodicities reflecting both seizure and alpha rhythms. This suggests a more elaborate, multi-factor structure in which two separate latent processes drive the data, i.e., a model of the form (5) in which $x_{1,t}$ is a TV-AR(2) "seizure" process and $x_{2,t}$ is a TV-AR(2) "alpha rhythm" process. Even with constant factor weights $\beta_{i,j,t} = \beta_{i,j}$ for all t, each channel i and factors $j = 1, 2$, this model is quite substantially more complex; accepting that time-varying factor weights may be of relevance too adds further complications. More formal approaches to analysis of these more complex but, as illustrated here, practically very relevant multivariate models is under current investigation. This development will involve generalisation of the framework, and resulting Bayesian simulation methods of analysis, in West (1996, 1997c). Nevertheless, the style of exploratory modelling and analysis illustrated here has been of key importance in elucidating the structure of the EEG series, as it is of similar utility in other application areas involving multiple, non-stationary time series.

4 References

[1] Dyro, F.M. (1989) *The EEG Handbook.* Little, Brown and Co., Boston.

[2] Gamerman, D., and Migon H.S. (1993) Dynamic hierarchical models. *Journal of the Royal Statistical Society, Series B*, 55, 629-642.

[3] Krystal, A.D. and Weiner, R.D. (1994) ECT seizure therapeutic adequacy. *Convulsive Therapy*, 10, 153-164.

[4] Krystal, A.D., Weiner, R.D., McCall, W.V., Shelp, F.E., Arias, R. and Smith, P. (1993) The effects of ECT stimulus dose and electrode place-

ment on the ictal electroencephalogram: An intraindividual crossover study. *Biological Psychiatry*, 34, 759-767.

[5] Peña, D., and Box, G.E.P. (1987) Identifying a simplifying structure in time series. *Journal of the American Statistical Association*, **82**, 836-843.

[6] Pole, A., West, M., and Harrison, P.J. (1994) *Applied Bayesian Forecasting and Time Series Analysis*. Chapman-Hall, New York.

[7] Weiner, R.D., and Krystal, A.D. (1993) EEG monitoring of ECT seizures. In *The Clinical Science of Electroconvulsive Therapy*, American Psychiatric Press, Inc., 93-109.

[8] West, M. (1995) Bayesian inference in cyclical component dynamic linear models. *Journal of the American Statistical Association*, **90**, 1301-1312.

[9] West, M. (1996) Some statistical issues in Palæoclimatology (with discussion). In *Bayesian Statistics 5*, (eds: J.O. Berger, J.M. Bernardo, A.P. Dawid and A.F.M. Smith), Oxford University Press.

[10] West, M. (1997a) Bayesian time series: Models and computations for the analysis of time series in the physical sciences. In *Maximum Entropy and Bayesian Methods 15*, (eds: K. Hanson and R. Silver), Kluwer.

[11] West, M. (1997b) Modelling and robustness issues in Bayesian time series analysis (with discussion). In *Bayesian Robustness 2*, (eds: J. Berger, F. Ruggeri, and L. Wasserman), IMS Monographs.

[12] West, M. (1997c) Time series decomposition. Under review at *Biometrika*.

[13] West, M., and Harrison, P.J. (1997) *Bayesian Forecasting and Dynamic Models* (2nd Edition). Springer-Verlag, New York.

Modeling Correlations Between Diagnostic Tests in Efficacy Studies with an Imperfect Reference Test

Yinsheng Qu
The Cleveland Clinic Foundation
United States

Alula Hagdu
Centers for Disease Control and Prevention
United States

ABSTRACT: In the Chlamydia trachomatis (CT) study, we compare five screening tests in terms of sensitivity and specificity for detecting CT in endocervical specimens. The five tests are correlated, and the reference test (cell culture test) is subject to error. The conventional method which ignores both the correlations between the tests and the misclassifications of the reference test cannot provide valid analysis. We propose a model by which one can evaluate and compare the sensitivities and specificities for correlated diagnostic tests with an imperfect reference test, or even without any reference test. We use a hybrid algorithm, which consists of the expectation maximization (EM) algorithm and the Newton-Raphson method, for its maximum likelihood estimation.

Key words and phrases: EM algorithm, finite mixture models, sensitivity, specificity.

1 Introduction

The purpose of an efficacy study is to evaluate and compare the sensitivities and specificities for several diagnostic tests. The disease status of each subject is diagnosed by using a reference test. The conventional method is based on two assumptions: (1) the diagnostic tests are independent of each other within the diseased and the non-diseased populations; (2) the reference test is error free. In reality, however, the diagnostic tests are often correlated within the diseased and the non-diseased populations, and the reference test is subject to error.

Using the CT data we compare three models. Model 1 is the conventional method based on the two assumptions; Model 2 is a random-effects model assuming the reference test is error free; Model 3 is the random-effects model assuming the reference test is subject to error.

2 The Chlamydia Trachomatis Study

Five thousand women attending family planning clinics were enrolled in the study. The specimens for Chlamydia testing were collected by taking six sequential swabs from the endocervix. The first of these swabs was placed into Chlamydia culture transport medium for the culture test, which was the reference test, and the remaining 5 swabs were randomized to one of five commercial nonculture tests, which are (1) Syva DFA, (2) Syva EIA, (3) Abbot EIA, (4) Pace 2 (Gen-Probe), and (5) Pathfinder EIA (Sanofi /Kalcstad).

3 Modeling Multiple Tests

We have $K = 4853$ subjects and $n = 5$ new diagnostic tests which are Y_1, Y_2, Y_3, Y_4, Y_5. The culture test Y_6 is the reference test. The true disease status is denoted by D. The random variables $Y_1, \ldots, Y_{n+1}$, and D are dichotomous, with 1 indicating a diagnosis of having the disease by the ith test($i = 1, \cdots, n+1$), and 0 a diagnosis of not having the disease.

For the kth subject, the vector $(y_{1k}, \ldots, y_{n+1,k})'$ denotes the test results. Also, the vector $D_k = (D_{0k}, D_{1k})'$ denotes the true disease status where the indicator D_{1k} equals 1 when the kth subject has the disease and D_{1k} equals 0 when the kth subject does not have the disease. The indicator $D_{0k} = 1 - D_{1k}$.

The test accuracy may depend on some covariates. In our example, the swab number t_{ik} is a test specific covariate, which is 1 if it is the third or earlier swab and 0 if it is the fourth or later swab. The first three swabs from an infected individual contain more infectious agents and thereby have higher true positive rate than the remaining swabs.

3.1 Model 1: The Conventional Method

This conventional method assumes that (1) the new tests are independent of each other conditional on the disease status, and (2) the reference test is error free. Here $D_{1k} = y_{n+1,k}$. So, the observation $(y_{1k}, \cdots, y_{nk}, y_{n+1,k})$, can be written as (y_k', D_k), where y_k denotes $(y_{1k}, \cdots, y_{nk})'$.

Let τ_1 be the prevalence of the disease, $\tau_0 = 1 - \tau_1$, and $\theta = \log(\tau_1/\tau_0)$, then the probability of D_k is

$$f(D_k) = \prod_{d=0}^{1} \tau_d^{D_{dk}} = \exp\left(D_{1k}\theta - \log(1+e^{\theta})\right).$$

The conditional probability of y_k given D_k is

$$f(y_k|D_k) = \prod_{d=0}^{1} f(y_k|d)^{D_{dk}}, \tag{3.1}$$

where $f(y_k|d)$ is the probability of y_k given $D = d$. Let $\mu_{ik|d}$ denote the probability that $y_{ik} = 1$ given the true disease status d and the covariate t_{ik}. This positive rate is related to a linear predictor through a link function g in the framework of the generalized linear model:

$$g(\mu_{ik|d}) = \eta_{ik|d} = a_{id} + c_{id}t_{ik}, \quad i = 1, \cdots, n, \quad d = 0, 1. \tag{3.2}$$

Because the test specificity does not depend on the swab order, $c_{0i} = 0$ for $i = 1, \cdots, n$. Let

$$\theta_{ik|d} = \log \frac{\mu_{ik|d}}{1 - \mu_{ik|d}}$$

be the logit scale of the positive rate $\mu_{ik|d}$, then

$$f(y_{ik}|d) = \exp\left(y_{ik}\theta_{ik|d} - \log(1 + e^{\theta_{ik|d}})\right), \quad d = 0, 1.$$

The five tests are assumed to be independent of each other given the disease status, therefore the joint probability of y_k given $D = d$ is

$$f(y_k|d) = \exp\left(\sum_{i=1}^{n} y_{ik}\theta_{ik|d} - \log(1 + e^{\theta_{ik|d}})\right).$$

From eq(3.1),

$$\log f(y_k|D_k) = \sum_{d=0}^{1} D_{dk} \log f(y_k|d) = \sum_{d=0}^{1} D_{dk} \sum_{i=1}^{n} \left[y_{ik}\theta_{ik|d} - \log(1 + e^{\theta_{ik|d}})\right].$$

The log likelihood $\log f(y_k, D_k)$ of the kth subject is given by

$$l_k = \sum_{d=0}^{1} D_{dk} \sum_{i=1}^{n} \left[y_{ik}\theta_{ik|d} - \log(1 + e^{\theta_{ik|d}})\right] + D_{1k}\theta - \log(1 + e^{\theta}). \tag{3.3}$$

This model is simple but inaccurate. In the culture positive population the observed pair-wise correlation coefficients are about 0.5, and in the culture negative population they are about 0.13 except the correlation between tests 2 and 3, which is 0.38. The differences between the observed and the expected pairwise correlations for $(Y_2, Y_1), \cdots, (Y_5, Y_4)$ are remarkably larger than zero. The data do not support the model.

3.2 Model 2: The Random-Effects Model

In this model, the five new tests are assumed to be correlated in both the diseased and the non-diseased populations, and the reference test is still assumed to be 100 per cent correct. The correlation between tests can be explained by some unobserved factors. For example, in the diseased population, the severity of infection for each subject is not observed, but it is an important factor influencing the test results. A patient with a severe infection is more easily to be detected by all the tests than a patient with a mild or moderate infection. This unobserved variable denoted by Z causes the apparent correlation between the tests in the diseased population. We assume that Z and D are statistically independent of each other and in the population of $D = d$ $(d = 0, 1)$ Z varies among subjects as a Gaussian variable with mean zero and unknown variance σ_d^2.

Using Gauss-Hermite quadrature, the standard normal distribution is approximated by a finite discrete distribution:

$$\begin{pmatrix} z_1, \cdots, z_J \\ p_1, \cdots, p_J \end{pmatrix},$$

where z_j is the jth mass-point and p_j is the corresponding probability ($j = 1, \cdots, J$). It seems that there are J subpopulations, where each subject belongs to one of them. For the kth subject, we use the vector $Z_k = (Z_{1k}, \ldots, Z_{Jk})'$ to indicate the membership to each of the J subpopulations: if the subject belongs to the jth subpopulation then $Z_{jk} = 1$ and $Z_{sk} = 0$ for all $s \neq j$. Notice that the random-effect indicator Z_k is unobservable.

In the diseased population, given $Z = \sigma_1 z_j$ the positive rate of the ith test $\mu_{ik|1j} = \Pr(y_{ik} = 1|d = 1, z_j)$ is :

$$g(\mu_{ik|1j}) = \eta_{ik|1j} = a_{i1} + c_{i1}t_{ik} + \sigma_1 z_j, \text{ for } i = 1, \cdots, n. \tag{3.4}$$

In the culture negative population the correlations between the five tests are not as high as those in the culture positive population, except the correlation between test 2 (Syva EIA) and test 3 (Abbot EIA), which is 0.38. A plausible explanation is that these two tests are based on very similar biological processes, so that if one test makes a false positive response, the other is more likely to make the same mistake. Thus we assume that the false positive rates $\mu_{ik|0j}$ for tests 2 and 3 are related to an unobserved random-effect:

$$g(\mu_{ik|0j}) = \eta_{ik|0j} = \begin{cases} a_{i0} + \sigma_0 z_j, & \text{for } i = 2, 3 \\ a_{i0}, & \text{for } i = 1, 4, 5 \end{cases}$$

The five tests are assumed to be independent of each other given the disease status and the random-effect Z, thus the joint probability of y_k given $D = d$ and $Z = \sigma_d z_j$ is

$$f(y_k|d, z_j) = \exp\left(\sum_{i=1}^{n} y_{ik}\theta_{ik|dj} - \log(1 + e^{\theta_{ik|dj}})\right),$$

where $\theta_{ik|dj}$ is the logit of $\mu_{ik|dj}$.

The log-likelihood for the observed data (y_k, D_k) is

$$l_k = \log(f(y_k, D_k)) = \log\left(\sum_{j=1}^{J} p_j f(y_k, D_k|z_j)\right).$$

This is a finite mixture with J components and the mixing proportions p_j are known.

Compared with Model 1, the log-likelihood increases by 154.069 (Table 1). The goodness of fit improves remarkably (Table 2).

However, the assumption that the culture test is one hundred per cent sensitive is not true. People believe that like other tests the culture test is also subject to error, e.g. a mild infection may turn out to be negative.

Table 1: The MLE(standard errors) of the parameters in three models

Parameter	Model 1	Model 2	Model 3
a_{10}	-6.189(.334)	-6.189(.342)	-6.570(.450)
a_{20}	-5.612(.251)	-12.635(2.346)	-11.559(1.873)
a_{30}	-5.339(.219)	-12.193(2.291)	-11.077(1.796)
a_{40}	-5.494(.236)	-5.494(.236)	-5.674(.273)
a_{50}	-5.551(.243)	-5.551(.243)	-5.699(.266)
a_{11}	1.012(.206)	1.940(.412)	1.535(.541)
a_{21}	0.873(.207)	1.893(.425)	1.532(.550)
a_{31}	0.383(.193)	0.904(.395)	0.492(.549)
a_{41}	0.936(.212)	2.128(.435)	1.730(.561)
a_{51}	0.452(.197)	1.069(.400)	0.699(.562)
a_{61}			5.163(1.169)
c_1	0.232(.359)	1.172(.577)	1.151(.559)
c_2	0.354(.345)	0.647(.537)	0.535(.524)
c_3	0.452(.316)	0.805(.513)	0.892(.508)
c_4	0.856(.389)	1.366(.592)	1.288(.572)
c_5	0.769(.333)	1.470(.538)	1.409(.524)
σ_0		4.329(1.006)	3.774(.789)
σ_1		2.912(.317)	3.233(.563)
τ_1	0.041(.003)	0.041(.003)	0.045(.004)
log-likelihood	-1859.743	-1705.674	-1680.260

3.3 Model 3: The Random-Effects Model With Missing Disease Status

In this model, everything is the same with Model 2 except the true disease status may not be identical with the diagnosis made by the reference test. A subject with mild infection may be culture negative. Therefore we assume that the disease status D_{dk} is missing for the subjects with negative cell culture. For the subjects with positive cell culture, we still believe that the culture is right, i.e., $D_{1k} = y_{n+1,k}$.

In this model, (3.4) becomes

$$g(\mu_{ik|1j}) = \eta_{ik|1j} = \begin{cases} a_{i1} + c_{i1}t_{ik} + \sigma_1 z_j, & \text{for } i = 1, \cdots, n \\ a_{i1} + \sigma_1 z_j & \text{for } i = n+1 \end{cases}$$

Here, $\mu_{n+1,k|1j}$ is the true positive rate for the reference test, which depends on z_j.

For the subjects whose D_{dk} is missing, the log-likelihood of the observed incomplete data $(y_{1k}, \cdots, y_{nk}, y_{n+1,k})'$ is

$$l_k = \log\left(\sum_{d=0}^{1}\sum_{j=1}^{J} p_j \tau_d f(y_k|d, z_j)\right)$$

which is a finite mixture with $2J$ components with unknown mixing proportions $\tau_d \pi_j$. With this model we can compare the accuracies of diagnostic tests even without a reference test (Qu et al., 1996).

Compared with Model 2, the log-likelihood increases by 25.414 (Table 1). The plot of the correlation residuals under Model 3 is similar to that under Model 2. The estimated sensitivity of the culture test is 0.919 with standard error of 0.066 (Table 3).

4 Maximum Likelihood Estimation

For Model 1, the n binary responses are independent of each other in both the culture negative and the culture positive populations, the maximum likelihood estimates can be obtained by using the Newton-Raphson method. In Model 2 and Model 3 there are missing values (in Model 2 Z is missing, in Model 3 both Z and D may be missing) the maximum likelihood estimates (MLE) can be obtained by using the EM algorithm (Dempster, Laird and Rubin, 1977) or the Newton-Raphson method. We use the EM algorithm in the beginning for four to five iterations and then change to the Newton-Raphson method to accelerate the convergence and to get the information matrix (Aitkin and Aitkin, 1994). The scores and the information matrix for the observed incomplete data are computed from the scores and information matrix for the complete data (Louis, 1982).

Table 2: The goodness of fit for the three models

Response pattern	Observed frequency	Expected frequency in Model 1	Model 2	Model 3
000000	4328	4315.59	4322.45	4328.31
100000	7	4.43	4.44	3.49
010000	9	11.04	6.24	6.28
001000	14	16.50	11.04	11.06
000100	16	15.96	15.99	14.24
000010	15	11.63	11.65	14.84
011000	5	0.02	2.09	1.49
111110	2	0.00	0.00	0.03
000001	17	0.20	11.06	15.41
100001	5	0.36	1.89	1.96
010001	2	0.19	0.78	0.75
001001	1	0.09	0.24	0.26
000101	4	0.41	1.98	2.02
000011	3	0.22	0.85	0.85
001101	1	0.33	0.32	0.34
000111	2	0.26	0.23	2.02
100011	2	0.37	0.22	0.23
110001	6	1.10	0.77	0.83
010101	5	1.74	1.69	1.77
101001	1	1.17	0.09	0.09
011001	1	0.30	0.21	0.23
100101	1	0.26	0.17	1.93
001111	2	0.92	0.28	0.31
110101	6	5.30	3.16	3.38
110011	1	0.55	0.15	0.16
010111	1	0.88	0.49	0.54
100111	4	2.73	1.36	1.46
011011	1	0.46	0.12	0.14
011101	1	0.75	0.31	0.32
011111	6	5.63	1.93	1.88
101111	7	8.48	3.17	3.04
110111	9	12.30	7.26	6.90
111011	2	2.61	0.90	0.87
111101	9	8.27	4.88	4.62
111111	87	33.73	87.58	86.81

5 Sensitivity and Specificity

The usual definition of sensitivity of a diagnostic test is the probability of positive response for a subject who has the disease. However, this probability may be a function of observed covariates and unobserved random variables. In the CT data, the subject specific sensitivity of the ith test given the swab number indicator t_i and the "severity of infection" $\sigma_1 z_j$ is

$$\Pr(y_i = 1 | d = 1, z_j, t_i) = g^{-1}(a_{i1} + c_{i1} t_i + \sigma_1 z_j),$$

where g^{-1} is the inverse of the link function g. The population-averaged sensitivity given the covariate t_i is

$$\Pr(y_i = 1 | d = 1, t_i) = \sum_{j=1}^{J} p_j \Pr(y_i = 1 | d = 1, z_j, t_i).$$

The standard errors for the sensitivities can be obtained by the delta-method. The calculation for specificity is similar. The specificity and sensitivity (population-averaged) for each test are listed in Table 3, and the pairwise differences in sensitivities are listed in Table 4.

Table 3: The MLE(standard errors) of the specificities and sensitivities in three models

	Model 1	Model 2	Model 3
Specificity			
# 1	0.998(.001)	0.998(.001)	0.999(.001)
# 2	0.996(.001)	0.996(.001)	0.997(.001)
# 3	0.995(.001)	0.995(.001)	0.996(.001)
# 4	0.996(.001)	0.996(.001)	0.997(.001)
# 5	0.996(.001)	0.996(.001)	0.997(.001)
Sensitivity (The fourth swab or later)			
# 1	0.733(.040)	0.716(.038)	0.662(.066)
# 2	0.705(.043)	0.711(.040)	0.662(.066)
# 3	0.595(.047)	0.605(.044)	0.553(.063)
# 4	0.718(.043)	0.734(.039)	0.681(.067)
# 5	0.611(.047)	0.623(.043)	0.575(.066)
Sensitivity (The third swab or earlier)			
# 1	0.776(.051)	0.820(.040)	0.767(.065)
# 2	0.773(.048)	0.772(.042)	0.713(.072)
# 3	0.697(.053)	0.693(.046)	0.647(.070)
# 4	0.857(.040)	0.847(.037)	0.793(.067)
# 5	0.772(.047)	0.772(.042)	0.717(.068)
# 6	1.000	1.000	0.919(.066)

6 Discussion

Table 4 shows that Model 3 is the most efficient model. For instance, the difference in sensitivity between test 4 and test 3 with the fourth swab or later has variances 0.0040 for Model 1, 0.0022 for Model 2, and 0.0021 for Model 3. If the efficiency of Model 3 is 1, then the efficiency of Model 1 is $0.0021/0.0040 = 0.519$, and the efficiency of Model 2 is 0.945. Model 2 is much more efficient for comparisons of test accuracy than the conventional method, because the pairwise correlations among the tests are addressed.

The correlation problem can also be addressed by using the generalized estimating equations approach (Smith and Hadgu, 1992), if the reference test is perfect. Otherwise we need Model 3, which works when the true disease statuses are missing partially or completely. If the true disease statuses are missing completely, Model 3 becomes an extended latent class model, which will reduce to the traditional latent class model if no random-effects and no covariates are involved.

Table 4: The MLE(standard errors) for the pairwise differences in sensitivities

Difference	Model 1	Model 2	Model 3
The fourth swab or later			
#2 - #1	-0.028(.059)	-0.005(.045)	-0.000(.044)
#3 - #1	-0.139(.062)*	-0.111(.046)*	-0.109(.045)*
#3 - #2	-0.111(.064)	-0.107(.048)*	-0.109(.046)*
#4 - #1	-0.015(.059)	0.018(.043)	0.019(.042)
#4 - #2	0.013(.061)	0.023(.045)	0.020(.044)
#4 - #3	0.124(.063)	0.130(.047)**	0.128(.046)**
#5 - #1	-0.122(.062)*	-0.093(.046)*	-0.087(.044)*
#5 - #2	-0.094(.064)	-0.088(.047)	-0.087(.045)
#5 - #3	0.017(.066)	0.019(.049)	0.022(.047)
#5 - #4	-0.107(.064)	-0.111(.047)*	-0.106(.045)*
The third swab or earlier			
#2 - #1	-0.028(.070)	-0.047(.052)	-0.054(.053)
#3 - #1	-0.079(.073)	-0.127(.054)*	-0.120(.054)*
#3 - #2	-0.076(.072)	-0.080(.053)	-0.066(.053)
#4 - #1	0.081(.065)	0.028(.048)	0.027(.051)
#4 - #2	0.084(.063)	0.075(.049)	0.080(.051)
#4 - #3	0.160(.066)*	0.155(.053)**	0.147(.053)*
#5 - #1	-0.004(.069)	-0.047(.051)	-0.050(.052)
#5 - #2	-0.001(.068)	-0.000(.051)	0.004(.051)
#5 - #3	0.075(.071)	0.080(.055)	0.070(.054)
#5 - #4	-0.085(.062)	-0.075(.049)	-0.077(.051)

* : $p < 0.05$ **: $p < 0.005$

References

[1] Aitkin, M. and Aitkin, I. (1994). Efficient Computation of Maximum Likelihood Estimates in Mixture Distributions, with Reference to Overdispersion and Variance Component Models, Proc 17th Internat Biometric Con, 123-135.

[2] Dempster, A.P., Laird, N. and Rubin, D.B. (1977). Maximum likelihood from incomplete data via the EM algorithm, J R Statist Soc B, 39, 1-38.

[3] Louis, T.A. (1982). Finding the observed information matrix when using the EM algorithm, J R Statist Soc B, 44, 226-233.

[4] Qu, Y., Tan, M. and Kutner, M.H. (1996). Random effects models in latent class analysis for evaluating accuracy of diagnostic tests, Biometrics, 52, 797-810.

[5] Smith, P.J. and Hadgu, A. (1992). Sensitivity and specificity for correlated observations, Stat Med, 11, 1503-1509.

Combining Standard Block Analyses With Spatial Analyses Under a Random Effects Model

Walter T. Federer, Elizabeth A. Newton, and Naomi S. Altman*

Cornell University
United States

ABSTRACT Spatial trends are often a significant source of variability in field trials. Since trends vary from block to block, they should be estimated as random effects. In this paper we propose to consider spatial covariates as post hoc random effects within the context of the experiment design. We demonstrate that making use of the spatial information leads to more efficient estimation of treatment effects. The models considered for spatial effects include block effects which are part of the experiment design, random gradients, regression trends, nearest neighbor analysis and smoothing. The analyses are applied to an example, which exhibits quite different results for the different methods. Since computations are tedious, programs for the various statistical procedures are presented.

Key words and phrases: ANOVA, gradients, field trials, trend analysis, nearest neighbor, random effects, REML, smoothing, spatial analysis.

1 Introduction

Spatial trend is often a significant source of variation among experimental units in field trials. We propose a number of methods for accounting for smooth spatial variation which varies randomly from block to block. We demonstrate that accounting for spatial variation can improve the efficiency of estimating treatment effects, and may improve on removing row and column effects, even when the experiment has been designed to account for

*The authors can be reached at the Biometrics Unit, 434 Warren Hall, Cornell University, Ithaca, NY 14853 or by e-mail at biometrics@cornell.edu.

such effects. As well, we provide sample SAS code to obtain the maximum likelihood estimators (MLEs) of the treatment effects in the context of the linear mixed model.

A number of features of a standard analysis may alert the scientist to the need to consider spatial variation. The most effective diagnostic is often mapping the residuals on the field design. Patterns of positive and negative residuals may indicate spatial gradients. When the data are counts or indicators, a mean square error that is too large, indicating extra-Poisson or extra-Binomial variation, may also indicate the need to remove spatial trends. For some responses, the order of magnitude of the coefficient of variation is well known. For example, depending on plot size, cereal yield experiments usually have a coefficient of variation of 4–8% and maize of 8–12%. Larger coefficients of variation may also indicate an uncontrolled source of variation. See Federer (1992) for other diagnostics.

In the next section, a number of spatial analyses are introduced in the context of a lattice square experiment (Table 12.5 of Cochran and Cox, 1957). The models presented will be for this lattice square experiment, but it is straight-forward to extend the procedures to other designs and situations. The key ideas are that spatial gradients should be smooth, and that the gradients vary randomly among blocks. A designed experiment should be analyzed with spatial effects taken into account, while retaining any restrictions to randomization that were part of the design. In addition, if the experimental design is not balanced with respect to the spatial gradients, treating the gradient as a random effect may substantially alter the MLEs of the treatment effects compared to their ANOVA estimators. The MLEs may be considered the "adjusted treatment means" in analogy with the adjusted treatment means obtained from classical incomplete block analyses.

1.1 The Data

The numerical example used for the analyses was presented by Wadley (1946) and is reproduced in Table 12.5 of Cochran and Cox (1957). The data are means of counts of three samples of 100 cotton squares indicating attack or not of boll weevils. The mean count for the experiment was 11. If the counts were distributed as a Poisson variable, one would expect the residual mean square to be near $11/3 = 3.667$, since the counts are means of three samples. The anticipated coefficient of variation would be $1.91/11 = 17\%$. The experiment design is a balanced lattice square with $v = 16$ insecticide treatments arranged in $r = 4$ rows and $c = 4$ columns within each of $b = 5$ complete blocks or replicates. The randomization is restricted in such a manner as to have every ordered pair of treatments appear together once in each row and once in each column. Restrictions on randomization of treatments must be taken into account when an analysis is made. SAS code for each analysis is presented in the appendix.

2 Models for Analysis of Field Trials with Spatial Gradients

A number of models can be devised for taking into account spatial effects in field trials. In this section, we present a few possibilities. In the next section, the results of these models are discussed for the example.

2.1 Standard Textbook (ANOVA) Model

The first form of a spatial analysis is the usual textbook response model for a lattice rectangle designed experiment (See e.g., Cochran and Cox, 1957, Federer, 1955, and Kempthorne, 1952.):

$$Y_{ghij} = \mu + \beta_g + \rho_{gh} + \gamma_{gi} + \tau_j + \epsilon_{ghij} \tag{1}$$

where μ is a general mean effect, β_g is the gth replicate effect distributed with mean zero and variance σ^2_β, ρ_{gh} is the ghth row effect distributed with mean zero and variance σ^2_ρ, γ_{gi} is the gith column effect distributed with mean zero and variance σ^2_γ, τ_j is the jth treatment effect, ϵ_{ghij} is a random error effect distributed with mean zero and variance σ^2_ϵ, g = 1, ..., b, h = 1, ..., r, i = 1, ..., c, and j = 1, ..., v = rc.

The standard intrablock effects analysis of variance (ANOVA) can be obtained by using, for example, SAS PROC GLM, treating replicate, row(replicate) and column(replicate) as fixed. To compute the MLEs of the treatment effects using REML (restricted maximum likelihood) solutions for the variance components, SAS PROC MIXED could be used. Sample SAS code is displayed in the appendix (5.1).

Sums of squares and intrablock means obtained are those presented in textbooks. Textbook analyses make use of ANOVA solutions for variance components when recovering interblock information, whereas the REML solutions automatically adjust for interblock information. The adjusted treatment means can vary considerably between the methods for some situations since the estimated variance components for REML and ANOVA can be quite different.

2.2 Differential Trends within Blocks (Rows)

Cox (1958) considered a situation wherein differential curvatures existed within the columns of a Latin square. Differential trends may also occur within each incomplete block of an incomplete block design or within each row (column) of a lattice rectangle (square) experiment (Federer, 1996). In such an event, equation (1) is an inappropriate response model. Instead, the following response model is used:

$$Y_{ghij} = \mu + \beta_g + \rho_{gh} + \pi_{gh}\alpha_{ghi} + \tau_j + \epsilon_{ghij} \tag{2}$$

where the column effects have been replaced by a linear trend within each row. In this model π_{gh} is the ghth linear regression coefficient of responses on the ordered and centered positions, a_{ghi}, within a block and the remaining terms are as defined for equation (1). The linear regression coefficients are random variates distributed with mean zero and variance σ_{π}^2. (See Federer, 1996, for other models.) If desired, additional polynomial regressions could be added to the model, depending upon the nature of the trends within blocks or rows (columns).

A continuous variable, a_{ghi}, for position in the row (column) needs to be added to the data. (For example, the coefficients of the corresponding linear contrast can be used.) The standard analysis using SAS PROC GLM and most other analysis of covariance (ANCOVA) software treats the regression coefficients as fixed effects. To compute the adjusted treatment means (MLEs) using the REML solutions for the random slopes, PROC MIXED or other general linear mixed model software must be used. Sample SAS code is displayed in the appendix (5.2). The code is readily generalized to polynomial trends.

2.3 Row and Column Regressions

The analysis above is readily generalized to the case of polynomials in both row and column. In this case, the spatial trend need not be aligned to the row and column design of the experiment. (This situation has been considered by several authors over the past 50 years or more; also, see Federer, 1996, for the random effects situation.). A response model for this type of variation is:

$$\begin{aligned} Y_{ghij} &= \mu + \beta_g + \tau_j + \pi_{g1} RL_{ghi} + \pi_{g2} RQ_{ghi} + \pi_{g3} CL_{ghi} \\ &\quad + \pi_{g4} CQ_{ghi} + \pi_{g5} LL_{ghi} + \pi_{g6} LQ_{ghi} + \pi_{g7} QQ_{ghi} + \epsilon_{ghij} \quad (3) \end{aligned}$$

where RL_{ghi} are the linear regression values of ordered row positions, RQ_{ghi} are the quadratic regression values of ordered row positions, CL_{ghi} and CQ_{ghi} are defined similarly, LL_{ghi} is the row linear by column linear interaction, LQ_{ghi} is the row linear by column quadratic interaction, QQ_{ghi} is the row quadratic by column quadratic interaction, and the remaining terms are as defined for (1). As in (2), the regression coefficients, π_{gk} are considered to be random effects. If appropriate, additional regression terms may be included or terms may be deleted from the model.

Once again, standard ANCOVA software can be used to remove such trends if they are considered fixed. More realistically, however, the trends should be considered random effects and may be estimated by use of PROC MIXED or other linear mixed model software. An example is in the appendix (5.4).

Note that other higher degree regression polynomials or other forms of regression could be used as well. This analysis preserves the design structure. The above analysis is a form of what has been called trend analysis in the spatial statistics literature. It is, however, a technique that goes back at least to R. A. Fisher over 60 years ago for the fixed effects case.

2.4 *Nearest Neighbor Analysis*

A response model equation for a nearest neighbor analysis (Papadakis, 1937) of a design laid out in a row-column arrangement is:

$$Y_{ghij} = \mu + \beta_g + \tau_j + \pi_{g1} R_{ghi} + \pi_{g2} C_{ghi} + \pi_{g3} P_{ghi} + \epsilon_{ghij} \qquad (4)$$

where $R_{ghij} = (\epsilon_{g(h-1)ij} + \epsilon_{g(h+1)ijk})$, $C_{ghij} = (\epsilon_{gh(i-1)j} + \epsilon_{gh(i+1)j})$ are the averages of adjacent row and column errors respectively, and P_{ghij} is the interaction (product) of these terms, π_{gk} are regression coefficients and the other terms are as defined in (1). This model induces a spatial covariance structure on the errors. Papadakis (1937) used a two-stage procedure in which the errors were estimated by the residuals from a RCB analysis, and the π_{gk} were estimated as fixed effects by using these residuals in an ANCOVA. The MLEs of all coefficients and treatment effects under a fixed effects model can be computed by iteratively fitting model (4), using the residuals from the previous iteration to estimate R_{ghi}, C_{ghi} and P_{ghi} (Papadakis, 1937). Alternatively, REML can be used to fit the covariance structure and obtain the MLEs of the treatment effects. An interesting discussion of this is in Cressie (1993, Chap. 5.7).

However, for random blocks the π_{gk} should be random effects. Discussion of fitting a covariance model with random parameters for the covariance structure is in Section 2.6. As a "quick and dirty" approximation, we used Papadakis' (1937) two-step procedure, using SAS PROC GLM to generate the RCB residuals and PROC MIXED to estimate the regression coefficients as random effects. The program is listed in the appendix (5.4).

2.5 *Smoothing*

Polynomial trends (equations 2 or 3) can be replaced by general smooth trends. If the trends are assumed to line up with the column (row) layout of the design, the polynomial trends in (2) can be replaced with the model:

$$Y_{ghi} = \mu + \beta_g + \rho_{gh} + \gamma_{ghi} + \tau_j + \epsilon_{ghij} \qquad (5)$$

where γ_{ghi} is a smooth trend within row ρ_{gh}. If the trends are not assumed to line up with the rectangular layout of the design, then polynomial trends of the type in model (3) can be replaced with the model:

$$Y_{ghij} = \mu + \beta_g + \gamma_{ghi} + \tau_j + \epsilon_{ghij} \qquad (6)$$

where γ_{ghi} now represents a 2-dimensional spatial curve. In either case, we now have a semi-parametric additive model, (Hastie and Tibshirani, 1990), sometimes termed a partial linear model (Heckman, 1986; Speckman, 1988), and a number of methods have been developed for simultaneously fitting the smooth and parametric terms in the fixed effect case. The smooth terms in the model are fitted using a tuning parameter (the bandwidth, span or smoothing parameter) which controls the smoothness of the spatial term. For the fixed effects case, the tuning parameter should be fitted adaptively in each block, as there is no a priori reason to expect the spatial trends to have the same degree of smoothness in different blocks.

Smoothing splines (Wahba, 1990) and least squares smoothing (Green, Jennison and Seheult, 1985; Jennison and Seheult, 1984) have natural extensions to the random effects case, as discussed in the papers cited. In this paper, we have followed the computational procedure outlined by Green et al (1985), using S-PLUS as the computational tool, to fit (5). A copy of the S-PLUS code is available upon request.

2.6 Covariance Models

Models (6) and (7) treat spatial gradients within a block as fixed in the sense that the gradient should persist under a new realization of the errors. Often spatial gradients are modeled as random correlated processes. A large literature exists for this approach in the spatial and geostatistics literature. See Cressie (1993) for a comprehensive treatment. The model is:

$$Y_{ghi} = \mu + \beta_g + \gamma_{ghi} + \tau_j + \epsilon_{ghij} \tag{7}$$

where all the terms are as in (5.2) except that γ_{ghi} is now the random realization of a spatially autocorrelated process $\gamma_{ghi} \sim (0, \Sigma(\theta_g))$ where θ_g are parameters defining the correlation structure. If the θ_g are considered fixed, this model may be fitted using REML to estimate the covariance structure. For θ_g random we plan to use Monte Carlo Markov Chain methods for fitting hierarchical models (Geyer, 1992). We have not yet explored the intricacies of fitting such a model.

3 Data Analysis

In this section we apply the methods above to the lattice square experiment described in Table 12.5 of Cochran and Cox (1957). As well, we present a randomized complete block design analysis which, however, is inappropriate as it ignores the restrictions to randomization imposed by the design and row and column effects for which the design should adjust.

In Table 1, Type III (partial) sums of squares are presented for treatments, spatial effects, and residual from each model. (The block mean has been removed from the data prior to analysis, accounting for 4 degrees of freedom in the model.) The spatial sum of squares is an average of all the blocking variables within replicates. The F-value is the ratio of treatment and residual mean squares.

In the RCB analysis, there appear to be significant treatment effects. However, a plot of the residuals within block shows that there is considerable within-block spatial pattern which does not align with the row/column layout of the treatments. As well, the residuals are quite skewed, possibly indicating confounding of treatment and residual effects. Finally, the residual mean square is much greater than we would expect from Poisson data.

The standard lattice square analysis, LSD(1), suggests that variation among treatments is less than the residual mean square. The residuals are somewhat smaller than those obtained from the RCB analysis, but the treatment mean square has also been considerably reduced. Spatial patterning of the residuals is also evident, but is less clear than in the RCB analysis.

The remaining analyses treat the spatial effects as continuous covariates with random coefficients. It is interesting to note that the treatment and residual mean squares differ considerably depending on the model.

RG(2), CG, CLGr and RCreg(3) are all models in which the spatial effects are considered to be polynomials in rows and columns with random coefficients. RG(2) is model (2), with a separate linear gradient in each column. CG has a separate linear gradient in each column. CLGr assumes a linear gradient across the columns in each block, and a linear gradient within each column. RCreg(3) is model 3. It is interesting to note that the F-ratio varies considerably among these models, as does the amount of variation ascribed to the treatment and spatial effects. However, the designs in which the gradient is assumed to be aligned with the row/column layout of the design (LSD(1), RG(2), CG and CLGr) all have about the same partial sum of squares for spatial effects, although they have different degrees of freedom. Conclusions drawn from these models range from "no significant treatment effects" (RG and CG) to "highly significant treatment effects" (RCreg(3)).

Of the linear models, model (3) appears to give the best fit, with a residual mean square of 11.9. However, this is still three times the variance which would be indicated if the counts were Poisson.

If the experimenter had used the standard textbook analysis, he would reach the conclusion that there were no differences among the 16 insecticide treatments. Using the RCreg(3) analysis, it would be concluded that there were significant differences at the 2% level. These two completely different conclusions demonstrate how spatial patterns can sometimes distort treatment differences and why it is essential that an appropriate analysis be selected.

Method of analysis	mean	median	range
Rows as incomplete blocks	124	112	91-270
Lattice square	147	136	95-312
1D row neighbors	138	124	96-282
column neighbors	117	108	98-211
maximum of row or column neighbor	144	133	98-282
Papadakis (2 covariates)	148	136	96-297

4 Discussion

For any given experiment design, a number of analyses are generally possible, besides the standard textbook one. Although the experiment design should, to the extent possible, control for known sources of variation, this is often not possible due to the inherent variability of the experimental material. When the experiment has a spatial component, this is particularly important, as field plots may have to adapt to existing field designs which have not been laid out taking spatial variability into account. Even when the field has been optimally oriented with respect to existing gradients, the gradients may not be orthogonal, so that row/column designs cannot fully control for spatial effects.

It is interesting to note the results presented by Kempton (1984) and Kempton and Howes (1981) on the relative efficiencies of standard textbook lattice square analyses and some spatial methods of analysis. They studied the results of 118 wheat variety trials all designed as five by five balanced lattice squares. See the results in the figure above.

In these trials, the experimental unit was three times as long as wide so that the distance between rows was three times larger than between columns. So analyses involving columns will not control as much variation as ones with rows. An interesting statistic not reported would be the number of experiments in which each of the above analyses had the highest efficiency. The table demonstrates clearly the need to remove row and column effects, although for these trials the lattice square analysis appears to be just as effective as the more complex spatial models.

A possible contender for the analysis RCreg(3) using response model equation (3) would be to replace LL, LQ, and QQ with first, second, and perhaps third principal components in the manner used for additive main effects and multiplicative interactions (AMMI) analysis (Gaugh, 1988). The interactions used in (3) may not maximize the sums of squares for variation whereas the principal components method would do this. Since this method is not for interpretive purposes but to control extraneous variation, there would be no problem in using an AMMI analysis.

As we have seen in our preceding numerical example as well as the example above, a number of a priori reasonable models can lead to very different interpretation of treatment effects. There is little guidance in the literature for choosing among non-nested models of the types presented here, beyond graphical analysis of the residuals. Serious concerns when choosing among several models are overfitting and bias. We are studying these via simulation studies. For the semiparametric methods such as nearest neighbors, smoothing and AMMI the appropriate degree of freedom adjustment to the error mean square also needs to be computed.

5 REFERENCES

[1] Cochran, W. G., Cox, G. M. (1957). *Experimental Designs*, 2nd edition. John Wiley & Sons, Inc. New York.

[2] Cox, C. P. (1958). The analysis of Latin squares with individual curvatures in one direction. *J. Royal Statistical Soc., Series B*, **20**, 193-204.

[3] Cressie, N.A.C. (1993)*Statistics for Spatial Data.* John Wiley & Sons: New York.

[4] Federer, W. T. (1992) Diagnostic Procedures for Analysis of Variance. In *New Progress in Probability and Statistics, Proceedings of the Conference "Nicolas Arriquibar", 4th International Meeting of Statistics in the Basque Country.* M.L. Puri and J.P. Vilaplana (eds.) International Science Publishers, Zeist, The Netherlands, pp 1-23.

[5] Federer, W. T. (1955). *Experimental Design - Theory and Application.* Macmillan Co., New York. (Republished by Oxford & IBH Publishing Co., Calcutta, 1967 and 1974).

[6] Federer, W. T. (1996). Recovery of interblock, intergradient, and intervariety information for incomplete block and lattice rectangle designed experiments. BU-1315-M in the Technical Report Series of the Biometrics Unit, Cornell University, Ithaca, NY 14853.

[7] Federer, W. T., Wolfinger, R. D. (1996). SAS PROC GLM and PROC MIXED for recovering inter-effect information. BU-1330-M in the Technical Report Series of the Biometrics Unit, Cornell University, Ithaca, NY 14853.

[8] Gauch, H. G. Jr. (1988) Model selection and validation for yield trials with interaction. *Biometrics*, **44**, 705-715.

[9] Geyer, C.J. (1992) Practical Markov Chain Monte Carlo (with discussion). *Statistical Science*, **7**, 473-502.

[10] Green, P., Jennison, C., Seheult, A. (1985). Analysis of field experiments by least squares smoothing. *J. Royal Statistical Soc., Series B*, **47**, 299-315.

[11] Hastie, T.J., Tibshirani, R.J. (1990) *Generalized Additive Models.* Chapman & Hall: London.

[12] Heckman, N.E. (1986) Spline smoothing in a partly linear model. *J. Royal Statistical Soc., Series B*, **48**, 244-248.

[13] Kempthorne, O. (1952) *The Design and Analysis of Experiments.* John Wiley & Sons, Inc., New York.

[14] Kempton, R. A. (1984). Comparison of nearest neighbor and classical methods of analysis. In *Spatial Methods in Field Experiments* (Editor: R. A. Kempton), University of Durham, pp 51-52.

[15] Kempton, R. A., Howes, C. W. (1981). The use of neighboring plot values in the analysis of plot trials. *Applied Statistics*, **30**, 59-70.

[16] Jennison, C., Seheult, A. (1984). Two dimensional (2D) least squares smoothing (LSS) analysis. In *Spatial Methods in Field Experiments* (Editor: R. A. Kempton), University of Durham, pp. 25-28.

[17] Papadakis, J. S. (1937). Methode statistique pour des Experiences sur Champ. *Bulletin Inst. Ameliorations Plantes Salonique*, **23**, 1-30.

[18] Speckman, P. (1988) Kernel smoothng in partial linear models. *J. Royal Statistical Soc., Series B*, **50**, 413-436.

[19] Stroup, W. W., Mulitze, D. K. (1991). Nearest neighbor adjusted best linear unbiased predictor. *American Statistician*, **45**, 194-200.

[20] Wadley, F. M. (1946). Incomplete block designs in insect population problems. *J. Economic Entomology*, **38**, 651-654.

Source of variation	df	Sum of squares	df	Sum of squares	df	Sum of squares
	RCBD		LSD(1)		RG(2)	
Treatment	15	1244	15	320	15	347
Spatial	0	0	30	1653	35	1650
Residual	60	2333	30	680	25	474
F-ratio		2.13		0.94		1.22
	CG		CLGr		RCreg(3)	
Treatment	15	514	15	614	15	435
Spatial	35	1645	25	1637	30	1761
Residual	25	614	35	695	30	357
F-ratio		1.39		2.06		2.43
	NN(4)		SMOOTH(5.2)			
Treatment	15	530	15	723		
Spatial	?	920	27.1	2147		
Residual	?	1151	36.9	738		
F-ratio		?		2.41		

TABLE 1. Partial sums of squares for treatment, spatial, and residual for various analyses: RCBD = randomized complete block; LSD(1) = lattice square, equation (1); RGr(2) = rows and gradients in rows, equation (2); CGr = columns and gradients in columns; CLGr = linear column effects within replicates with differential gradients in columns; RCreg(3) = linear and quadratic regressions and interactions as in equation (3); NN(4) = nearest neighbor within replicates as in equation (4); SMOOTH(5.2)=Least squares smoothing as in equation 5.2; F-ratio = treatment / residual.

6 Appendix - SAS Programs

6.1 Lattice Square (Model 1)

ANOVA

```
data lsgr;
  infile 'lsgr1645.dat';
  input count rep row column treat;
proc glm data = lsgr;
  class rep row column treat;
  model count = rep row(rep) column(rep) treat;
  random rep row(rep) column(rep);
  lsmeans treat;
run;
```

Using REML to Obtain MLE of Treatment Effects

```
data lsgr;
  infile 'lsgr1645.dat';
  input count rep row column treat;
proc mixed data = lsgr;
  class rep row column treat;
  model count = treat;
  random rep row(rep) column(rep);
  lsmeans treat;
run;
```

6.2 *Random Gradients within Row (Model 2)*

The created variable "grad" is the coefficients of the linear contrast of columns, within each row.

ANOVA

```
data lsgr;
  infile 'lsgr1645.dat';
  input count rep row column grad treat;
proc glm data = lsgr;
  class rep row column treat;
  model count = rep row(rep) grad*row(rep) treat;
  random rep row(rep);
  lsmeans treat;
run;
```

Using REML to Obtain MLE of Treatment Effects

```
data lsgr;
  infile 'lsgr1645.dat';
  input count rep row column grad treat;
proc mixed data = lsgr;
  class rep row treat;
  model count = treat;
  random rep row(rep) grad*row(rep);
  lsmeans treat;
run;
```

6.3 *Row and Column Regressions (Model 3)*

RL and RQ are the linear and quadratic within row variables. CL and CQ are the linear and quadratic within column variables.

ANOVA

```
data lsgr;

infile 'lsgr1645.dat';
```

```
   input count rep  treat RL RQ CL CQ;
LL = RL*CL;
LQ = RL*CQ;
QQ = RQ*CQ;

proc glm data = lsgr;

class rep  treat;
model count = rep RL*rep RQ*rep CL*rep LL*rep LQ*rep QQ*rep treat;
random rep;
lsmeans treat;

  run;
```

Using REML to Obtain MLE of Treatment Effects

```
data lsgr;

infile 'lsgr1645.dat';
input count treat RL RQ CL CQ;
LL = RL*CL;
LQ = RL*CQ;
QQ = RQ*CQ;

proc mixed data = lsgr;

class rep treat;
model count =  treat;
random rep RL*rep RQ*rep CL*rep LL*rep LQ*rep QQ*rep;
lsmeans treat;

run;
```

6.4 Two-step NN Analysis

```
data lsgr;  infile 'a:backslash lsgr1645.dat';
input count rep row column treat;

proc sort; by rep row column;      sort data
proc glm data = lsgr;              generate RCB residuals

class rep treat;
  model count = rep treat;
  output out = lsgr2  r = res;
  data lsgr3;
   merge lsgr lsgr2;

proc iml;                          generate R, C and P, taking edge effects
use lsgr3;                         into account

  read all var {rep row column res};
  n = nrow(res);
```

```
rnn = J(n,1,0);
cnn = J(n,1,0);
nr = max(row);
nc = max(column);
nb = max(rep);
ind = 0;
do k = 1 to nb;

do i = 1 to nr;
        do j = 1 to nc;
        ind = ind + 1;
                if i = 1 then rnn[ind] = res[ind + nc];
                else if i = nr then rnn[ind] = res[ind - nc];
        else rnn[ind] = 0.5*(res[ind - rc] + res[ind + nc]);
                if  j = 1 then cnn[ind] = res[ind + 1];
                else if j = nc then cnn[ind] = res[ind - 1];
        else cnn[ind] = 0.5*(res[ind - 1] + res[ind + 1]);
        end;
end;

end;
create lsgr4 {rnn cnn};
append;
quit;
data lsgr5;
merge lsgr3 lsgr4;

proc mixed data = lsgr5;                    Compute REML estimators.

class rep treat;
model count = treat;
random rep rnn*rep cnn*rep rnn*cnn*rep;
run;
```

Spatial and Longitudinal Data Analysis : Two Histories with a Common Future?

Peter J. Diggle
Lancaster University
United Kingdom

ABSTRACT A historically oriented review of spatial and longitudinal data analysis is presented. It is argued that these two branches of statistical research developed separately for good historical reasons, but that their common foundation in the analysis of correlated data, coupled with modern computing developments has encouraged their convergence. Current research in generalized linear mixed models and, more generally, in highly structured stochastic systems, exemplifies this convergence.

Key words and phrases: Correlation; dropout; generalized estimating equations; generalized linear mixed models.

1 Introduction

Spatial and longitudinal statistical methods have each evolved to address problems concerning the analysis of correlated data, yet despite this common thread their developments have been largely independent. A partial explanation from a theoretical standpoint is that the contrast between the ordered character of time and the unordered character of geographical space has had a major impact on the way in which stochastic models for the two kinds of data have been formulated. Perhaps a more fundamental explanation is that the two methodologies were motivated by different kinds of scientific question. Spatial applications typically concern the analysis of a single realisation of an underlying process, often observed in its natural state, whereas longitudinal studies almost always involve replicated data, and often in the context of a designed experiment.

In recent years, there have been signs that the two methodologies are converging as a consequence of an explosive expansion in both the variety of models amenable to statistical analysis and the range of applications which call for their use. In the remainder of this paper I will first summarise some methodological developments from spatial statistics which seem to me especially relevant to longitudinal studies. I will then give a brief account of the development of longitudinal statistical methodology, emphasising the gradual emergence of explicit models for the stochastic dependence which is an inherent feature of longitudinal data. Finally, I will suggest that recent work on generalized linear mixed models (Breslow and Clayton, 1993) and, more generally, on what have come to be known as *highly structured stochastic systems* justifies my claim that the two sub-disciplines are converging.

2 Spatial Statistics

This section draws heavily on Diggle (1996), where spatial statistical methods are discussed under three broad headings: continuous spatial variation, discrete spatial variation and spatial point processes. Note that Cressie (1991) adopts essentially the same classification, but with different terminology.

2.1 Continuous spatial variation: geostatistical models and methods

Continuous spatial variation is concerned with phenomena which can be described by a stochastic process of the form $\{Y(x) : x \in \mathbb{R}^2\}$. The most commonly studied special cases are those in which $Y(x)$ is a Gaussian process, giving one possible theoretical framework for the applied topic known as geostatistics (Matheron, 1963; Journel and Huijbregts, 1978).

In this area, the basic format for a set of data is

$$(y_i, x_i) : i = 1, ..., m$$

where y_i is a measurement of some phenomenon of interest and x_i a spatial location associated with y_i. For example, in the original context of mining, y_i might represent the grade of a sample of ore from the location x_i. A fundamental concern of geostatistics is to use data of this kind to predict the value of the phenomenon at arbitrary locations within a defined spatial region, eg an area being surveyed prior to mining. Although this prediction problem can be articulated without declaring an explicit stochastic model for the data, from a classical statistical perspective the standard geostatistical prediction method known as kriging can be obtained as the solution to the following problem: given an unobserved stationary Gaussian process $S(x) : x \in \mathbb{R}^2$ and data generated according to the model

$$Y_i = S(x_i) + Z_i : i = 1, ..., m \tag{1}$$

where Z_i are mutually independent $N(0, \tau^2)$ random variables, evaluate $\hat{S}(x) = E[S(x)|Y_1, ..., Y_m]$, the minimum mean square error predictor for $S(x)$. The Z_i are a formal expression of what is known in geostatistics as the *nugget effect*, a colourful expression whose contextual origin is clear! Its literal interpretation in (1) is as a random measurement error. In practice, it also takes indirect account of very small-scale spatial variation, in the following sense. The covariance structure of $S(x)$ is intended to model the spatial variation in the data, but the data only provide information about this on the scale of the observed range of distances between pairs of sample locations x_i. Any spatial variation at smaller scale is then indistinguishable in practice from uncorrelated measurement errors.

Likelihood-based inference for the model (1) is now computationally feasible for quite large values of m, say of the order of several hundred, but would have been quite impractical in the 1960's when geostatistical methods were developed, largely at École des Mines, Fontainebleau (Matheron, 1963). Partly for this reason, partly through a reluctance to adopt an explicitly model-based approach, and partly reinforced by doubts which were later voiced about the performance of maximum likelihood estimators in this context (Warnes and Ripley, 1987), more ad hoc methods of inference have been developed. In particular, geostatistical applications have popularised the *variogram* as a tool for exploring the correlation structure of spatial (and, more recently, longitudinal) data and for parametric estimation.

A spatial stochastic process $Y(x)$ is said to be *stationary* if $E[Y(x)]$ is a constant and the covariance $\text{Cov}\{Y(x), Y(x')\}$ depends only on $u = x - x'$. The *variogram* of a stationary process is defined as $\gamma(u) = \frac{1}{2}\text{Var}\{Y(x) - Y(x-u)\}$. When the process $S(x)$ in (1) is stationary with covariance function $\sigma^2\rho(u)$, the variogram of data generated by the model (1) is

$$\gamma(u) = \tau^2 + \sigma^2\{1 - \rho(u)\}.$$

Thus, the intercept of the variogram corresponds to the nugget variance, τ^2, whilst the asymptote, sometimes called the *sill*, is $\tau^2 + \sigma^2$ and the correlation function $\rho(u)$ determines the mode of progression from the nugget to the sill with increasing spatial separation.

The variogram can be used to estimate a parametric model of the form (1), by matching the theoretical variogram to the empirical variogram. The *empirical variogram*, $\tilde{\gamma}(u)$, consists of one half the sample mean squared difference between pairs of observations at spatial separation u. Methods of this kind are compared with likelihood-based estimation under Gaussian assumptions in Zimmerman and Zimmerman (1991) and in Barry, Crowder and Diggle (1997). For likelihood-based estimation under Gaussian assumptions, there is a concensus that restricted maximum likelihood, or REML, estimation (Patterson and Thompson, 1971; Harville, 1974) is preferable to maximum likelihood.

Standard prediction intervals for $S(x)$ ignore the variability in the estimates of model parameters. This additional variability can, however, be accommodated by adopting a Bayesian approach, as in Handcock and Stein (1993).

Recent research in this area includes the embedding of (1) within the framework of the generalised linear mixed model (Breslow and Clayton, 1993). This provides one way of extending the model to non-Gaussian settings. For example, Diggle, Harper and Simon (1997) describe an application to the assessment of residual radioactive contamination on a South Pacific island, following the nuclear weapons testing programme during the 1950's. In that context, each observation y_i is the number of photon emissions recorded by a gamma camera and can be modelled as a Poisson count, conditional on the underlying concentration of radionuclide at (or close to) the corresponding location x_i. One possible specification of a probability model for the spatial variation, $\lambda(x)$ say, in concentration is that $\lambda(x) = \exp\{\mu + S(x)\}$ where $S(x)$ is a stationary Gaussian process. For further discussion, see Section 4 below.

2.2 Discrete spatial variation: Markov random fields

Discrete spatial variation deals with stochastic processes defined on a finite or countable index-set, say $\{Y_i : i \in \mathcal{I}\}$. In practice, models of this kind have been widely used to describe phenomena which strictly exist in continuous space; for example, in image analysis (Geman and Geman, 1984; Besag, 1986) where $\mathcal{I}$ represents an array of pixels, or in epidemiology (Clayton and Kaldor, 1987; Clayton and Bernardinelli, 1992) where $\mathcal{I}$ indexes a partition of a geographical region into sub-regions. However, it turns out that the distinction between continuous and discrete spatial variation has a major impact on the way in which explicit models are formulated.

The restriction to a countable index set encourages the specification of a model in terms of conditional, rather than joint, distributions and, almost incidentally, diminishes the focus on the Gaussian case. During the early development of spatial statistical methods there was vigorous debate on the relative merits of the conditional and joint approaches. See, for example, Besag (1974) and the associated discussion. At that time, a conditional specification appeared to provide the only feasible approach in the non-Gaussian setting. It also spawned the whole area of multivariate statistics now known as graphical modelling (Darroch, Lauritzen and Speed, 1980; Whittaker, 1990). Using the conditional approach, models are specified implicitly in terms of their full conditional distributions, $\mathrm{P}(Y_i|Y_j : j \neq i)$. Typically, simplifying assumptions about the spatial dependence amongst the Y_i are expressed by imposing a form of local, or Markovian dependence as follows. For each $i \in \mathcal{I}$, we define a set of *neighbours* as a subset $N_i \subset \mathcal{I}$ such that $\mathrm{P}(Y_i|Y_j : j \neq i) = \mathrm{P}(Y_i|Y_j : j \in N_i)$. For example, when $\mathcal{I}$ is a regular two-dimensional square lattice, a natural definition for N_i might be the four nearest neighbours of i. Models of this kind are called Markov random fields.

At the time they were introduced, an obstacle to progress using conditional models was that, except in the Gaussian case where there is a a one-to-one correspondence between joint and conditional formulations, the likelihood is generally intractable. The full conditional distributions determine the joint distribution of $Y_1, ..., Y_m$ up to a normalising constant, evaluation of which is extremely difficult. The initial solution to this problem was to use sensible but ad hoc methods of estimation such as maximum pseudo-likelihood (Besag, 1975), the pseudo-likelihood function being defined as the product of the m full conditionals. Nowadays, the method of choice might well be a Markov Chain Monte Carlo (MCMC) method (Gilks, Richardson and Spiegelhalter, 1996). In fact, it would be fairer to say that MCMC methods were introduced to the mainstream of statistical methodology for complex stochastic systems through their earlier application to models of discrete spatial variation, in the particular context of image processing (Geman and Geman, 1984).

2.3 Spatial point processes

A spatial point pattern is a set of data consisting of locations $x_i \in \mathbb{R}^2 : i = 1, ..., n$, presumed to have been generated by some underlying two-dimensional point process. This sub-area nicely illustrates one of the fundamental differences between spatial and longitudinal statistics. For the longitudinal counterpart of points occurring at random in time, the ordered nature of time means that in building stochastic models it is natural to think in terms of the conditional hazard for a point at time t, given the history of the process up to that point. A classic example is the Cox (1972) regression model which is the foundation of present-day methods of survival analysis. Except in very special circumstances, this ordering is lost in the spatial setting, and the most widely used statistical descriptors of spatial point patterns are second moment measures and so-called nearest neighbour distributions, with the conditional hazard playing only a limited role, albeit an important one in the context of the particular class of models known as Markov point processes (Ripley and Kelly, 1977).

Models and methods developed for spatial point patterns have so far had a limited impact on the analysis of point patterns in time. Cross-fertilisation in the opposite direction is beginning to occur, driven by the needs of neuroscience applications. Modern developments in microscopy have led to widespread collection of neuroanatomical data in the form of images of spatial point distributions, each point representing the nucleus of an individual cell within a tissue section. A typical data set consists of a large number of such images, involving both replicated images within subjects and multiple subjects, often allocated amongst different experimental treatments and with the objective of investigating the effect of the experimental treatments on the spatial organisation of the cells. One approach to analysing data of this kind is to use spatial point process methods to summarise each image, and analysis of variance techniques to investigate variability between subjects or experimental groups (Diggle, Lange and Benes, 1989; Baddeley, Moyeed, Howard and Boyde, 1993). Which brings us to the origins of present-day methodology for longitudinal data.

3 Longitudinal Statistics

The essence of a longitudinal study is that a time-sequence of measurements is taken on each of a number of subjects. A generic notation for a set of longitudinal data is therefore

$$(y_{ij}, t_{ij}) : j = 1, ..., n_i; i = 1, ..., m$$

in which y_{ij} is the jth measurement on the ith of m subjects, and t_{ij} the time at which y_{ij} is taken. Typically, this basic array of measurements is supplemented by covariate information at either or both of two levels: individual observations (time-dependent covariates); and individual subjects (time-independent covariates). Time-dependent covariates may include time itself, or transformations of time, whilst time-independent covariates typically include subject-specific characteristics (eg sex) and design variables (eg treatment allocation in a randomised clinical trial).

Longitudinal data analysis can be viewed, according to taste and purpose, as a branch of the analysis of variance, multivariate analysis or time series analysis. In reality, it is all three and, to a first approximation, its historical development represents a progression from the first, via the second, to the third.

3.1 Early days

The earliest approaches to the analysis of longitudinal data were constrained by the need to offer computationally feasible solutions to the practical questions posed by the data. These questions typically concerned the effect of experimental interventions on functions $\mu_i(t)$ which determine the set of mean responses, $E(Y_{ij}) = \mu_i(t_{ij})$. A reasonable approach was therefore to focus on the experimental design (completely randomised, randomised block or whatever) and reduce the time-sequence of responses on each subject to one or more univariate measures which addressed the questions of primary interest. A classic example is the paper by Wishart (1938) which introduced the strategy of analysing such *summary measures.* Wishart's specific concern was with studies of growth in pigs, in which context it is natural to focus on directly interpretable summary measures such as the weight-gain over the duration of the experiment.

In a perhaps excessively formal notation, the method of summary measures can be expressed as a preliminary transformation of the data to $s_i : i = 1, ..., m$ where $s_i = \mathcal{F}(y_{i1}, ..., y_{in_i})$. The subsequent analysis typically assumes that, apart from the influence of design variables between subjects, the s_i are replicates. Our notation emphasises that in general this is strictly justifiable only if the set of observation times, $t_{ij} : j = 1, ..., n_i$, is common to all m subjects. The approach also leaves an uncomfortable feeling that the chosen summary measure may not make the best use of all the available information – to take an extreme example, if weight gain over the experiment was the whole story, there would be no point in taking intermediate measurements.

Reservations of this kind may have been a motivating factor behind the methodological developments of the 1950's and 1960's which viewed longitudinal data from the standpoint of multivariate analysis. This brought to the foreground the question of how to describe the correlation structure amongst the repeated measurments within a subject, and how to incorporate this structure into the analysis of the data. On the assumption that the time-sequence of measurements is common to all subjects (often true at the design stage if not after the event – but more of this anon), and provided that the sequence length, n, is small relative to the number of subjects, m, the assumption of a general covariance structure, i.e., an arbitrary $n \times n$ covariance matrix V, is feasible and leads to analysis by standard multivariate methods including the multivariate analysis of variance. See, for example, Hand and Taylor (1987). A different approach is to pretend, temporarily, that the data are univariate and treat time as an experimental factor. We could then construct the usual univariate analysis of variance table, but adjust the nominal significance levels of the F-ratios in the ANOVA table to allow for the non-independence of measurements within subjects (Geisser and Greenhouse, 1958; Greenhouse and Geisser, 1959). This method remains popular in some areas of application, presumably because it allows the analysis to be carried out very easily using simple and familiar univariate calculations. However, it is limited in what it can achieve beyond tests of hypotheses about treatment effects.

A third early approach, very firmly in the tradition of design-based inference, was to consider longitudinal data as analogous to a split-plot experiment in which the subjects are the primary plots, and times within subjects the sub-plots. Indeed, the split-plot ANOVA is still called *repeated measures* ANOVA in some text-books. See, for example, Winer (1977). However, it makes no sense to treat time as a factor whose allocation can be randomised and the validity of the split-plot *analysis* therefore rests on a model-based assumption, namely that the data y_{ij} can be decomposed as

$$y_{ij} = \mu_{ij} + U_i + Z_{ij} \tag{2}$$

where $\mu_{ij} = \mathrm{E}(y_{ij})$, the U_i are random subjects effects, mutually independent with zero mean and variance ν^2, and the Z_{ij} are random measurement errors, mutually independent with zero mean and variance τ^2.

3.2 Gaussian linear models

The split-plot *model* (2) could be advanced in its own right as a model for the covariance structure of longitudinal data. It implies that for all i and all $j \neq k$, $\text{Corr}(y_{ij}, y_{ik}) = \rho = \nu^2/(\nu^2 + \tau^2)$, and is perhaps more properly called the uniform correlation model.

The assumption that the correlation between a pair of measurements does not depend on their time separation is anathema to a time series analyst, and the uniform correlation model was duly challenged as soon as time series methods began to exert an influence on longitudinal methodology. The fundamental tool of classical time series analysis is the serial correlation function, $\rho(u)$, which describes the correlation between a pair of measurements as a function of their time separation. The earliest explicit depiction of empirical serial correlation for a set of longitudinal data which I have found is in Danford, Hughes and McNee (1960). Their Figure 3 shows a pattern of serial correlation instantly recognisable to any student of time series, namely a convex, exponential-like decay towards zero with increasing time-separation. However, and crucially, this behaviour only manifested itself after subtraction of a mean response for each subject. What this implies is that simply replacing the superficially implausible uniform correlation model (2) with a standard time series model, for example

$$y_{ij} = \mu_{ij} + W_{ij}$$

where $W_{ij} = \alpha W_{i,j-1} + Z_{ij}$ is a first-order autoregressiveprocess, would be throwing the baby out with the bathwater by denying the possibility of random variation between subjects. This question only arises, of course, because of the replication between subjects which is inherent to longitudinal studies, but rare in classical time series or spatial statistics.

Another consideration in modelling correlation structure is whether the correlation between a pair of measurements should be forced to approach unity as their time-separation approaches zero. Clearly, this need not be the case if the measurements are themselves subject to random error; one example would be measurements representing chemical determinations from blood-samples. To accommodate this, we need to recognise an analogue of the geostatistican's nugget effect.

Combining the above considerations leads to model of the form

$$y_{ij} = \mu_i(t_{ij}) + U_i + W_i(t_{ij}) + Z_{ij} \tag{3}$$

in which $\mu_i(t)$ denotes the mean response for subject i at time t, U_i and Z_{ij} have the same meaning as in (2) and $W_i(t) : i = 1, ..., m$ are independent copies of a stationary random process with mean zero and covariance

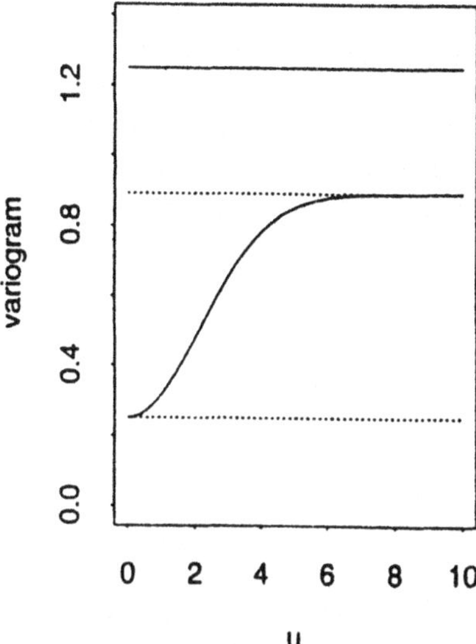

FIGURE 1. The theoretical variogram of the lonigtudinal model (3). The solid curve is the function $\gamma(u) = \tau^2 + \sigma^2[1 - \exp\{(u/\alpha)^2\}]$, the solid horizontal line is at height $\tau^2 + \sigma^2 + \nu^2$ and the two dotted horizontal lines are at heights τ^2 and $\tau^2 + \sigma^2$. Parameter values are $\tau = 0.5$, $\sigma = 0.8$, $\nu = 0.6$ and $\alpha = 3$.

function $\text{Cov}\{Y(t), Y(t-u)\} = \sigma^2\rho(u)$. The model (3) gives an explicit decomposition of the random variation into three components: between subjects, between times within subjects, and measurement error. So far as I am aware, it was first expressed in this form in Diggle (1988), but similar ideas were at least implicit in earlier papers, notably the seminal one of Laird and Ware (1982) which included a more general specification of the variation between subjects through a linear random effects model, $d'_{ij}U_i$, where U_i is now a vector of zero-mean random variables and d_{ij} a vector of covariates.

The model (3) provides a ready explanation of why the uniform correlation model often works well in practice. The theoretical variogram of the model (3) is shown in Figure 1. The role of the serially correlated process $W_i(t)$ is to describe how the variogram progresses from its intercept, $\gamma(0) = \tau^2$, to its asymptote, $\gamma(u) \sim \tau^2 + \sigma^2$, which in turn falls short of $\text{Var}\{Y(t)\}$ by an amount ν^2. If $\tau^2 + \nu^2 >> \sigma^2$, this is of little practical importance, and the uniform correlation model, which results in the limit as $\sigma^2/(\tau^2+\nu^2) \rightarrow 0$, will do very well as a first approximation. However, for inference I would still advocate formal, likelihood-based methods based on the uniform correlation *model* rather than a split-plot analysis of variance.

Inference for models of the kind exemplified by (3) typically use likelihood-based methods. The models are similar (apart from the reduction to one temporal dimension) to the geostatistical models described in Section 2.1 above, but the evaluation of the likelihood function is computationally less demanding because of the assumption that measurements are only correlated within subjects. This means that the matrix manipulations involved are of order n_i, the number of measurements on a single subject, which is typically small. As in the spatial setting, the concensus is that REML estimation is to be preferred over classical maximum likelihood.

3.3 Generalized linear models

Many longitudinal studies generate discrete or categorical responses, rather than the continuous measurements for which the models of Section 3.1 above might be appropriate. The long association of longitudinal studies with replicated, designed experiments and the recognition that models for continuous longitudinal data are no more than linear models with correlated errors led naturally to the following line of inquiry: how can and should generalized linear models (McCullagh and Nelder, 1989) be extended to deal with correlated data? This question has been answered in three essentially different ways. The first two are analogous to continuous and discrete spatial variation models, respectively, whilst the third is a moment-based method which directly exploits the replication in longitudinal data in order to estimate the correlation structure nonparametrically.

For the purposes of this article, it is convenient to focus attention on an important special case, namely linear logistic models for a binary response variable, and to assume a common set of observation times for each subject, although this latter simplification is not necessary in practice. The response data can therefore be represented as an array $Y_{ij} : j = 1, ..., n; i = 1, ..., m$ of n binary observations on each of m subjects, with the jth observation on each subject taken at time t_j. A linear logistic model for these data which ignored the correlations between repeated measurements on a subject might then take the form

$$\log\{\mu_{ij}/(1-\mu_{ij})\} = x'_{ij}\beta \tag{4}$$

where $\mu_{ij} = \mathrm{P}(Y_{ij} = 1)$, x_{ij} is a vector of explanatory variables attached to each subject, β is a vector of associated regression parameters and the Y_{ij} are assumed to be mutually independent.

3.3.1 Random effects models

In a random effects model, we seek to account for the correlation between repeated measurements by recognising sources of random variation between subjects. A simple example would replace (4) by

$$\log\{\mu_{ij}/(1-\mu_{ij})\} = x'_{ij}\beta + U_i \tag{5}$$

where $U_i : i = 1, ..., m$ are mutually independent, $N(0, \nu^2)$ random variables, and $\mu_{ij} = P(Y_{ij} = 1|U_i)$. Adding stochastic terms to the linear predictor seems intuitively natural if we regard the U_i as a manifestation of variation between subjects which, in principle, could be explained by identifying and measuring the appropriate subject-specific characteristics. However, it is important to remember that the interpretation of β is different in (5) than in (4). In (5) it measures the effect of the explanatory variables on an individual subject's probability of a positive response, which will vary substantially between subjects when ν^2 is large, whereas in (4) β measures the effect of the explanatory variables on the proportion of positive responses in the population.

3.3.2 Transition models

In a transition model, we seek to explain the correlation by postulating a direct dependence of the present response on past responses. A simple example of a transition model extension of (4) would be

$$\log\{\mu_{ij}/(1 - \mu_{ij})\} = x'_{ij}\beta + \alpha Y_{i,j-1} \tag{6}$$

where now $\mu_{ij} = P(Y_{ij} = 1|Y_{i,j-1})$. One question to consider in choosing between random effects or transition models is whether they seems scientifically reasonable in the context of the specific application. From a statistical point of view, both kinds of model generate dependence amongst the time-ordered responses on each subject: transition models do this by assuming that the past directly influences the present, whereas random effects models assume that the dependence is a by-product of random variation betwen subjects. Note also that the substantive meaning of β in (6) is again different from its meaning in (5) or (4). Also, (6) is not a natural model if the observation times t_j are not equally spaced.

3.3.3 Marginal models

In a marginal model, we seek to preserve the interpretation of β in (4), i.e., as a measure of the effect of explanatory variables on the proportion of positive responses in the population, whilst making allowance for correlation structure in forming inferences about β. To achieve this, we assume that (4) holds unconditionally, or *marginally*, and add the assumption that the repeated measurements on a subject are correlated to an unknown extent.

In the non-Gaussian setting, specifying the first two moments falls short of a full specification of the joint distribution of $Y_{i1}, ..., Y_{in}$. It follows that likelihood inference is not always available for models of this kind. Nor would we necessarily wish to use likelihood-based methods, as one motivation for using marginal models is that they address relevant questions about mean responses without requiring precise specification of higher order moments. The usual method of inference is to construct consistent estimates of the marginal parameters, β, and their large-sample standard errors, using an iteratively weighted least squares algorithm introduced in the present context by Liang and Zeger (1986) and known as generalised estimating equations, or GEE. The GEE algorithm incorporates a weighting matrix which is derived from a specifed form for the correlation structure, usually called the *working correlation structure*, but does not rely on the correctness of this specification for inference about β. Instead, the empirical correlation structure is used to estimate the true structure, and a mis-specification between the working and true correlation structures may compromise efficiency but does not affect the asymptotic validity of the inference about β.

In discussing the relative merits of the three approaches to generalized linear modelling of longitudinal data, it is important to remember that the regression parameters, β, have different interpretations in the three approaches. My own opinion is that the choice of approach should be determined primarily by the scientific objectives of each application.

3.4 Dropouts

In practice, most longitudinal studies encounter the following problem: not all subjects supply the intended sequence of measurements, ie some measurements are missing. The term *dropout* is used to describe a particularly common and important form of this problem, in which some subjects leave the study prematurely so that all of their intended measurements beyond some point, the dropout time, are missing.

The methodological challenge of longitudinal studies with dropout is how to make valid inferences which recognise that the processes governing the dropouts may be stochastically related to the measurement process which is of primary interest; for example, in a longitudinal clinical trial the willingness of a subject to continue may depend on their perception of the effectiveness of their treatment. For a recent review of this area, see Little (1995). An emerging general conclusion is that when the dropout process is non-ignorable in the sense of Rubin (1976), which in the present context means that the dropout time is stochastically dependent on the measurement which would have been observed had the subject not dropped out, inferences are highly sensitive to model assumptions which are difficult, or even impossible, to validate from the observed data (see, for example, several contributions to the discussion of Diggle and Kenward, 1994). This points to the desirability of conducting sensitivity analyses over a range of assumptions about the dropout process, rather than relying on the inferences from the notionally best-fitting single model.

On the face of it, the dropout problem has no direct counterpart in spatial statistics. However, there is a connection which I suspect occurs frequently but is often ignored. In geostatistics, a fundamental assumption is that the sampling locations x_i are chosen without reference to the spatial process

$S(x)$ which is the inferential focus. If, on the contrary, the x_i reflect an expert's judgement as to where, say, $S(x)$ might be large (as, for example, in taking exploratory drillings in a prospective oil field), then the absence of a measurement at a location x might in itself convey information about the corresponding value of $S(x)$. Under this scenario, as in the case of dropouts in longitudinal studies, inferential difficulties arise because the data are *informatively censored*, but so far as I am aware, the resulting problems of interpretation have not been considered explicitly in the spatial statistics literature.

4 Generalized Linear Mixed Models: A Unifying Framework

A generalized linear mixed model is a generalized linear model with one or more stochastic terms added to the linear predictor. Breslow and Clayton (1993) summarise the theory associated with this class of models and describe a range of applications.

Random effects models for longitudinal data, of the kind illustrated in Section 3.3.1 above, provide examples of GLMM's in which the stochastic terms are used to describe random variation between subjects. Diggle, Harper and Simon's (1997) model for residual radioactive contamination is also a GLMM, but one in which the stochastic term, $S(x)$, describes spatially correlated variation within a single replicate. The GLMM framework has also been used to model discrete spatial variation, for example in the production of cancer atlases (Clayton and Kaldor, 1987; Clayton and Bernardinelli, 1992); here, estimates of cancer risk within administrative sub-regions, eg UK Counties or French Départements, are obtained by combining data on the numbers of reported cases for each sub-region with an assumption that spatially adjacent sub-regions might be expected to have similar underlying levels of risk. This assumption is formally expressed by specifying a Markov random field model for the set of underlying risks in all sub-regions.

The GLMM is an extremely flexible class of models, which at the same time is highly structured in at least two different senses: the "generalized linear" part of the formulation allows specific and physically natural sampling distributions such as the binomial or Poisson to be incorporated; and the "mixed" part can be chosen to reflect the particular spatial or longitudinal context for whch the model is required. Furthermore, inference for this class of models is now feasible for quite large data-sets using Markov Chain Monte Carlo (Gilks, Richardson and Spiegelhalter, 1996), reducing the need for approximations whose accuracy is sometimes less than we might wish.

I would therefore claim that the increased flexibility of modelling options, as exemplified by the GLMM class, coupled with the ever-increasing practicability of Monte Carlo methods of inference, has brought our subject to the point where it can address many, although not yet all, of the scientific problems posed by spatial *or* longitudinal studies within a common framework. The essential feature of the statistical methodology required for this task is that it must tackle the problem of stochastic dependence amongst large numbers of physically commensurate responses by parsimonious modelling of high-dimensional correlation structures. This general specification of a class of statistical problems, which sometimes goes under the banner of *highly structured stochastic systems*, clearly embraces both spatial and longitudinal studies, and convinces the author, if not the reader, that the question mark in the title of this article is redundant.

5 References

[1] Baddeley, A.J., Moyeed, R.A., Howard, C.V. and Boyde, A. (1993). Analysis of a Three-dimensional Point Pattern with Replication. *Applied Statistics*, **42**, 641–668.

[2] Barry, J.T., Crowder, M.J. and Diggle, P.J. (1997). Parametric estimation of the variogram. *Lancaster University Technical Report.*

[3] Besag, J.E. (1975). Statistical analysis of non-lattice data. *The Statistician*, **24**, 179–95.

[4] Besag, J. (1986). On the statistical analysis of dirty pictures (with Discussion). *Journal of the Royal Statistical Society*, B **48**, 259–302.

[5] Breslow, N.E. and Clayton, D.G. (1993). Approximate inference in generalized linear mixed models. *Journal of the American Statistical Association* **88**, 9–25.

[6] Clayton, D. and Bernardinelli, L. (1992). Bayesian methods for mapping disease risk. In *Geographical and Environmental Epidemiology*, eds. P. Elliott, J. Cuzick, D. English and R. Stern, 205–20. Oxford University Press: Oxford.

[7] Clayton, D. and Kaldor, J. (1987). Empirical Bayes estimates of age-standardised relative risks for use in disease mapping. *Biometrics* **43**, 671–81.

[8] Cox, D.R. (1972). Regression models and life tables (with Discussion). *Journal of the Royal Statistical Society* B, **34**, 187–220.

[9] Cressie, N.A.C. (1991). *Statistics for Spatial Data.* Wiley: New York.

[10] Danford, M.B., Hughes, H.M. and McNee, R.C. (1960). On the analysis of repeated-measurements experiments. *Biometrics*, **16**, 547–65.

[11] Darroch, J.N., Lauritzen, S.L. and Speed, T.P. (1980). Markov fields and log linear interaction models for contingency tables. *Annals of Statistics*, **8**, 522–39.

[12] Diggle, P.J. (1988). An approach to the analysis of repeated measurements. *Biometrics* **44**, 959–71.

[13] Diggle, P.J. (1996). Spatial analysis in biometry. In *Advances in Biometry*, eds P. Armitage and H.A. David, 363–84. Wiley: New York.

[14] Diggle, P., Harper, L. and Simon, S. (1997). Geostatistical analysis of residual contamination from nuclear weapons testing. In *Statistics for the Environment 3*, eds V. Barnett and F. Turkman. Wiley: Chichester.

[15] Diggle, P.J. and Kenward, M.G. (1994). Informative dropout in longitudinal data analysis (with Discussion). *Appl. Statist.* **43**, 49–93.

[16] Diggle, P.J., Lange, N. and Benes, F.M. (1991). Analysis of variance for replicated spatial point patterns in clinical neuroanatomy. *J. Amer. Statist. Assn.* **86**, 618–25.

[17] Geman, S. and Geman, D. (1984). Stochastic relaxation, Gibbs distributions and the Bayesian resoration of images.*IEEE Transactions on Pattern Analysis and Machine Intelligence*,**PAMI-6**, 721–41.

[18] Gilks, W.R., Richardson, S. and Spiegelhalter, D.J. (eds) (1996). *Markov Chain Monte Carlo in Practice.* Chapman and Hall: London.

[19] Geisser, S. and Greenhouse, S.W.(1958). An extension of Box's results on the use of F distributions in multivariate analysis.*Annals of Mathematical Statistics*, **29**, 885–91.

[20] Greenhouse, S.W. and Geisser, S.(1959). On the methods in the analysis of profile data.*Psychometrika*, **24**, 95–112.

[21] Handcock, M.S. and Stein, M.L.(1993). A Bayesian analysis of kriging.*Technometrics*, **35**, 403–10.

[22] Harville, D.A. (1974). Bayesian inference for variance components using only error contrasts.*Biometrika*, **61**, 383–5.

[23] Journel, A.G. and Huijbregts, C.J.(1978). *Mining Geostatistics*.London : Academic Press.

[24] Laird, N.M. and Ware, J.H.(1982). Random-effects models for longitudinal data.*Biometrics*, **38**, 963–74.

[25] Liang, K-Y and Zeger, S.L.(1986). Longitudinal data analysis using generalized linear models*Biometrika* **73**, 13–22.

[26] Little, R.J.A.(1995). Modelling the drop-out mechanism in repeated-measures studies. *Journal of the American Statistical Association*,**90**, 1112–21.

[27] McCullagh, P. and Nelder, J.A.(1989). *Generalized Linear Models* (second edition). London : Chapman and Hall.

[28] Matheron, G.(1963). Principles of geostatistics. *Economic Geology*, **58**, 1246–66.

[29] Patterson, H.D. and Thompson, R.(1971). Recovery of inter-block information when block sizes are unequal.*Biometrika*, **58**, 545–54.

[30] Ripley, B.D. and Kelly, F.P.(1977). Markov point processes.*Journal of the London Mathematical Society*,**15**, 188–92.

[31] Rubin, D.B.(1976). Inference and missing data. *Biometrika*,**63**, 581–92.

[32] Warnes, J.J. and Ripley, B.D.(1987). Problems with likelihood estimation of covariance functions of spatial Gaussian processes.*Biometrika*, **74**, 640–2.

[33] Whittaker, J.C.(1990). *Graphical Models in Applied Multivariate Statistics.* Chichester : Wiley.

[34] Winer, B.J.(1977). *Statistical Principles in Experimental Design* (2nd edition). McGraw-Hill, New York.

[35] Wishart, J.(1938). Growth-rate determinations in nutrition studies with the bacon pig, and their analysis.*Biometrika*, *30*, 16–28.

[36] Zimmerman, D.L. and Zimmerman, M.B.(1991). A Monte Carlo comparison of spatial semivariogramestimators and corresponding ordinary kriging predictors.*Technometrics*, **33**, 77–91.

Lecture Notes in Statistics

For information about Volumes 1 to 46 please contact Springer-Verlag

Vol. 47: A.J. Getson, F.C. Hsuan, {2}-Inverses and Their Statistical Application. viii, 110 pages, 1988.

Vol. 48: G.L. Bretthorst, Bayesian Spectrum Analysis and Parameter Estimation. xii, 209 pages, 1988.

Vol. 49: S.L. Lauritzen, Extremal Families and Systems of Sufficient Statistics. xv, 268 pages, 1988.

Vol. 50: O.E. Barndorff-Nielsen, Parametric Statistical Models and Likelihood. vii, 276 pages, 1988.

Vol. 51: J. Hüsler, R.-D. Reiss (Editors). Extreme Value Theory, Proceedings, 1987. x, 279 pages, 1989.

Vol. 52: P.K. Goel, T. Ramalingam, The Matching Methodology: Some Statistical Properties. viii, 152 pages, 1989.

Vol. 53: B.C. Arnold, N. Balakrishnan, Relations, Bounds and Approximations for Order Statistics. ix, 173 pages, 1989.

Vol. 54: K.R. Shah, B.K. Sinha, Theory of Optimal Designs. viii, 171 pages, 1989.

Vol. 55: L. McDonald, B. Manly, J. Lockwood, J. Logan (Editors), Estimation and Analysis of Insect Populations. Proceedings, 1988. xiv, 492 pages, 1989.

Vol. 56: J.K. Lindsey, The Analysis of Categorical Data Using GLIM. v, 168 pages, 1989.

Vol. 57: A. Decarli, B.J. Francis, R. Gilchrist, G.U.H. Seeber (Editors), Statistical Modelling. Proceedings, 1989. ix, 343 pages, 1989.

Vol. 58: O.E. Barndorff-Nielsen, P. Bl¾sild, P.S. Eriksen, Decomposition and Invariance of Measures, and Statistical Transformation Models. v, 147 pages, 1989.

Vol. 59: S. Gupta, R. Mukerjee, A Calculus for Factorial Arrangements. vi, 126 pages, 1989.

Vol. 60: L. Gyorfi, W. Härdle, P. Sarda, Ph. Vieu, Nonparametric Curve Estimation from Time Series. viii, 153 pages, 1989.

Vol. 61: J. Breckling, The Analysis of Directional Time Series: Applications to Wind Speed and Direction. viii, 238 pages, 1989.

Vol. 62: J.C. Akkerboom, Testing Problems with Linear or Angular Inequality Constraints. xii, 291 pages, 1990.

Vol. 63: J. Pfanzagl, Estimation in Semiparametric Models: Some Recent Developments. iii, 112 pages, 1990.

Vol. 64: S. Gabler, Minimax Solutions in Sampling from Finite Populations. v, 132 pages, 1990.

Vol. 65: A. Janssen, D.M. Mason, Non-Standard Rank Tests. vi, 252 pages, 1990.

Vol 66: T. Wright, Exact Confidence Bounds when Sampling from Small Finite Universes. xvi, 431 pages, 1991.

Vol. 67: M.A. Tanner, Tools for Statistical Inference: Observed Data and Data Augmentation Methods. vi, 110 pages, 1991.

Vol. 68: M. Taniguchi, Higher Order Asymptotic Theory for Time Series Analysis. viii, 160 pages, 1991.

Vol. 69: N.J.D. Nagelkerke, Maximum Likelihood Estimation of Functional Relationships. V, 110 pages, 1992.

Vol. 70: K. Iida, Studies on the Optimal Search Plan. viii, 130 pages, 1992.

Vol. 71: E.M.R.A. Engel, A Road to Randomness in Physical Systems. ix, 155 pages, 1992.

Vol. 72: J.K. Lindsey, The Analysis of Stochastic Processes using GLIM. vi, 294 pages, 1992.

Vol. 73: B.C. Arnold, E. Castillo, J.-M. Sarabia, Conditionally Specified Distributions. xiii, 151 pages, 1992.

Vol. 74: P. Barone, A. Frigessi, M. Piccioni, Stochastic Models, Statistical Methods, and Algorithms in Image Analysis. vi, 258 pages, 1992.

Vol. 75: P.K. Goel, N.S. Iyengar (Eds.), Bayesian Analysis in Statistics and Econometrics. xi, 410 pages, 1992.

Vol. 76: L. Bondesson, Generalized Gamma Convolutions and Related Classes of Distributions and Densities. viii, 173 pages, 1992.

Vol. 77: E. Mammen, When Does Bootstrap Work? Asymptotic Results and Simulations. vi, 196 pages, 1992.

Vol. 78: L. Fahrmeir, B. Francis, R. Gilchrist, G. Tutz (Eds.), Advances in GLIM and Statistical Modelling: Proceedings of the GLIM92 Conference and the 7th International Workshop on Statistical Modelling, Munich, 13-17 July 1992. ix, 225 pages, 1992.

Vol. 79: N. Schmitz, Optimal Sequentially Planned Decision Procedures. xii, 209 pages, 1992.

Vol. 80: M. Fligner, J. Verducci (Eds.), Probability Models and Statistical Analyses for Ranking Data. xxii, 306 pages, 1992.

Vol. 81: P. Spirtes, C. Glymour, R. Scheines, Causation, Prediction, and Search. xxiii, 526 pages, 1993.

Vol. 82: A. Korostelev and A. Tsybakov, Minimax Theory of Image Reconstruction. xii, 268 pages, 1993.

Vol. 83: C. Gatsonis, J. Hodges, R. Kass, N. Singpurwalla (Editors), Case Studies in Bayesian Statistics. xii, 437 pages, 1993.

Vol. 84: S. Yamada, Pivotal Measures in Statistical Experiments and Sufficiency. vii, 129 pages, 1994.

Vol. 85: P. Doukhan, Mixing: Properties and Examples. xi, 142 pages, 1994.

Vol. 86: W. Vach, Logistic Regression with Missing Values in the Covariates. xi, 139 pages, 1994.

Vol. 87: J. Müller, Lectures on Random Voronoi Tessellations.vii, 134 pages, 1994.

Vol. 88: J. E. Kolassa, Series Approximation Methods in Statistics.viii, 150 pages, 1994.

Vol. 89: P. Cheeseman, R.W. Oldford (Editors), Selecting Models From Data: AI and Statistics IV. xii, 487 pages, 1994.

Vol. 90: A. Csenki, Dependability for Systems with a Partitioned State Space: Markov and Semi-Markov Theory and Computational Implementation. x, 241 pages, 1994.

Vol. 91: J.D. Malley, Statistical Applications of Jordan Algebras. viii, 101 pages, 1994.

Vol. 92: M. Eerola, Probabilistic Causality in Longitudinal Studies. vii, 133 pages, 1994.

Vol. 93: Bernard Van Cutsem (Editor), Classification and Dissimilarity Analysis. xiv, 238 pages, 1994.

Vol. 94: Jane F. Gentleman and G.A. Whitmore (Editors), Case Studies in Data Analysis. viii, 262 pages, 1994.

Vol. 95: Shelemyahu Zacks, Stochastic Visibility in Random Fields. x, 175 pages, 1994.

Vol. 96: Ibrahim Rahimov, Random Sums and Branching Stochastic Processes. viii, 195 pages, 1995.

Vol. 97: R. Szekli, Stochastic Ordering and Dependence in Applied Probability. viii, 194 pages, 1995.

Vol. 98: Philippe Barbe and Patrice Bertail, The Weighted Bootstrap. viii, 230 pages, 1995.

Vol. 99: C.C. Heyde (Editor), Branching Processes: Proceedings of the First World Congress. viii, 185 pages, 1995.

Vol. 100: Wlodzimierz Bryc, The Normal Distribution: Characterizations with Applications. viii, 139 pages, 1995.

Vol. 101: H.H. Andersen, M.Højbjerre, D. Sørensen, P.S.Eriksen, Linear and Graphical Models: for the Multivariate Complex Normal Distribution. x, 184 pages, 1995.

Vol. 102: A.M. Mathai, Serge B. Provost, Takesi Hayakawa, Bilinear Forms and Zonal Polynomials. x, 378 pages, 1995.

Vol. 103: Anestis Antoniadis and Georges Oppenheim (Editors), Wavelets and Statistics. vi, 411 pages, 1995.

Vol. 104: Gilg U.H. Seeber, Brian J. Francis, Reinhold Hatzinger, Gabriele Steckel-Berger (Editors), Statistical Modelling: 10th International Workshop, Innsbruck, July 10-14th 1995. x, 327 pages, 1995.

Vol. 105: Constantine Gatsonis, James S. Hodges, Robert E. Kass, Nozer D. Singpurwalla(Editors), Case Studies in Bayesian Statistics, Volume II. x, 354 pages, 1995.

Vol. 106: Harald Niederreiter, Peter Jau-Shyong Shiue (Editors), Monte Carlo and Quasi-Monte Carlo Methods in Scientific Computing. xiv, 372 pages, 1995.

Vol. 107: Masafumi Akahira, Kei Takeuchi, Non-Regular Statistical Estimation. vii, 183 pages, 1995.

Vol. 108: Wesley L. Schaible (Editor), Indirect Estimators in U.S. Federal Programs. iix, 195 pages, 1995.

Vol. 109: Helmut Rieder (Editor), Robust Statistics, Data Analysis, and Computer Intensive Methods. xiv, 427 pages, 1996.

Vol. 110: D. Bosq, Nonparametric Statistics for Stochastic Processes. xii, 169 pages, 1996.

Vol. 111: Leon Willenborg, Ton de Waal, Statistical Disclosure Control in Practice. xiv, 152 pages, 1996.

Vol. 112: Doug Fischer, Hans-J. Lenz (Editors), Learning from Data. xii, 450 pages, 1996.

Vol. 113: Rainer Schwabe, Optimum Designs for Multi-Factor Models. viii, 124 pages, 1996.

Vol. 114: C.C. Heyde, Yu. V. Prohorov, R. Pyke, and S. T. Rachev (Editors), Athens Conference on Applied Probability and Time Series Analysis Volume I: Applied Probability In Honor of J.M. Gani. viii, 424 pages, 1996.

Vol. 115: P.M. Robinson, M. Rosenblatt (Editors), Athens Conference on Applied Probability and Time Series Analysis Volume II: Time Series Analysis In Memory of E.J. Hannan. viii, 448 pages, 1996.

Vol. 116: Genshiro Kitagawa and Will Gersch, Smoothness Priors Analysis of Time Series. x, 261 pages, 1996.

Vol. 117: Paul Glasserman, Karl Sigman, David D. Yao (Editors), Stochastic Networks. xii, 298, 1996.

Vol. 118: Radford M. Neal, Bayesian Learning for Neural Networks. xv, 183, 1996.

Vol. 119: Masanao Aoki, Arthur M. Havenner, Applications of Computer Aided Time Series Modeling, ix, 329 pages, 1997.

Vol. 120: Maia Berkane, Latent Variable Modeling and Applications to Causality, vi, 288 pages, 1997.

Vol. 121: Constantine Gatsonis, James S. Hodges, Robert E. Kass, Robert McCulloch, Peter Rossi, Nozer D. Singpurwalla (Editors), Case Studies in Bayesian Statistics, Volume III. xvi, 487 pages, 1997.

Vol. 122: Timothy G. Gregoire, David R. Brillinger, Peter J. Diggle, Estelle Russek-Cohen, William G. Warren, Russell D. Wolfinger (Editors), Modeling Longitudinal and Spatially Correlated Data, x, 402 pages, 1997

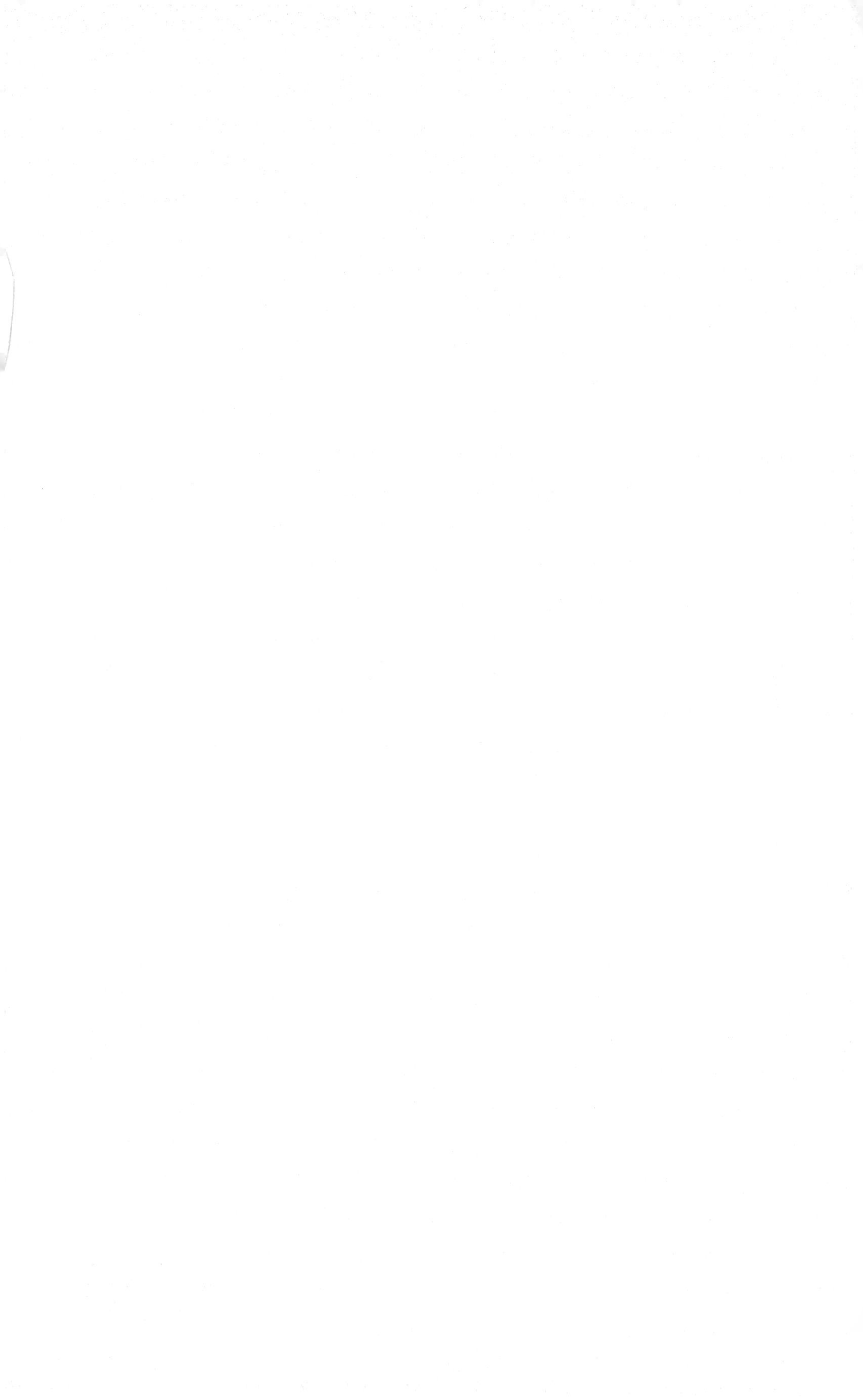

9 780387 982168